D0422157

Consciousness in Four Dimensions

Consciousness in Four Dimensions

Biological Relativity and the Origins of Thought

Richard M. Pico, Ph.D., M.D.

McGraw-Hill
New York Chicago San Francisco
Lisbon London Madrid Mexico City Milan
New Delhi San Juan Seoul Singapore
Sydney Toronto

Library of Congress Cataloging-in-Publication Data

Pico, Richard M.
Consciousness in four dimensions : biological relativity and the origins of thought / Richard M. Pico.
p. cm.
ISBN 0-07-135499-9
1. Consciousness. 2. Brain—Evolution. I. Title.

QP411 .P535 2001
612.8′2—dc21

2001026634

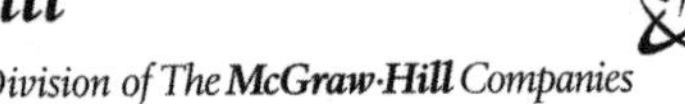

A Division of The McGraw-Hill Companies

1 2 3 4 5 6 7 8 9 0 DOC/DOC 0 7 6 5 4 3 2 1

ISBN 0-07-135499-9

Printed and bound by R. R. Donnelley & Sons Company.

This book is printed on recycled, acid-free paper containing a minimum of 50% recycled de-inked fiber.

For Alexander
Son, colleague, and fellow explorer

Contents

Part Five: Infinite Reflection

Acknowledgments

Thinking about thought, mind, and consciousness is a human phenomenon. As such, in my personal life I have failed to encounter many who do not want to know more about our brain functions; and in my professional life I have likewise failed to find a scientist or physician who does not desire to understand these concepts. The young history and current chapters of neuroscience and the medicine of brain disorders is that of devoted research scientists and clinicians who attend to focused areas of study: from the amino acid to the cell, from the synapse to the system. And it is the findings from these specialized investigations that will illuminate the path to our understanding of the human mind. Thus, it must be acknowledged here that the significant influences on my thinking about consciousness have come from the scientific and medical communities, and less so from purely social, psychological, or philosophical writings.

There are many mentors, colleagues, and friends to thank for their contributions and help in realizing this work, but I will mention only a few who have been most near and influential during my basic science and clinical careers. In the brain and behavioral sciences, Joel L. Davis, Christine Gall, Edward G. Jones, Gary Lynch, and Charles Ribak have all provided guidance, insight, and set high standards of scientific excellence. Joel Davis has also been a greatly valued source of encouragement and a good friend, engaging in late night discussions on computational models, memory, and thought.

In medicine, Thomas M. Brown, Travis Nobles, Peter T. Fox, Jack Lancaster, Robert Trestman, Eileen DiFrancesco, and John Edgar, along with the nursing staff and residents at The Mount Sinai Medical Center challenged my models of the human mind and supported me in the development of research programs into human thought disorders, and in the teaching of biological relativity as it applied to the diagnosis and treatment of brain-related illnesses. An unwavering supporter and colleague, Tom Brown embodies the best of science, medicine, and humanity in his energetic approach to the study of the biological basis of brain diseases. His deep insights into medication effects on nervous system function will have profound influence on the future of neuromedicine and on our ability to alleviate the suffering of those with nervous system disorders.

To effectively halt a career path to conduct the necessary research and devote the time needed to produce this book could have proved a most difficult task. I am fortunate to have several friends and colleagues who helped create a supportive environment within which I could bring together twenty-some years of writings and teachings into a formal model of brain function. Stuart Z. Levin, a technology visionary and humanitarian provided unqualified encouragement and support throughout the writing process. S. Robert Levine gave of his time regularly to review and discuss portions of the manuscript. Parker Ladd has been steadfast in his representation of my work and ideas since the beginning of the project. Robert Kinberg worked with me early on to set the writing style and scope of this volume, and to outline the next three books of the series. Julie Johnson created a stable work environment and conducted business relationships with tireless professionalism.

A special acknowledgment must be made to Amy Murphy who, as editor of this work, understood the value of the ideas and the potential impact that biological relativity may have on neuroscience and medicine. Amy's dedication of many long days of reading and editing each chapter is truly appreciated. Her ability to bring clarity and style to the writing without detracting from the basic scientific subject matter was remarkable. It was a pleasure to have my words read better through her efforts. The McGraw-Hill team of Ruth Mannino, Elizabeth Strange, Sue Gerber, and Wendy Beth Jakelow brought the manuscript to its final form with impressive sensitivity and enthusiasm. I could not have been in better hands.

One of my guiding principles for the study of brain and mind is that in order to understand the limits of human consciousness, we must know how disorders of brain function alter its expression. To this end, I have been privileged to treat hundreds of children, men, and women with disruptions of brain function affecting thought, mood, and memory. While I endeavor to provide each patient the best of care, it must be acknowledged that each patient has brought me a deeper understanding of human emotion and consciousness through our interactions. I am grateful to each individual for sharing his or her unique experiences in thought. The model of consciousness presented in this work would not be as rich or meaningful without their contributions. Perhaps, the ideas contained herein will lead to treatments that will prevent suffering and relieve disorders of consciousness in others.

Richard M. Pico
New York City
2001

Consciousness in Four Dimensions

Introduction
Toward a Framework for Consciousness

We live in a four-dimensional universe that bounds our existence and determines our reality. All that we may perceive, feel, think, and imagine occurs within the four dimensions of space and time. Our experience of consciousness, mind, and the human spirit is a local, earthly phenomenon forged across billions of light years in the evolution of matter and energy. Yet in today's discourse, it is considered radical to propose that we are the stuff of such a straightforward, unadorned universe, the product of one biological evolutionary time line, living and being in the absence of mysterious forces.

It is my hope that in the uncomplicated formulation presented in this book, we may indeed find a perspective into the structure and function of the brain as it relates to the generation of thought and consciousness that is consistent with the known physical reality. Thus, the central idea in this book may challenge and affect the reader in many ways. This work will offer an understanding of what it means when we look into a mirror and wonder about our sense of "self"—that is when we ask, "How is it possible to think about my own thoughts, my self, my life in the past, present, and future?" Relatedly, it will present an explanation for the way in which the brain creates our *sixth* sense, the sense of time. In looking at our self-image and our personal sense of time in this manner, we may discover a new way of thinking about the nature and evolution of emotions, memories, language, math, and music. The overarching concept in this book reflects a humanistic position that embodies an appreciation for all life around us and our responsibility to care for it. Finally, a unique perspective by which we may celebrate the emergence of thought and consciousness in each of our children is presented.

The point of view established in this book may be stated as follows: Just as planets move around the Sun and galaxies move out from a common origin, so may all living things likewise move through seasons of existence—without choice, control, or willful consideration. Our sensations of an uncertain future and our perceived dominion over nature may both be illusions of information in the flow of time—illusions of random events and powers of choice produced by a nervous system that is limited in its ability to react to the matter and energies of the cosmos at large. All we may experience, think, and remember is a product of a parochial nervous system that evolved in the relatively microscopic, sheltered environment of Earth.

The emergence of a biological system that produced thought and consciousness may be understood through an examination of the basic operating principles of evolution, viewed herein as local entropic shifts of matter and energy across vast scales of time. The threshold from pre-life to life is thus intimately related to the threshold from pre-consciousness to consciousness, when these thresholds are examined at the level of evolutionary modification of organic systems as they attain an organization that captures all four dimensions of existence within their structure and function. The production of an internal dimension of time defines the emergent evolutionary event. I postulate that it is this threshold event that brought thought and consciousness to the nervous system. Importantly, I define this emergent property of consciousness as an exclusively human condition, with limits and constraints that may be examined, understood, and thereby systematically influenced. A singularly beneficial outcome of adopting this understanding of human brain function may be the development of effective medical treatments for disorders of thought, emotion, memory, and mind.

I therefore propose that the essential link between the complex pathways through space and time of each inorganic particle of matter and each organic plant and animal (including humans and all their thoughts, hopes, and dreams) is found in the unified view of the three spatial dimensions and one temporal dimension that form irreducible four-dimensional referent systems. In special and general relativity, Albert Einstein developed the frame of reference approach and postulated that, in fact, every arrangement of matter and energy creates four-dimensional systems. The model offered in this book extends Einstein's vision of the universe into the world of organic systems, and postulates that the process of evolution created three independent frames of reference in space and time: the inorganic universe of matter and energy, organic systems of life, and the reference system of consciousness. This model of biological relativity provides the foundation for establishing and investigating quantitative parameters across qualitative thresholds for emergent systems in nature.

One may ask, what does it matter if we view nature in this way or another way? And, if there are such constraints on our existence, why should we care? As we tend our gardens, care for our animals, raise our children, and love our partners, this may not have an obvious importance. However, within each of these human activities—and more particularly within the science and medicine of the nervous system and brain function underlying thought and consciousness—it may have profound implications and consequences for all of us.

We currently conduct our daily routines with an incoherent concept of the brain structure and function that generate thought and consciousness. In fact, for several decades now, experts in the computer sciences have proposed that calculating machines do think and that machine consciousness has already arrived or is just around the programming corner. Moreover, since the beginning of human written history, it has been acceptable to postulate that nature includes a special force of free will or volition that supersedes the spatial and temporal dimensions and provides humans (and perhaps plants and animals) with a unique perspective and an ability to control the course of events. Misperceptions about thinking machines, willful minds, and the force of consciousness have a direct influence on the way in which we conceptualize nature and, in turn, on the way in which we develop new devices, conduct experiments, and diagnose and treat patients with disorders of the central nervous system. The incorporation of illusions, along with accurate knowledge, into our daily thoughts and actions influences the paths we take into the future. Our lack of a consistent biophysical model of thought and consciousness threatens to relegate us to an ungrounded free fall into the unknown future.

In childhood, we each discover the laws of nature through experience and education. We learn about force, energy, gravity, and behavior through interaction with the world throughout the duration of our lives. All the hypotheses that we may generate in science and medicine are thereby uniquely personal and ultimately are derived from individual experience. The origins of biological relativity, as a unifying model of emergent systems in organic evolution, can thus be traced to the thoughts of a particular child (this author) contemplating space and time. In my preteen years, I was intently interested in the dimensions of nature. When I was learning to draw perspectives and volume objects such as cones and cubes (Figure I-1), I wondered where the perceived dimension of depth came from. I was captivated by the fact that any three drawn lines intersecting at a common point would evoke a sense of volume. Once, when I was idly staring at a tiled ceiling (Figure I-1) I crossed my eyes so that my relaxed, unfocused vision effectively overlapped and fused two separate square tiles. To my amazement, when one flat tile was visually moved atop another, a full-depth cubic structure emerged. Where was that dimension created? Was it real or an illusion? I later learned about the stereoscope, through which three-dimensional depth perception is induced by special lens arrangements that overlap two two-dimensional fields; the principle used in all 3D-movies. I also began to read about the history of Gestalt psychology and the research field of psychophysics.[1]

I explored the fourth dimension, time, as an equally inducible phenomenon through the work of Edweard Muybridge.[2] In 1872, Muybridge created the original photographic evidence that a galloping horse leaves the ground as it moves. He used photography, which at the time was quite new, to take serial images of a horse in motion. His photographs clearly showed that at certain moments, all four hooves are off the ground. The fascinating consequence of Muybridge's work became apparent when his images of serial, discrete moments in time were viewed in rapid succession (Figure I-2). When a set of images was *flickered* at a rapid (critical threshold) rate, a

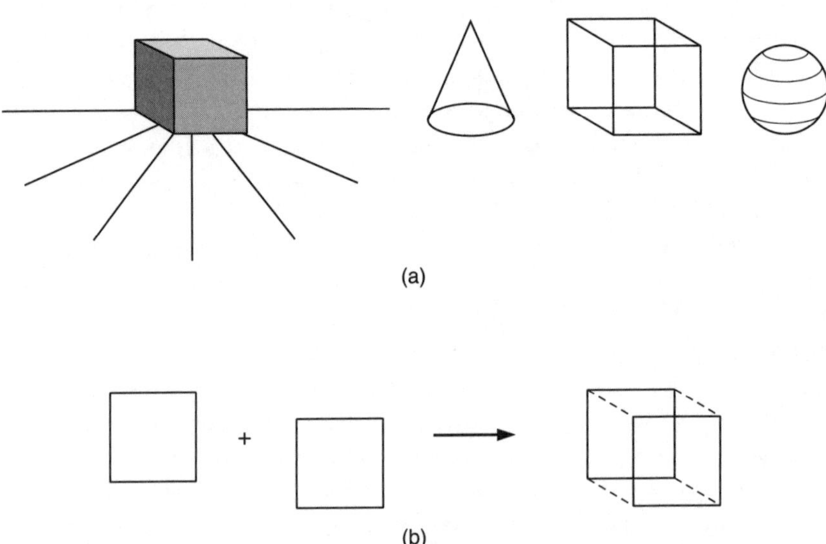

Figure I-1 (*a*) Examples of simple drawings that evoke a sensation of the three spatial dimensions. (*b*) The illusion of depth is created by visually overlapping two 2-dimensional squares.

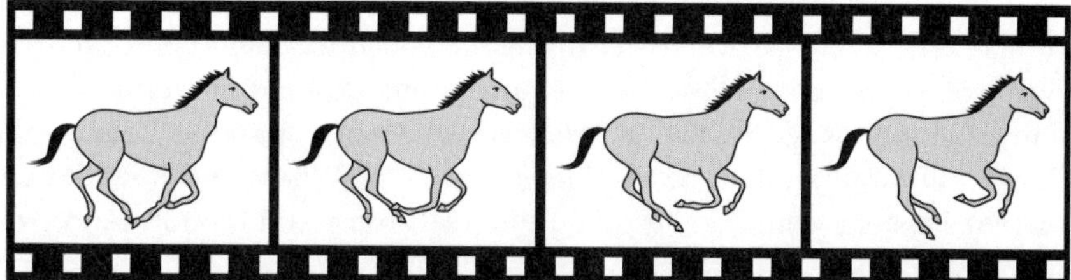

Figure I-2 Example of a sequence of images that evokes a sensation of motion, and thus time, if shown in rapid succession. The original demonstration of this "flicker-fusion" technique for photographic images was produced by Edweard Muybridge in 1872.

fusion of moments was induced in the viewer's mind, and one saw a singular scene that appeared to include motion. Thus the temporal dimension appeared to actually be embedded in a series of static, timeless, images, when viewed in this manner. This relatively simple technique formed the basis for all motion picture and television technologies.

As a fledgling grade-school athlete who dedicated innumerable hours to "perfecting" a jump shot, the high jump, and other basic skill techniques, I began to experience an exhilarating sensation of frozen time during moments of explosive physical execution. I began referring to this as a *flow* moment, and I wrote my first paper on this experience a few years later. I now saw the world in its four dimensions, but I perceived two distinct systems: the one that the *real* physical world produced, and the sensation of depth and time-through-motion that was created internal to my biological being—a personal reality that seemed relative to my experience.

I finally found someone who spoke to me about space and time in this manner at the age of 12, when I read my first biography of Albert Einstein.[3] Through his writings and those of his biographers and contemporaries, the philosophical, psychological, and material constructs of space and time—of reality and illusion—began to take new form in my thoughts. Standing on the shoulders of many great scientists and thinkers, Einstein saw through the illusions of the so-called luminiferous ether and the mysterious force of gravity and produced a novel vision of the fabric of the universe. He applied a conceptual construct, the four-dimensional frame of reference, that treated all dimensions as valid coordinate components of our existence; and it changed forever the way we understand nature.

At the deepest level of insight produced by Einstein and his colleagues was the explicitly articulated belief that everything that we may perceive and know about nature comes through our human sensory abilities and that it may reflect only a severely narrow and clouded fragment of a larger universe of matter and energy. Thus, in my young thoughts, I started formulating questions about the internal generation of space and time—the biological interpretation of the inorganic reality. Where and how did our nervous system generate the perception of volume and motion from two-dimensional objects presented in particular arrangements? Where and how did Einstein's brain permit his imagination to see the wave-particle duality of nature, the speed limit of the universe, and the profound reality of matter-energy transformations? And, more importantly, if the four-dimensional universe of Einstein was a valid material construct, then why did it not have a direct influence on the way in which we spoke about and taught biology? I searched for the application of relativity theory to the understanding of organic systems, from the living cell to the thinking brain. I sought after the book, the teacher, the class that would show me the relationship. I wanted to understand how our internal sensations of four dimensions related to the larger universe of matter, energy, entropy, and evolution. Was there a biological relativity?

By the time I was 14, I lived and loved the integrated view of space and time that Einstein postulated as the fabric of the electromagnetic field. For instance, I could never again shoot a basketball without visualizing a spinning planet plunging into a vortex of curved space-time, created in my imagination by the rim and net; and, I thoroughly enjoyed the sensation of altered personal time during focused physical activity such as a tennis serve. In my early twenties, I developed a conceptual model that I called *biological relativity* that related our internal world of sensory experience and brain function to the frame of reference viewpoint of inorganic nature. Through the subsequent 25 years, I continued to devote my professional life to the study of the physics, psychology, biology, and medical psychiatry of nervous system structure and function, to conduct basic and clinical investigations, and to care for patients with disorders of mood, thought, and memory. My experience in neuroscience and neuromedicine, through teaching, lectures, publications, and clinical practice, has served to refine and reinforce the utility and applicability of the model. This book contains the very first presentation of the complete biological relativity model.

The current state of our knowledge must not be overestimated: There is absolutely no accepted model of brain structure and function underlying the concepts of higher-brain function. We conduct our science and medicine concerning thought and mind in a great void, lacking a guidebook or consensus opinion, and the related fields of study are filled with hypotheses delineating dramatically disparate biases, many of which have no basis in science. The model of biological relativity presents a set of operational definitions and their logical foundations in an effort to bring a consistency and focus to the relationship between inorganic and organic systems, including the nervous system, in nature. My goal is to provide a framework that we can use to peer more deeply into the nature of our unique personal experiences in thought and consciousness, and to understand the inescapable connection with the larger supporting background of living systems—and ultimately with the four-dimensional inorganic field of matter and energy. The utility of a model that strives to bridge mind and matter is that it generates a wealth of testable hypotheses that may lead to better theories of brain function, and thereby promote advances in the diagnosis and treatment of disorders of the mind.

Einstein's relativity model forced us to give up long-standing, deeply felt beliefs—in absolute dimensions, engulfing ethers, a mysterious force of gravity, and unlimited concepts of infinite space and time. At the cost of destroying the status quo, his frame of reference approach brought a vision of an immensely dynamic, but constrained, universe that stands virtually unchanged today. The four-dimensional space-time continuum envisioned by Einstein generated testable hypotheses, many of which have been confirmed. The new point of view created in his theories of special and general relativity has resulted in quantitative measures of changes in spatial dimensions that occur with reference systems in relative motion. We have demonstrated that time is a relative dimension as well and that the temporal functions of all systems, including biological ones, are altered with acceleration. We have built telescopes that view the universe across a wide range of the electromagnetic spectrum (from microwave to gamma ray) and look for evidence of extreme gravitational distortions, the black holes predicted by Einstein, that may inhabit the center of each galaxy. Devices are being constructed to detect ripples in space-time, which were also an element of Einstein's vision of the universe. There is no end in sight to the knowledge that we will gain about our existence as a direct effect of a frame of reference perspective that accepts limits and boundaries to the universe.

Throughout the history of humanity, a succession of certain strongly felt beliefs have been shattered by new knowledge and replaced by a new point of view that provided a deeper insight into nature. We see virtually the same process recapitulated in each child during development. The belief that all matter is alive (animism) gives way to the separation of inorganic from organic systems. The belief that all living things, from cells to plants to animals, are aware of their existence and are infused with thought and intent (anthropomorphism) has to some degree been relinquished through an understanding of nervous systems, brain function, and an evolutionary progression across the species. It is in this phase of our knowledge development that we currently stand, uncertain as to the nature of nervous system function and the abilities it bestows upon humankind.

The model of biological relativity challenges deeply entrenched beliefs about thought and consciousness as they relate to concepts of self-control, free will, animal and artificial intelligence, cognitive theory, and mentalism. Perhaps, if we can relinquish our cherished biases regarding the forces of life and mind, we will see more deeply into nature and discover a rich world of new insights. With study and testing of the model's hypotheses, we may develop a more revealing approach to the study of brain function and a more successful, if not more humanistic, approach to the diagnosis and treatment of patients with disorders of mood, thought, memory, and mind. Biological relativity may reflect a step along the road toward our collective childhood's end.

Part One

DIMENSIONS OF SPACE AND TIME

1

Einstein's Vision of the Universe I: Relativity and Reference Systems

This book presents a point of view, a model, a framework. The model of biological relativity that it contains focuses on the relationships among space, time, dimension, and order in nature's biological systems. It is based on the integrated framework developed by Albert Einstein, whose discoveries provided a critical understanding of how our concepts of space, time, and dimension are truly inseparable.[1] Einstein's profound and beautifully articulated insights into the grand order of nature that underlies all the dimensions and organizations of matter and energy, as we understand them today, were themselves predicated upon a unique perspective that was forged in his early thoughts and that shaped the structure of his logic across decades of time.

Einstein's theory of relativity is, of course, recognized as one of the great tenets of modern physics, and he is remembered as well for his specific contributions regarding the speed of light (c), the quantitative relationship between energy and matter ($E = mc^2$), the bending of light as it passes near gravitational sources, and the photoelectric effect (for which he won the Nobel Prize). However, the deeper structure in Einstein's thoughts, from which these individual insights emerged, dealt with the understanding that all natural occurrences are four-dimensional (4D) events. That nature, as it plays through our senses, is composed of irreducible 4D moments of space and time is at once the most important and the least appreciated or understood aspect of Einstein's vision of the universe. It is this singular principle upon which our new model of the biological systems underlying thought and consciousness is constructed. Thus, to accurately present our biological model, we must first see the universe through Einstein's eyes: We must understand the deep fundamental structure of relativity theory.

The presentation of relativity and its core element, the 4D frame of reference, contained in this book is unlike that of most, if not all, textbook and popularized approaches. Our view of relativity theory provides the necessary tools with which to understand how the principles that apply to the inorganic universe of particles and planets also underlie the organic structures of molecules and brains. It is our hope that by examining the interface of relativity and biology, we can ultimately gain a profound understanding of our human experience in thought and mind.

A Relativistic Perspective

To begin this exploration, we must acknowledge the simple fact that it is through our human senses that we perceive all of nature. Also, one individual's perception will not always, if ever, completely correspond to another's perception. Thus, a dynamic dichotomy of subjectivity and objectivity permeates all attempts to understand our existence—and, parenthetically, has plagued our discourse though the ages. That very quest for understanding, perhaps the only unique function of our human experience, must eternally refine the distinctions at the interface of subjective (individual) perception and objective (consensus) reality. Along the path of time's arrow, the interplay between the external world and our senses creates a never-ending process by which an individual's subjective experience is continually modified by enduring objective understanding. In other words, while each person experiences the world from a unique point of view, collectively we have derived an agreed-upon, learned, impersonal, or shared, perspective of natural processes. Thus, an event or process in nature is relative to the individual experience: Each individual may experience what is recognized as the same event or process a little differently, depending upon many factors. *At the foundation of scientific exploration (and Einstein's vision) is the understanding that any objective knowledge is relative to the point of view of the observer, the one experiencing nature's behavior.* This position does not negate the establishment of an objective source of stable events or processes; it just acknowledges the unique point of view of each observer and how this point of view alters the observer's perspective of the event.

One of Einstein's greatest insights was to recognize that this general relativistic perspective applies not only to our common experiences in relationships, conversations, and opinions, but also to our basic understanding of the physical interactions of all things that surround us. Thus, it extends to our experience of the infinitesimal interactions of energies, quarks, electrons, protons, and neutrons; of the intermediate-scale actions of all particles and objects; and of the vast structure of our expanding universe. Einstein's theory of relativity in its special and general formulations rang a resounding death knell to the classical view of an objective reality of absolutes, of *a priori* knowledge, of a stable universe that reassured us of its single clockwork design, order, and certainty.

Moreover, in a world-shattering synthesis of information that merged an understanding of the universal electromagnetic field, the behavior of matter objects that perturb its structure, the duality of wave and particle, Newtonian theories of absolute space and time, the motion of inertial systems in the hypothetical ether, and the powerful equations of Poincaré and Lorentz, Einstein created in his fertile imagination a relativistic frame of reference perspective that produced a fusion of the three dimensions (3D) of space with one dimension (1D) of time.[2] In other words, when Einstein concluded that nature operated on principles of relativity, he was able to peer more deeply through the obfuscating collage of contradictory facts, findings, and feelings about space and time to behold a profound reality: that all four dimensions of nature's order are relative to the local systems within which they are embodied.

Relativity becomes manifest in a universe of 4D referent systems. The two perspectives became one in Einstein's imagination, and subsequently have become the bedrock of our understanding of all reality. In the special and general theories of relativity, Einstein operationalized nature's basic unit of existence, the building block of all phenomena, as the indivisible 4D referent system, composed of the three dimensions of space plus the fourth dimension, time. At all scales of organization that we may perceive, measure, and understand, the independent 4D referent frame essentially creates its own unique reality, relative to any other referent frame. Observations of one 4D referent system made from any number of other local systems in motion relative to it would all vary, and thus each observation would be unique to the particular system making the observation. Furthermore, none of the observations or measures would be exactly what was being measured within the referent system of observation! Thus the reality of the space and time dimensions, indivisible to each system, is relative to the point of view of the observer. What makes this vision so extraordinarily insightful and revolutionary is that it is not a semantic nuance, not a metaphoric philosophical or mathematical conceptualization, but as real as anything we may understand.

In his introductory comments to *Einstein's Theory of Relativity*, the renowned physicist Max Born explained the far-reaching consequences the theory of special relativity would have following its publication in 1905:

> *The reason Einstein's name alone is usually connected with relativity is that his work of 1905 was only the initial step to a still more fundamental "general relativity," which included a new theory of gravita-*

> *tion and opened new vistas in our understanding of the structure of the universe. The special theory of relativity of 1905 can be justifiably considered the end of the classical period or the beginning of a new era.*[3]

This new way of thinking was derived from Einstein's fearless frame of reference approach, a relativistic approach, to the accepted absolutes of his time. Special relativity presents a point of view about the structure-function of nature. It provides a logical and internally consistent framework for the many concepts and definitions of space, time, energy, matter, mass, field, and dimension. It may not ultimately be the final organizing principle for our universe, but it certainly has accomplished much, and there is no successor in sight.

In nature, then, each and every referent system of matter and energy, relative to all others, is defined as a 4D space-time organization. The universe may therefore be visualized as a field containing a near-infinite number of referent systems, dynamically interacting. Each system has its own unique temporal dimension, but all of these unique temporal dimensions are limited in magnitude to the flow of the background, universal pace of expansion. In other words, no 4D system can have an internal pulse of time that is outside the physical boundary of the electromagnetic field of existence that gave rise to all referent systems. Einstein saw that there is no absolute space (no *luminiferous ether*) within which we may find eternal landmarks of dimensional measurement, and no absolute, single time dimension.

The crowning culmination of the point of view that brought relativity together with a frame of reference approach resulted in an utterly transforming understanding of the relationship between the universal background field of electromagnetism, all the emergent 4D systems of matter that arise from nonmatter origins, and the fundamental threshold transition between the two frames of reference, a relationship that Einstein expressed mathematically as $E = mc^2$. This relationship changed everything.

> *The influence of the theory of relativity goes far beyond the problem from which it arose. It removes the difficulties and contradictions of the field theory; it formulates more general mechanical laws; it replaces two conservation laws by one; it changes our classical concept of absolute time. Its validity is not restricted to one domain of physics; it forms a general framework embracing all phenomena of nature.*[4]

Operational Definitions

In order to proceed with the presentation of relativity theory and its extension into biological processes, we must place in our tool kit a set of operational definitions covering basic scientific concepts. In a universe devoid of absolutes, a relativistic universe, it is not easy to give even commonplace terms absolute definitions; nevertheless, we can agree on precise, objective designations.

As Max Born stated it, "The physical problem presented by space and time consists in fixing numerically a place and a point of time for every physical event, thus enabling us to single it out, as it were, from the chaos of the coexistence and succession of things."[5] *Space*, then, has no particular existence in and of itself; it is defined only as an inherent property of *dimension* within an organization of objects or matter. *Time*, similarly, is a powerful subjective experience that each of us has regarding the flow of a past, the present *now*, and a potential future. Objectively, it is the dimension of the duration between two events, between points in a process, or along a path of motion. The objective measure of time is accomplished by a clock, which is any artificial device or natural process that has a repeating periodicity within its function. Atomic clocks set a measure of objective time based on the rate of nuclear decay, and the standard of the second was derived from the motion of the Earth around the Sun. Thus, *motion* is the relative change in the position of an object, and its measure has both a spatial and a temporal component.

Energy and *matter* may be defined as manifestations of the background electromagnetic field. Energy is the process of electromagnetic waves that may exert force and perform work. At a larger-scale organization of objects, energy may be also measured as the potential for work resulting from the relative position of objects in an energy field, or as the action of an object in kinetic motion.

Force is any influence that can cause an object to deviate from its present position or acceleration, and *work* is the action of force over a duration of time [work has the same unit of measure as energy: the joule, equal to 1 kilogram-meter^2 per second^2 ($1 kg\text{-}m^2/s^2$)]. Matter is the state of energy that may be measured as a particle and thus possesses the four physical dimensions; examples are subatomic particles, atoms, elements, planets, and all organic materials. *Mass* is a property of matter that varies with its state of acceleration. The conversion factor that relates energy and matter is the speed of light, or c [3.0×10^8 meters per second (m/s)]. Thus, each particle of matter contains c^2 amount of energy, and each packet or quanta of energy has $1/c^2$ amount of matter.

A *metric* in general is a standard of measure for a particular set of relationships. A *field* in general is a region of space that has a particular set of values or a metrical system assigned at each point comprised in the region. A *frame of reference* in relativity is a set of coordinates in each of four dimensions that has a unique metrical system relative to all other referent frames and to the general background field. *Dimension* in nature is the property of an object with respect to its background field, or the property that is inherent in an arrangement of objects (thus, space and dimension are very similar concepts). We say that space is one-dimensional (1D, the line of any path or the line of a circle drawn on paper), two-dimensional (2D, a plane surface or a sphere surface like that of the Earth), three-dimensional (3D, the interior of a sphere or a cube), or 4D (expressed in the concept of space-time as an independent frame of reference; Figure 1-1).

The Relativistic Effect

Our universe is a 4D space-time structure. In our thoughts, pictured in our minds, we may experience the 4D nature of existence manifested in our

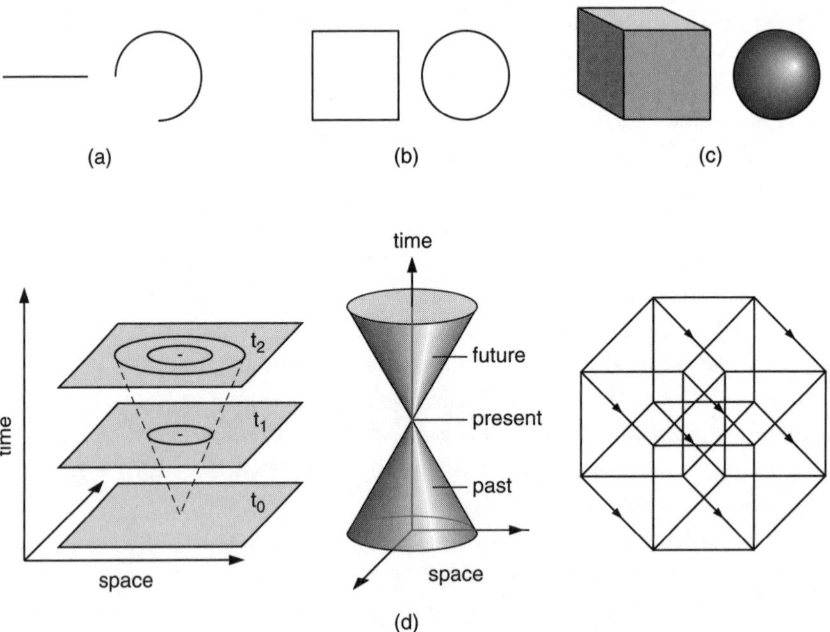

Figure 1-1 Illustrations of the three spatial dimensions and the one temporal dimension. (*a*) One-dimensional lines. (*b*) Two-dimensional surfaces. (*c*) Three-dimensional volumes. (*d*) Common attempts to infer the one time dimension by indicating motion or movement: (*left to right*) a series of stacked surfaces indicating a spreading event over time; a traditional light-cone model of events in time; a so-called hypercube, indicating time by a change in position of the elemental cubic shape.

subjective sense of a serial, flowing temporal dimension. When we observe the world, we see processes in inorganic and organic nature that involve objects in arrangements that have three spatial dimensions, and whose motion is caused by energy forces across a time interval (the fourth dimension). Thus, from our frame of reference, we may apply a metric to a physical system in nature and measure spatial dimensions, measure quantities of energy as force, and track the system's time course, all relative to the larger background field in which the system is interacting or behaving. In our minds we can put the whole scene together as a 4D construct.

Any attempt to represent this internal 4D experience in words, equations, or drawings, however, will always result in the loss of the temporal dimension. Indeed, it is the collapsing of the temporal dimension of any process of nature to zero that allows that process to be expressed outside of our thoughts. Our language may express the three spatial dimensions with words like *cube, sphere,* or *cone,* and we can represent such three-dimensional volumes with two-dimensional drawings that utilize three sets of coordinates, but any higher dimensions, such as the fourth dimension of time or any other imaginary conceptualization of *n*-dimensional spaces, may not be so expressed. The hypercube, the stacked planes, and the light cone in Figure 1-1 represent some of the ways in which we attempt to impart the reality of our 4D existence outside of our minds. These actual figures are 3D or less in their dimensionality. Time is not there. We may reconstruct it in our minds, but it is not in the depictions or in any set of equations. This reality is the first limit and constraint to be noted here for the human nervous system as it processes and experiences space, time, and dimension.

Anything in 4D, a referent frame or biological process, can be expressed only when the temporal dimension is collapsed to zero and a one-, two-, or three-dimensional representation is produced. For example, we may conceive of an entire plane flight from New York to Los Angeles as a 4D event, yet we cannot express it unless we decompose the unitary referent system of space and time (the flight) and present it as a series of 3D, 2D, or 1D *freeze-frames* (represented by words, equations, or drawings) that, put together in stacks or overlays or aligned in some manner, allow us to infer the 4D process. The 4D system, the full event in time, must be reconstructed in our thoughts before its complete nature can be known or remembered. Thus, although we are constrained in our ability to express it, we instinctively experience the world as a four-dimensional extension, what Einstein called the *space-time continuum*:

> *Indeed, not two, but four, numbers must be used to describe events in nature. Our physical space as conceived through objects and their*

> *motion has three dimensions, and positions are characterized by three numbers. The instant of an event is the fourth number. Four definite numbers correspond to every event; a definite event corresponds to any four numbers. Therefore: The world of events forms a four-dimensional continuum. There is nothing mysterious about this, and the last sentence is equally true for classical physics and the relativity theory.*[6]

The importance of the space-time continuum becomes apparent when we consider two independent coordinate systems (referent systems) moving relative to each other—that is, when the relativistic effect is observed by applying a frame of reference approach. If we observe a room in motion (a referent system), then from our perspective (as a separate referent system)

> *The room is moving, and the observers inside and outside determine the time-space coordinates of the same events. Again, the classical physicist splits the four-dimensional continua into the three-dimensional spaces and the one-dimensional time-continuum. The old physicist bothers only about space transformations, as time is absolute for him. He finds the splitting of the four-dimensional world-continua into space and time natural and convenient. But from the point of view of the relativity theory, time as well as space is changed by passing from one [referent system] to another.*[7]

To envision the application of a frame of reference approach to all laws of nature, Einstein imagined an elevator moving through space, occupied by a person who would measure her experience—her reality—within the referent frame of the elevator. An observer outside of the elevator would make a different set of measurements according to the metrics of his local frame of reference. The outside observer would note the following changes: As the speed of the elevator accelerates along a gently increasing curve of rate change, the mass inside the elevator eventually increases to infinity, and the energy required to produce this effect is on the same curve; the spatial dimension of length reaches zero at the acceleration limit; and time, measured as the interval between the ticks of a clock or the cycle of any process, also becomes infinite.

At the same time, the profound and bizarre reality of nature provides a different experience for the observer within the accelerating system. She cannot measure, feel, or understand the changes that the outside observer sees from his frame of reference. From her relative point of view, the clock is running as it always has, and the measuring stick shows the same distance between any two points. Inside the elevator—her unique, independent region of space-time—all dimensions retain an internal consistency relative to one another, regardless of the system's momentary velocity. All her biological processes are ticking along the same inherent temporal dimension as the clock she observes; thus, from her perspective, the rate does not change. The measuring ruler she holds conforms to the contraction of the spatial dimension, and thus she can detect no change in its units.

However, in the final few moments before the elevator reaches the speed of light, all mass dramatically increases toward infinity, and the elevator's occupant is squashed into a very tiny space. If the elevator were to remain below about 95 percent of the speed of light, and eventually were to return to Earth safely, the occupant would find that the slowing of her clocks, external and biological, had in fact really happened! Those whom she left behind during her trip would have aged more quickly than she. During her travels, there was no way for her to measure her contracting length and slowing clock, but nevertheless these changes were real. This is special relativity as it applies to the unification of space and time within 4D referent systems and the limits of our universal frame of reference. Our concepts of 4D space, matter, energy, and time likewise come to an abrupt end at this thermodynamic barrier of the speed of light (c), as does our language. We are constrained within this boundary condition, and no matter how hard we think, there is nothing that we can imagine, say, draw, or symbolize that represents what would happen at or beyond this barrier in 4D nature. We will revisit this line of thought in Chapters 10, 11, and 12.

In any referent system, three space dimensions and one temporal dimension internal to the system create an indivisible 4D referent frame. One, a few, or many atomic particles, atoms, elements, and all their arrangements may be a part of one referent system, such as the entire system of the elevator and its occupant or the planet Earth. However, it is important to note that within each large-scale frame of reference, all smaller particles retain their 4D individuality; that is, we cannot transform an atom of hydrogen into an atom of carbon simply by rearranging its components. Though ultimately both are made of the same stuff and both exist as part of Earth, each of these atoms retains a unique structure and function, one that can be broken only by powerful methods that tear atomic-level referent systems apart. Such a fission reaction would result in the creation of a new product with its own unique 4D existence and thermodynamic order. The final point is that if Earth were accelerated to a speed near that of light, like our imaginary elevator, all the component referent systems going along for the ride would experience similar relativistic effects, as they too would be being accelerated at essentially the same rate. Einstein showed that we truly cannot accurately talk about any phenomena in the universe except in relativistic terms, that is, as 4D processes between referent systems.

The Application of Relativity to Biology

This book is about space, time, dimension, and order in nature's systems. Our focus is on the biological systems that evolved on this planet. Our approach is to apply a frame of reference perspective to observations of the space-time order in independent, individual systems of biological components—in other words, to construct a model of biological relativity as a framework within which to view the emergent processes that organic evolution has created. *Relativistic effects* as we learn of them in basic physics texts refer to the behavior of 4D systems moving at a speed near that of light. But, as Einstein showed, relativistic effects are basic processes of nature for all 4D systems at any acceleration. It is just that we tend not to notice that a clock runs slightly more slowly in a spaceship as it orbits Earth or heads out toward the planets. The relativistic effects between reference systems at slower velocities are subtle, but they are always a part of the full context of the local environment. This is as true of biological systems as it is of nonbiological ones. To identify minute relativistic effects and appreciate their profound influence on biological systems, we may just have to look at our nature from a slightly different perspective.

As we move into the world of biology, we must continue to remain acutely aware of the fact that everything that we read, view, hear, think about, remember, and know is created in our minds. *We* as humanity provide an organization, an order, to all our knowledge, and the same processes that create order and knowledge may also at times create illusions. Illusions of space, time, dimension, and cause and effect that arise from the temporal order of information, as it flows through our minds, also form information in our physical memories. Einstein and his contemporaries were acutely aware of these human limitations and their role in the efforts to understand the new small universe of quantum probabilities, waves, and atomic particles and the new big universe of neutron stars, galaxies, nebulas, and novas. They all knew very well that at the interface of our senses with the infinitesimal world of the electromagnetic field or the grand-scale cosmic structures and distances, we make errors and create illusions of relationships, of cause and effect:

> *For man is enchained by the very condition of his being, his finiteness and involvement in nature. The farther he extends his horizons, the more vividly he recognizes the fact that, as the physicist Niels Bohr puts it, "we are both spectators and actors in the great drama of existence." Man is thus his own greatest mystery. He does not understand himself. He comprehends but little of his organic processes and even less of his unique capacity to perceive the world about him, to reason, and to dream. . . . Man's inescapable impasse is that he himself is part of the world he seeks to explore; his body and proud brain are mosaics of the same elemental particles that compose the dark, drifting clouds of interstellar space; he is, in the final analysis, merely an ephemeral conformation of the primordial space-time field.*[8]

Einstein's view of the universe emerged from his understanding of the irreducibility of the four dimensions in each and every particle of nature. All manifestations of inorganic systems have an inherent 4D referent frame. The model of biological relativity proposes that unique organic systems evolved that created novel 4D frames of reference and led to the emergence of consciousness. In the chapters that follow, we will explore the evolutionary processes that brought the system of life out of the background field of nonliving inorganic and organic substances. For it is from the basic 4D system of life that brain, thought, mind, and ultimately consciousness came into being.

Part Two

DIMENSIONS OF LIFE

2
Evolution and the Emergence of Life

Just as all matter and the properties of space, time, and dimension emerge from a background field of electromagnetic energies, so do the same properties for life and consciousness emerge from the background field of inorganic and organic substances. And just as an evolutionary view may be applied to the formation of elementary particles and enormous constellations of the universe in order to provide an overarching framework within which to conceptualize the current structure of space-time and its myriad reference systems, so may an evolutionary view be applied to the formation of life and consciousness to achieve an understanding of them as four-dimensional (4D) systems that ultimately emerge from the same fundamental fabric of the cosmos.

Arising from a prebiological phase of the Earth's evolution, living systems were created with the cell as the basic unit of existence. It is in the structure and function of the living cell that we find a new, emergent frame of reference that is qualitatively different from the referent systems of atoms, molecules, or planets. By following the path along which prebiological nature advanced, we may observe a progression among chemical reactions that ultimately produced living cells, and thus gain a critical insight into the basic patterns of organization upon which evolution plays. We have seen how Einstein revealed that the transition between energy and matter defines the formation of 4D reference systems, albeit by an unknown path of emergence. In our model of biological relativity, the equally mysterious transition between pre-life and life likewise defines the formation of 4D reference systems—cells. When we can materially conceptualize this threshold event in nature's organization, we will have constructed the necessary perspective from which to view the final evolutionary threshold: the emergence of consciousness from the collective activity of specialized cells that compose the nervous system.

The Primordial Earth

We can only imagine the actual events whereby life first arose from inorganic matter and energy in a choreographed display of chemical reactions four billion years ago. For, while many of the basic organic building blocks of life remain present within the current biosphere of the Earth, the vast majority of the complex structures and functional products of pre-life chemical systems have long since been recycled and hence lost in the living world. An impressive multidisciplinary body of research on the early phases of the Earth's organic maturation has produced many logical hypotheses consistent with known information about evolutionary processes preceding the dawn of life,[1] but we must admit that many pieces of the story are still missing. It is not surprising, then, that there are many significantly dissimilar theories about the origins of life and that no single viewpoint has achieved the position of an accepted model around which the relevant scientific fields of study might organize themselves.[2]

Having said that, we note that the evolutionary pathways to the emergence of a living cellular system that we propose are as speculative as any others. That the Earth has cellular life is an easy proposition to defend, but defining or determining the path to the emergence of cellular life is not as easy. The questions of why cells evolved as they did and for what purpose are merely the organic extensions of the same questions that are posed for all particle systems of matter and energy. These imponderables will remain intact, but we may achieve a new perspective on the threshold events in the evolution of matter, cells, and consciousness by application of a dimensional analysis within the frame of reference approach.

In the catastrophically violent condensation of star elements that formed the Earth, a gradual settling occurred as energies of motion and heat dissipated into the void, leaving a more stable spheroid mass. Our planet became a cauldron of complex mixtures of atoms, elements, molecules, and compounds, with a cooling outer layer forming around a molten iron and nickel core. The processes of planetary evolution included millennia of eruptions of core materials through the outer crust in the form of volcanic activity and the unpredictable impacts of meteoric masses screaming into our primordial gravity field. As the crust or mantle layer of the Earth continued to take shape as silicate rock, molecules of water began to be unleashed (outgassed) from their bound states. Water as gas condensed to liquid in torrential rains and collected in pools, ponds, streams, rivers, and oceans over the globe, interacting with the rock to form all the surface muds, clays, and soils of the Earth. The rotating primeval planet was further encased in an atmosphere of gaseous particles of methane, carbon dioxide, ammonia, hydrogen, nitrogen, and water. During the first several hundred million years, the available oxygen molecules were entombed in gas, liquid, and solid compounds. This was the Earth around four billion years ago, but before the next billion years had passed, it was abundantly rich with diverse life.

Constraints on the Evolution of Life

On the primordial planet, *thermodynamics* and *entropy* as manifested in *chemical reactions* defined the vital processes of the biosphere (more accurately, the pre-biosphere).[3] These finite parameters and interactions determined the evolutionary dance of nature that led to life.

Thermodynamics is the study of how chemical reactions occur and the energy conditions that determine their likelihood. The two basic propositions of thermodynamics are conservation of energy (first law) and entropy (second law). Together, these rules of nature determine the processes of all the chemical reactions that became life and all the biological functions that have followed thereafter. Most simply, we may note that for any chemical reaction to take place—that is, for any set of elements or molecules to be rearranged into a different product set (Figure 2-1)—certain conditions of force (thermal, mechanical, or radiant energy) must be present. If the local conditions affecting the reactants do not achieve a threshold level of energy, sometimes referred to as the *activation energy*, within a critical period of time, the reaction will not take place. However, the critical period of time may range from picoseconds (10^{-12} second) to millions of years, depending upon the chemical reactants and the reaction conditions (for instance, the critical period for the conversion of iron to iron oxide is much shorter than that for the transformation of elemental carbon to diamond crystals). When conditions are favorable and the reaction takes place, an accounting will show that all matter and energy associated with the reactants, the reaction process, and the resultant products will equal the matter and energy present prior to the reaction event. This is the basis of the first law of thermodynamics, conservation of matter and energy.

Of course, Einstein showed the equivalence of matter and energy, which explains the loss of mass in very energetic reactions (e.g., atomic fission or fusion). In chemical reactions, the transformation of matter (nearly undetectable in most reactions) is measured by the heat (light or motion

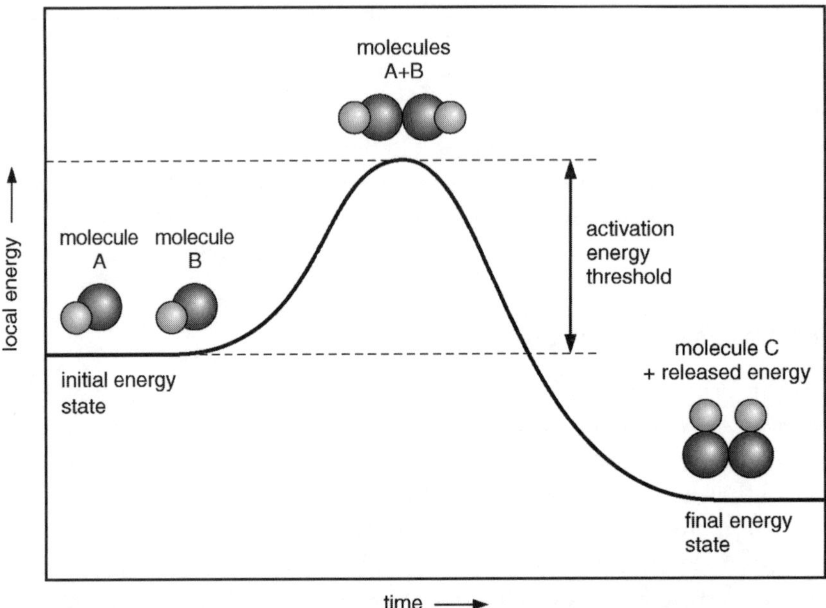

Figure 2-1 All chemical reactions must overcome a natural barrier in order to form new molecules. The *activation energy* defines the threshold energy necessary to accomplish either the synthesis of larger molecules from smaller ones or the breakdown of molecules into smaller constituents. An energy-releasing reaction is illustrated in this figure.

energy) of the reaction. The chemical reactions contained in a fire produce a rapid generation of heat energy that reflects the rate of reaction. The ashes left by the reaction processes do not add up to the original mass quantities because the missing matter was transformed into the energy of the event (each atom releases c^2 in energy force).

Two basic types of chemical reactions take place in nature. In general, these are classified as *exothermic* reactions, which release energy (heat), and *endothermic* reactions, which consume energy (heat). Many reactions between molecules take place spontaneously as a result of the relative energy and positional states of the reactants. Thus, the combination of *kinetic* energy (the energy of motion or action possessed by a molecule) and *potential* energy (the energy that is possessed by a molecule as a result of its position in the reaction space) may achieve or exceed a threshold activation energy, allowing the reaction to proceed.

The scientific study of nature's thermodynamic processes usually takes place under controlled conditions in *closed systems*. When we attempt to account for all energies of a reaction, determine the threshold activation energy, and measure the kinetic and potential energies of the products, it is much easier to do so when the reactants are contained within closed chambers that minimize outside influences. The simple example of measuring the change in heat energy in the spontaneous reaction of the state or phase transition from water ice to liquid water (one that most students perform in basic chemistry class) demonstrates the benefit of a closed-system approach. If the measurement of energy change were performed when the ice was exposed to the surrounding environment, the investigator would have no way to determine if some of the energy variation occurred as a result of influences other than those involved in the basic chemical reaction. This example indicates the potential for *bookkeeping errors of cause and effect* that is present at every moment of observation for any system in action, whether it is a chemical reaction, planets in motion, or people in thought.

The quantification of the energy relationships for chemical reactions in closed or equilibrium systems, an approach developed by J. Willard Gibbs (a pioneering American mathematician and physicist, and one of the greatest minds in the history of science), led to a set of basic equations that allows one to predict whether a defined reaction is likely to proceed spontaneously or not.[4] The *Gibbs free energy equation*, $\Delta G = \Delta H - T \Delta S$, is found in any book on chemical reactions and provides one of our great insights into nature's operating parameters. All progress in analyzing more complicated processes involving multiple simultaneous reactions in nonclosed systems (e.g., biological systems) stands upon Gibbs's original principles. The ΔG term relates the quantity of free energy change that occurs during a given chemical reaction in a defined thermodynamic environment. The variable ΔH indicates the change in the heat (*enthalpy*) of the system during the reaction, T is the absolute temperature, and ΔS indicates the *entropy* change of the system. If ΔG is calculated to have a negative value, then the chemical reaction will occur spontaneously under the defined conditions of the system (i.e., the activation energy demands have been met or exceeded, and therefore the reaction is exothermic). If ΔG has a positive value, additional energy is needed to drive the chemical reaction to completion, and thus the process is endothermic.

Entropy (represented by S in Gibbs's equation) as it applies to chemical reactions and molecular states may be defined as a measure of the amount of disorder or randomness in a given system. A change toward more order or less randomness in a thermodynamic system is a negative change in the entropy term, a *negative entropy*. A change toward more disorder or randomness is reflected as a positive change in the entropy term.

We may view the expansion and cooling of the universe at large as an ongoing change toward less order or more randomness. The ultimate outcome of this process would be a dispersed, cold, random nothing. However, in the universe and in earthly chemical reactions, there are regional organizations of matter and energy that move to a more ordered, less random state; thus, there is a negative entropy change. The energy necessary to drive a local system to more order must come from the surrounding region or universe. Thus, the organization of matter into particles, planets, and galaxies may be viewed as the formation of local regions of order that come as a drain on the background universe. Similarly, the chemical reactions that create new compounds utilize energy from the larger surround, leaving the overall system (the local region or universe as a whole) in a more disordered, more random state. And in local regions where conditions permit, new structures and thus new functions are derived during these matter and energy exchanges across long time scales. This concept of entropy provides the basis for our understanding of the emergence of life across thresholds of order in nature's ongoing dynamic transformation.

James Clerk Maxwell was the first to formalize our understanding of the unaided progression toward randomness (entropy) as it pertains to chemical reactions.[5] His famous thought experiment described the motion of gas particles contained in a sealed two-chambered box with a microscopically small passageway between the two compartments. In the imaginary gas mixture, some particles (on average) would be moving faster than others (i.e., would have more kinetic, and thus heat, energy). If no energy was allowed to escape from the box, the question then would be, how would the molecules of gas behave if left alone? Would they segregate themselves into the two chambers on the basis of their individual rates of motion (fast, heated particles in one chamber and slow, cooler ones in the other), or would their motions and interactions attain a state of purely random association (a final mixture of average heat)?

Maxwell surmised that the only way to gather all the fast, energetic particles into one chamber and leave the slower ones in the other would be to place a special door between the two chambers and have an all-knowing being control the action. When a fast particle was nearing the door, the omnipotent being (later known as Maxwell's demon) would open the door and allow the particle to enter. On the other side of the door, when a slower particle happened to move in the appropriate direction, the demon would again open the door to allow the slower particle to move into the other chamber. Only in this manner could the gas be segregated into a more ordered, and thus less random, state. Maxwell understood that this process does not reflect nature in most situations; there is no demon that preferentially guides chemical reactions. In other words, systems tend toward a more random state, with higher entropy. That is why a cube of ice melts when placed in a warm location. There is no force of nature that holds the molecules of ice together in the face of entropy.

We may, however, make note of local reactions that are driven by the processes of nature (including those initiated by human action) that do create more order, and accordingly take into account the cost of these events in terms of the increase in background entropy. Throughout the following chapters, we refer to the cost of creating order or negative entropy (as it applies to chemical reactions or information), when it happens, and where it exists in the local context. The course of a reaction toward a new state of organization, at the cost of less order in the larger system, becomes the jumping-off point for many discussions as to the true nature of order, randomness, entropy, systems, and information. There are many hypotheses and theories related to these considerations.[6] The details of these theories are too far removed from the focus of this current work, but we refer to them at key points in the presentation where they have application. In general, we must note that our model does not vary from the basic operational definition of entropy that comes from its use in the thermodynamics of chemical reactions as established by Gibbs and Maxwell.

One final comment should be made here as it relates to basic thermodynamic study, the derivation of the laws, and their application in more complex systems. As mentioned, thermodynamic theory initially applied to closed, controlled conditions of reaction. As we move toward open or semiclosed systems that exchange matter and energy during reaction events (e.g., cells and systems of cells such as nervous systems), the linear equilibrium equations of classic thermodynamics become inadequate to the analysis. To perform the bookkeeping functions necessary to account for all sources of energy, the reaction processes, the product states, and the changes to the larger background system, we must use nonlinear, nonequilibrium hypotheses and their accompanying mathematics. The current explosion of research into these conceptually and computationally very difficult areas was made possible only by the advent of high-speed computers.[7] The extraordinary number of variables and parallel activities that accompany even the simplest of metabolic pathways created in living organisms must truly humble us before the grandeur of nature and the understanding of what evolutionary processes may devise when billions of years are involved.

The Chemistry of Life

The basic distinction between inorganic and organic reactions is made at the carbon atom. All living systems are based on carbon-based compounds, of which there are more than a million known. The other central atoms involved in organic compounds include phosphorus, oxygen, and nitrogen. Only hydrogen is utilized in more molecules than is carbon, and these molecules include many of the several hundred thousand inorganic compounds on Earth.

From the theoretical work of A. I. Oparin and the experimental demonstrations of Harold C. Urey, Stanley L. Miller, and others after them, we can make educated guesses about what molecules could have existed in the prebiotic solutions of four billion years ago, under methane skies and the harsh glare of unabated radiation.[8] In 1953, Miller conducted a classic experiment under the direction of Urey in which he circulated four gases thought to resemble the primordial atmosphere (methane, water, ammonia, and hydrogen) in a glass chamber while exciting them with electrical discharges (to resemble lightning) for a week.[9] His analysis of the condensations in the chamber revealed dramatic results. Miller found that many organic compounds had formed, including amino acids, urea, acetic acid, and lactic acid. Many other researchers have replicated and extended his results.

Suitable niches for the formation of the primary compounds necessary for life may have been created in a variety of regions on the young Earth. Likely places would have been muddy shorelines, clay surfaces, hydrothermal vents deep in bodies of water, and rocky surfaces rich in catalytic compounds containing reactive metals like iron pyrites, magnesium, or zinc.[10] All such niches may be functionally viewed as interface regions where watery solutions of reactive compounds could be brought into close proximity at surface edges. At shorelines and other interfaces of solid surfaces and water, new compounds (with different elements, novel shapes, or new properties) could form, and catalytic substrates could function to make possible certain reactions that otherwise could not have occurred. In some regions, aqueous compounds could be formed and then dried as the liquid receded or evaporated, providing a dynamic niche where chemical, mechanical, thermal, and radiant energy could alternately drive reaction processes. A. G. Cairns-Smith has proposed an elegant theory of crystalline clay surfaces providing detailed structural scaffolding to guide the formation of early complex arrangements of molecules.[11] Alternatively, Sidney Fox has conducted decades of insightful research into the prebiotic formation of complex molecules and polymers (longer and more complex molecules) and has hypothesized that shorelines and pond edges might have been important regions where the mechanical forces of hydration, evaporation, and radiation could have directly contributed to the pathway to life.[12]

Another crucial prebiotic process might have involved the formation of polymers of ribonucleic acid (RNA), composed of sequences of purines (adenine and guanine) and pyramidines (cytosine and uracil) combined with sugar and phosphorus molecules. These dynamic molecules may have functioned as an organic catalyst or enzyme, acting to lower the activation energy hills in a reaction without being consumed by the reaction, and thus precluding the need for additional heat energy. This would have allowed many so-called cold reactions, whose thermal dynamics would not have disrupted nearby reaction pathways, to take place simultaneously in close proximity. The most important functions of RNA (and later of deoxyribonucleic acid, DNA, a more stable, double-helix molecule in which the pyramidine thymine is substituted for uracil) would have been its role in the formation of polypeptides and proteins by supporting the sequential coded binding of amino acids on long strands of nucleotide chains and its ability to produce copies of its own base sequence by a unique, thermodynamically favorable process called complementary templating. RNA may have thus formed the first proto-genes and proto-genomes in the primordial molecular solutions.[13]

In locations where elements, molecules, and complex compounds had the necessary spatial setting to interact and enough energy was available to overcome local entropy, new species of molecules and compounds were created through chemical transformation. Novel chemical products that were stable over time could now become new participants in the evolutionary dance and be paired with additional reactant partners. The changing probabilistic outcomes of this thermodynamic interplay forged novel and sustained products that possessed new structural and functional properties through moments of chemical choreography.

In this dance toward life, the fiddler, or entropic energy demands, was paid from the vast wealth of the background universe of mass in kinetic motion and radiant energy sources. Again, we must stress that in this retrospective view of organic evolution, the dynamic processes of chemical reactions, constrained by local thermodynamic and entropic parameters, produced new products, some of which tended to persist longer than others. This changing distribution of substances within each local region of chemical activity *is* the evolutionary path. The specific reactants, reactions, and products and what role they each had in the formation of the first cell could not be known until that cell emerged from this background of nonrandom activity.

A Structure for Life

Among the most fascinating and common phenomena of spontaneous formations that we may observe in natural chemical systems is the formation of tiny spheres or bubbles by soap and water. Phospholipid molecules similar to those in soap bubbles may also have formed the earliest enclosures in the preorganic world (Figure 2-2).[14] When dispersed in water, these molecules will spontaneously form spherical bilayers in which their charged ends are directed toward the water interface (*hydrophilic* layer) and the neutral chains are positioned within the sphere (*hydrophobic* layer). These structures will also spontaneously fuse with others or divide into smaller spheres; they can even be dehydrated and then regain their original shape when hydrated. All cells of living organisms have a high percentage of their membranes com-

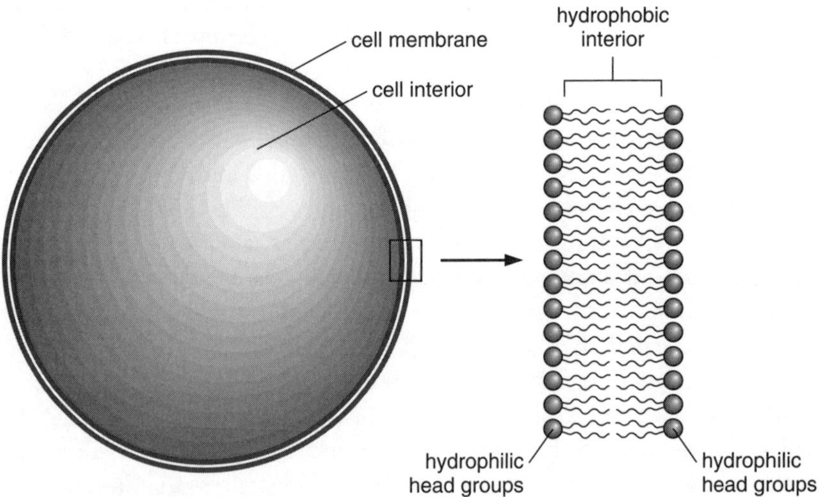

Figure 2-2 Phospholipid molecules spontaneously form spherical bilayered structures in aqueous solutions. Such molecular structures may have functioned as primitive protocellular membranes.

posed of phospholipid, and all have the basic bilayer design. This is a design constraint of life. Each cell is a system of chemical reactions taking place inside a bilayered phospholipid membrane.

Phospholipids are stable molecules and are virtually insoluble in water. Such naturally occurring spheres may have formed the basis of the first independent *protocells*, semiclosed volume spaces that could have survived in aqueous solutions of the primordial Earth. The phospholipid protocell, or a similar structure, would have provided a charged boundary, a barrier that created within its walls the first internal organic environment by capturing a tiny volume of the local aqueous solution. Thermodynamically, this can be viewed as a semiclosed (nonequilibrium) system that would have permitted the exchange of energy as well as matter through its semipermeable membrane of phospholipid strands, while being held in a three-dimensional spatial formation by the interaction of phosphate charge with the surrounding water molecules.

We will employ this model of the primordial protocell as a hypothetical vehicle for the transition from pre-life to life. Thus, we can begin to imagine how a unique collection of molecules, with their interrelated chemical reactions and products contained within the walls of phospholipid membranes, may have formed the first living cells. But what critical threshold conditions, created in evolutionary time, enabled the emergence of the first cell from the background of nonliving protocells?

The Protocell World

In a variety of local solutions, when a threshold concentration of phospholipid molecules was present, protocell membranes whose internal contents of potential reactive chemicals found moments of partial isolation from the larger external environment may have appeared spontaneously. These events would have marked a critical crossroads in the evolution of life: A separation had begun between the background flux of all possible energy sources (molecular, thermal, and radiant) and the fleeting existences of captured chemicals, molecules, and energies within the boundaries of the protocells. It is through this historic division of the primordial biosphere into dichotomous regions of internal and external structures and functions, and their dynamic interactions, that we may observe the emergence of a new form of 4D existence.

We may imagine that, in the protocell, the dynamic dance of evolution moved inside to a new ballroom and out of the harsh rain of the external surrounds. In this speculative pre-life world of tens, thousands, perhaps millions of local niches with relatively stable environmental conditions, the early protective phospholipid spheres came in many sizes and forms. Those that had very dense, tightly packed lipid molecules would have shut out the energy and matter of the outside solution to such an extent that it doomed any internal solution of reactants to a quick demise (an entropic stabilization in the absence of additional energy and material input). At the other extreme, porous spheres of phospholipid may have formed that allowed a constant flood of energy and matter to move into and out of the interior, rendering any *private* activity among the reactants unlikely (a low probability of any unique internal reactions persisting over time). In addition, a certain percentage of membrane spheres would have been physically torn apart by the dynamic forces of materials and energies within their local microniches.

Between the extremes of highly impermeable and highly permeable membrane structures, however, interesting things may have occurred. In local niches that were rich with inorganic and organic compounds (and whose background thermal and radiant energies fluctuated between maximal and minimal levels that were neither too intense nor too weak), phospholipid spheres possessing a moderate level of structural integrity and permeability could have contained solutions of reacting molecules that were provided with energy and protection at a level adequate to permit the formation of new chemical reaction pathways and new products that would not have been possible in the outside environment.

It is here, in these particular primordial protocells, that the processes of evolution for organic compounds and their reaction pathways might have been able to create new order, new regions of negative entropy, and new organizations of the background matter and energy during brief, fleeting moments of existence. These just-right conditions (analogous to the fairy tale of the three bears) could have led to the extended existence of increasingly novel 3D systems of reactive molecules inside a protective membrane. The existence of any protocell, however, would still have been tied closely to the rise and fall of the background energy environment. Thus, at this point in the dance of evolution, if the local energy levels dropped below a critical threshold, protocell activity also soon ceased. The internal and external divisions of the primordial biosphere (all the protocell volumes and biochemical niches) were still defined by only one independent and all-encompassing temporal dimension; there was effectively one planetary chemical system supporting protocell formation, existence, and destruction.

Inside the early protocells, chemical reactions may have lasted for only brief moments, but perhaps this was long enough for even just one new product or compound to form—just long enough for one series of reaction steps to be completed in a protected region that brought together in space and time a collection of molecules and energies that statistically or physically could not have encountered each other in this manner outside of such a place. For example, perhaps in certain types of protocells RNA strands and solutions of amino acids could form specific polypeptides, which in turn engaged in chemical reactions with nearby carbohydrate molecules to produce additional energy release within the confines of the membrane. This interior release of new energy may then have initiated additional chemical reactions that in effect extended the time that the protocell's internal activity maintained its own unique existence relative to background energy fluctuations.

If this process of nonrandom juxtapositions of solutions containing reacting compounds within semipermeable phospholipid spheres occurred in enough spheres over enough time, the resultant production of novel active compounds might have reached critical concentration thresholds. As these new molecules attained such density levels, they would themselves become significant to the processes of protocell creation and internal energy-producing reactions; such a feedback cycle of reactions, forged over eons of time, would have promoted self-sustaining activity within protocells. In effect, the process of extended internal time of protocell existence would further separate it from the external time of the larger biosphere.

We may imagine ourselves watching a view of ponds, pools, rivers, shorelines, and oceans of activity, wherein protocells flicker into physical and biochemical existence. Across wide expanses of time, in bioenergetically dynamic local regions around the planet, the statistical shifts in the populations of phospholipid spheres, their duration of existence, and the content of their internal solutions would begin to approach a critical threshold level of 3D spatial order and persistence in time. The process of organic evolution would thus be creating very small semiclosed systems whose structure and internal energy function would become more complex and would derive novel order relative to the background levels of entropy. The local relative order inside the protocell would of course come at the cost of disorder in the background environment, extracted as energy and energy compounds flowed across the phospholipid membrane. And the entropic balance sheet of the local region would be maintained by the larger influx of energy and matter provided by the supporting biosphere.

In the prebiotic environment, the process of evolution was unfolding through tiny, unique protected environments of novel reaction pathways to develop and produce new products of organic structure and function. The interaction within protocells probably included the construction of longer polymers (branching chains) of carbohydrates, proteins, nucleotides, and phospholipids. The reactions between any two or more of these basic compounds within these protective shells might have led to combination products such as the nucleic acid–protein complexes of ribosomes developing, or to small and large proteins becoming inserted into the phospholipid membrane and functioning as channels and receptors. Thus, during the time that a protocell could survive, novel chemical reactions and their products could be generated. The fusion and/or destruction of protocells further promoted the evolutionary process, as it allowed compounds produced within one protocell to be captured by another protocell. The cumulative results of this cannibalization were new and increasingly complex and energetic internal environments producing products that may have caused some protocells to last longer than their predecessors.

Evolution, the nonrandom statistical shift in structures over time, resulted in regions of the biosphere where protocells were maintaining longer existences, creating more interrelated pathways of energy exchange reactions, and involving more energy and more molecules: A protometabolism was emerging. To the extent that background conditions permitted, protocells continued to evolve, to extend their own time of the dance. However, we must again note a likely, and critical, limiting factor to this process. If the source of energy and material in the microenvironment surrounding a group of protocells declined below a critical minimal threshold level for a sufficient period of time, the thermodynamic pathways within the affected protocells would invariably lose a necessary amount of energy and begin an irreversible decay to an equilibrium state. Even protocells of high structural integrity and finely tuned permeability would not have survived the loss of driving energy and energy-supplying molecules as the local background flux reached a minimal state. However, the products of their demise could be recycled into other protocells in nearby microenvironments that had maintained a sufficient level of energy.

As the dance of the flickering protocells in the pre-life world continued in microniches around the planet, the internal protocell environments also may have begun to produce increasingly longer chains of nucleic acid sequences. These in turn would interact with amino acids to produce more peptide and protein products. Proteins that functioned as enzymes or channels may have served to further extend protocell existence by forming more efficient energy transfer pathways and molecular exchange mechanisms between the external and internal solutions. Again, in a statistical fashion, protocell populations were becoming more efficient in their ability to utilize the external flow of energy across the membrane to drive internal reactions. Finally, at some point along this probable evolutionary pathway, the internal collection of RNA and/or DNA would have reached a critical length and coding sequence such that by translation to peptide and protein products the necessary structural constituents that formed the protocell could be replicated within that same environment.

A *reiterative* and *recombinant* process wherein one new chemical reaction, one new phosphate bond, one additional polymeric-chain link, one new folding pattern in a sequence of amino acids, one new combination of carbohydrate and nucleic acid, and so on, continued to take place over millions of years in uncountable numbers of protocells on the primordial Earth. All this began with fleeting moments of structural and functional integrity, evolving to ever more enduring protocellular existences that served to bring quantities of the external organic solution into protected proximity, all under the driving and sustaining energies of the background biosphere. New molecular products created new reaction pathways, which, through feedback mechanisms, created additional new products. As the internal spatial arrangement of molecules became more complicated and the number of pathways increased, and as the length of time that a protocell could exist also increased, the protocell produced more of the products that it could produce. Of course, the library of internally generated products included the molecules that constituted the protocell.

From a perspective high above the local niches of protocell activity, we can imagine that the flicker fields of protocell existence began to glow more brightly as the proto-metabolic environments grew more and more complex and energetic. We might even observe new protocells forming inside of protocells. However, in any given area, we would ultimately see the fluctuations of background energy fall below a critical sustaining threshold for the increasingly energy-hungry reaction pathways inside the protocells, causing the spheres of bright energy transfer activity to begin their fade into the background energy glow and nonexistence.

We can thus watch in wonderment this dance of organic evolution as it creates specialized local environments, each containing a grand colorful waltz of unique but fleeting protocell existence. Each niche is a complete world of bioenergetic processes, whose maximum and minimum energy flux pace the private dance taking place in each and every protocell ballroom, imagined as a metronome of pulsating light timing and limiting each performance. Each microworld devises its own costumes, colors, and motions, as protocell diversity explodes with the numerical expansion. The protocell populations' presence and products likewise shape the very environments that gave rise to them. This is an extremely important part of the feedback process of evolution in organic systems. All reiterative and recombinant changes hold for the nourishing background as well as for the protocells within it. It is this fully dynamic and interrelated process that determined the course of biological existence and brought life into being.

As we move closer to the threshold of life, just prior to the final moments in the individual dance of the protocell, as its internal light fades into equilibrium with the background flux, we begin to observe the replication of the set of molecules to form a near-duplicate structure within the boundaries of the growing membrane. When the background conditions reach a state of maximal availability of energy and molecules, we may even see an amazing event occur: Within certain biosphere regions and in highly organized protocells that have created a copy of their structure, we note the first fission of massively bloated protocells into two separate entities. Under the permitting conditions of the local environment, a critical mass of materials disrupts the integrity of the stretched and misshapen outer membrane and creates a division of the protocell. The violated membranes fold back into a spheroid shape under the mechanical and electrostatic forces created by the surrounding solution.

At first, we may see the great majority of protocells destroyed by this overweight condition, as their internal environment is exposed to the background. However, in time some protocells may reorganize and continue to conduct other reactions before they lose integrity, time-locked to periodic declines in background energy. Perhaps some of the protocell-like products, the new offspring, survive the destructive event and exist in moments of internal activity before entropy draws them into the background as material for use in other protocells. This hypothetical state of protocell activity may have existed in thousands or millions of local regions scattered around the planet more than three billion years ago (Figure 2-3).

This description of protocell activity, for all its complexity, does not define life. We have walked right to the edge of life and now stand on a stepping-stone along the evolutionary path that started at the inorganic world of nonliving systems of matter and energy in relative motion. We have stepped across to the primordial biosphere and watched the evolutionary processes shape the local background conditions and the protocells within. We are now ready to take one more step and observe the emergence of life as a unique 4D reference system of organic existence.

The Emergence of Life

We survey an imaginary niche of protocells flickering into and out of existence, riding the tides of energy and matter supplied by the background

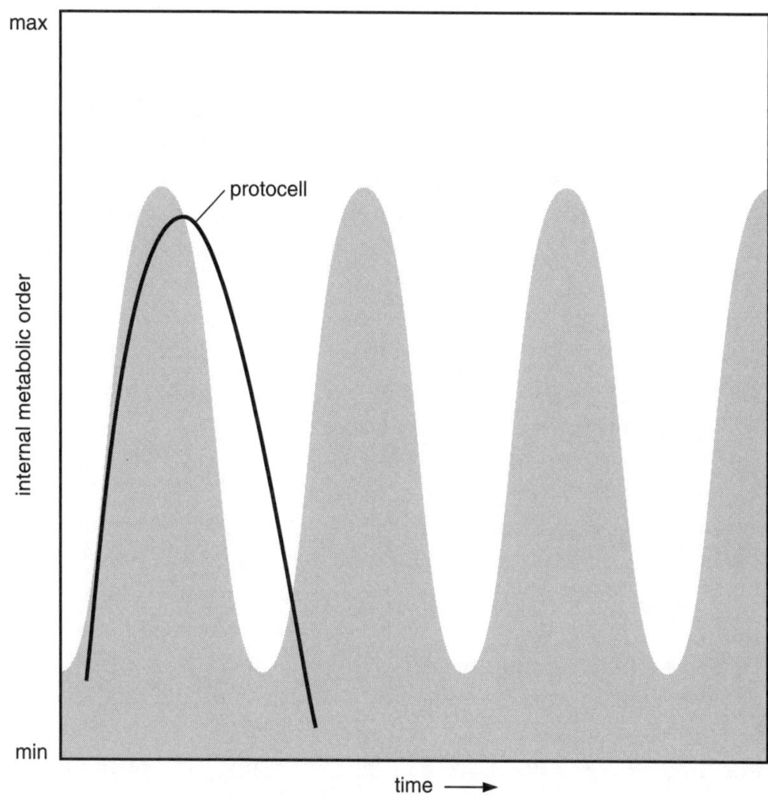

Figure 2-3 Protocell internal metabolic activity relative to available energy sources in the prebiotic environment. All protocells degraded to background levels of thermodynamic order and were incapable of propagating offspring that sustained sufficient internal metabolic order. The shaded area represents background energy flux.

flux. As the evolutionary clock marks the passage of time, we have the privilege of witnessing the swan song of pre-life in the final moments before the emergence of a new system. The dance of chemical reactions over millions of years has led to progressively more complex and stable intra-protocell environments, and finally to the complete replication of the protocell's own structure. We must now remain acutely aware of several factors as life emerges from this lifelike activity.

First, the background system of matter and energy (the active biosphere) has played the role of conductor in evolution's orchestra. That is, the temporal dimension that has set the pace for all reactions along the shorelines of the oceans, on the clay surfaces of ponds and lakes, and in the interior solutions captured by protocell membranes was the single clock of the entire Earth in action. The rise and fall of all fluctuations of radiant energies and the energies contained in molecular bonds determined the measure of time, the measure of existence for each and every chemical reaction, and thus the measure of existence for each and every protocell. As we described in this scenario, when the level of energy flux across the membranes of protocells fell below a critical level to a lower equilibrium state, a state of positive entropy, the thermodynamic pathways of reaction within the affected protocells would follow a path of decay from which they could not recover. For us to witness the emergence of life, we must bring our focus of attention to the process of evolution that was slowly separating the thermodynamic properties of the external background environment and the internal chemical reactions of the protocells.

The reiterative, recombinant refinement of the chemical pathways within protocells, their products, and, in turn, the entire aqueous solution of the background niche was slowly changing the structural arrangements of molecules in newly generated protocells. The evolution of novel enzymes, coupled reactions, and oscillatory pathways of electron energy transport (wherein one decaying path of reaction energy would provide the fuel to help another reaction over its activation hill) was achieved by the unique 3D spatial array of the collective materials within the internal environments of the protocells. The structure of the protocell determined its functional parameters. What we had been watching as private ballroom dances, the activity of internal environments of the protocells, was in reality the evolution of structure and function that was leading to longer and more complicated dance routines. Thus, in innumerable variations on the basic design of the ballroom and steps of the dance, unique populations of protocells around the planet began to extend their existence in protocell time—the flickering moments of bioenergetic light that we see in the oceans of a singular thermodynamic flow of planetary time.

Inside the protocell ballroom, a new conductor was anxiously tapping his baton and awaiting the moment when a new orchestra would attain a threshold level of musicians, instruments, and sheet music so that he could begin to set the rhythm of a new private, internal dance. The application of a frame of reference approach to the evolution of organic systems can have utility only if we remain continually aware of the structure-function (the 4D nature) of the background referent system, relative to the behavior of any other systems with a different structure-function existing within that field of matter and energy. The protocells that we watch seem to be fighting against the pace of the background thermodynamic dance, struggling to climb a collective activation energy hill against the pull of entropic gravity and to create a sustained rhythm of their own making. But ultimately they fall into step and become subject to the background pulse of time, destined to decay to the lowest level of equilibrium, to randomness and disorder. *This is the swan song of the protocell.* However, this momentary dance of death is actually a prelude to the emergent shape of things to come.

The *first living cell* was a semiclosed membrane-bound system of interdependent chemical reactions whose structure and function maintained an internal integrity, a nonequilibrium ordered existence, for a critical time relative to the periodicity of available external energy in the background field (Figure 2-4). To propagate the cellular system and the new order of structure and time, it was necessary for the binary fission products of self-replication, the newly created cells, to retain a similar threshold level of structure and function. Thus, each new cell possessed a minimal order of organic organization (a threshold negative entropy) and proceeded to produce additional cells of near-equal order—and therein the propagated organic system existence we call life emerged on the Earth.

The protocells reached the edge of life, became more and more stable, and thus existed for longer durations. A minute, subtle, and seemingly insignificant modification created the first living cell that maintained its threshold level of internal order—a novel internal temporal dimension, a thread of time across a threshold duration as the background energy flux cycled between its minimal and maximal states (its own independent thermodynamic clock of activity). From our imaginary point of view, as we stand above an ocean of flickering protocellular existence, the time-limited internal lights grow progressively brighter and more enduring relative to the fluctuating glow of the background thermodynamic pulse. In evolutionary time, we thus begin to notice small regions where the flickering becomes a fused, constant radiation; this is the temporal signal of life against the background noise of nonliving chemical reactions.

In discrete systems of thermodynamic stability, first one cell, then local groups, then oceans of living cells inherited the capability to maintain an internal order of structure and function across the periodic fluctuations of background energy that continued to flow through their membranes and reaction pathways. A new temporal dimension of organic existence was created in the activity of novel 3D molecular structures. The internal pace of thermodynamic reactions crossed a critical threshold of duration and order that caused a disconnection from the background temporal dimension. A new timeline for organic processes emerged as the biological field of cellular life, and was propagated as a constant glow in generations of new cells:

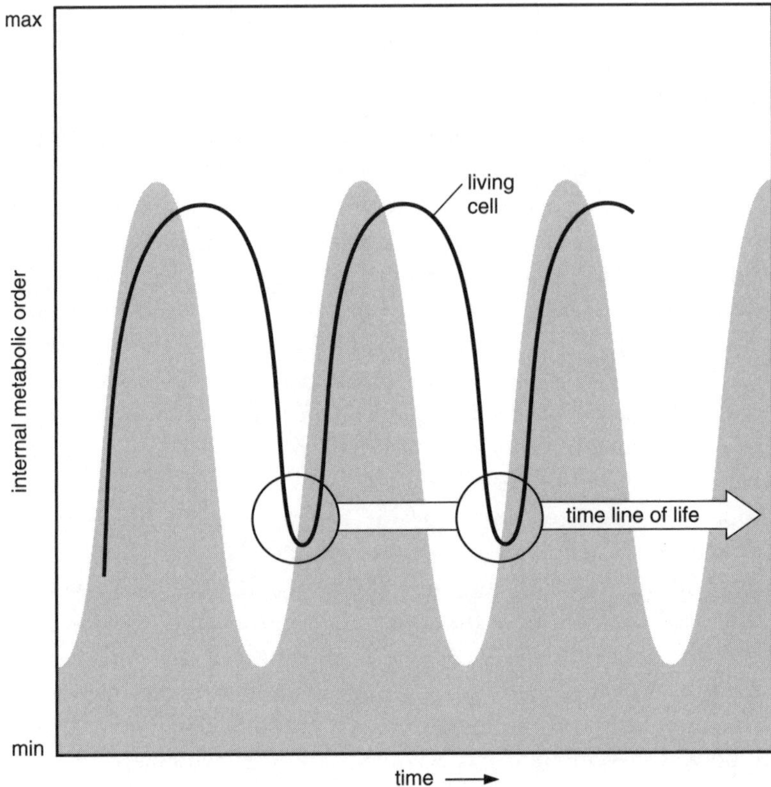

Figure 2-4 Emergence of cellular life from the hypothetical protocellular world. The arrow shows the time line of life. A threshold level of sustained internal metabolic order relative to the available background energy permitted the living cell to persist across external energy minima and propagate a critical level of order in binary fission offspring. A new 4D coordinate system whose temporal dimension is measured in generations emerged from the prebiotic environment.

as 4D organic referent systems behaving relative to the originating and sustaining biosphere field and creating a geometric explosion of new life around the planet. In generations of propagated order, 4D order, the life field of cells now existed temporally distinct from the pulse of the external environment—wholly dependent upon it for continued existence, but independent of it because of the cells' novel internal structural and functional organization. The protocell world thus came to an end, usurped and enveloped by the new order of structure and function, of space and time.

3

The Reference System of Life

Before we proceed further down the road of life and evolutionary change, along the path of stepping-stones that led to consciousness, let us formalize the model of biological relativity. Throughout the speculative discussion of the primordial conditions that generated the first living cell, we have been purposefully constructing a particular point of view, a model, by which to observe and define cellular life in terms of an evolutionary process of increasing thermodynamic order in small organic systems. This is a process that has played out over great expanses of time through reiterative, recombinant activities, ultimately leading to an emergent referent system whose internal structure-function can be defined as a unique four-dimensional (4D) entity.

An operating principle of this model is relativity, as it is used to examine and relate referent systems within a background continuum or field. We have defined two frames of reference in describing the emergence of life: the intracellular molecular environment of the cell and the extracellular environment of the planet. The essential *properties*, *processes*, and *products* of an observed 4D organic system may be understood only when they are defined relative to the surrounding referent environment. The molecular reactions of intracellular systems may be described as emergent only when they are related as a collective system to the flux (the rate of energy transfer) present in the larger, supporting local environment.

A second operating principle relates to the concept of dimension. It is imperative that we maintain an awareness of the 4D nature of our existence. In this model, we define a referent frame as an independent and irreducible 4D system. And time, along with the spatial dimensions, exists only as a relative quantity whose reality and thus meaning is determined by the frame of reference.

We may now present a conceptual model of biological relativity, the principle of emergence in organic evolution manifest in 4D referent systems. *When the process of evolution creates a sufficiently ordered organic system, such that its structure and function possess a threshold temporal dimension relative to the background field, an independent four-dimensional coordinate system emerges. This emergent system is defined as a new level of organic existence and, if propagated, functions as an irreducible frame of reference. By this we propose that unique properties and processes emerge that may be defined only by reference to the collective 4D coordinates of the system. Furthermore, we propose that only two emergent organic frames of reference have evolved in biological existence, and we refer to them in general as life and consciousness. As particles of matter organize energy in an interrelated existence to produce 4D referent systems in inorganic nature, so do molecules of matter organize energy in an interrelated existence to produce 4D referent systems in organic nature.*

Properties, Processes, and Products in Referent Systems

In the background environment of the biosphere, we may identify an enormous number of properties, processes, and products. For example, the noun *volcano* describes the property of a collective set of processes (geothermal activities). Likewise, *ocean* is the property of all the processes that we classify to give it meaning. Thus, properties are names for frames of reference; they do not have unique units of measure or force, and thus they have no effect on the processes of the system that defines them, or on any other system. The Earth, a volcano, or an ocean has an effect only because of its defining processes and their products.

Processes, then, are the 4D operations, cycles, or events that are unique in their coordinate systems, have their own units of measure, and create force and products. The Earth has a process of angular and linear motion in space, and this is associated with units of measure (distance, time, acceleration) and thus force (mass, work, energy). A volcano has many defining processes, such as an eruption. The process of an eruption has mass (steam, rocks, lava), velocities of ejection and flow, and thus force. Oceanic processes would include waves, tides, and pressures of depth and mass. Properties and processes reflect our observation of 4D events.

Products, however, are the 3D outcomes of processes, and are also uniquely created in individual referent systems. A cubic meter of soil, a ton of lava, and a gallon of salt water are products of the 4D systems. At the level of chemical reactions in the background field of the biosphere Earth, for example, we find the oxidation of iron, the formation of stalactites and stalagmites from mineral compounds deep inside of caves, and the creation of ozone by the reaction of radiation with oxygen in the atmosphere.

Life as the property of all the referent systems of cells in action has many processes and products that exist only within its 4D framework. All the chemistry of life—biological processes and products—is generated only within the internal environments of cells or in the collective processes of multicellular organisms. All metabolic pathways are 4D processes, and all new compounds that result from these processes are the unique products of life and may not be created in any other location in the biosphere. Molecular oxygen, hormones, peptides, blood, sweat, and tears are but a few of the multitude of novel products created by the myriad processes of living cells and organisms. Life is the frame of reference, the only 4D system within which these things are possible.

Relativity Effects in Biological Systems

Relativity effects may be subtle for inorganic systems at slow rates of motion and for biological systems, but they are always there as an inseparable aspect of the system's existence. For example, in a controlled setting we can make a solution and place just two cells in it. We select two cells that are as nearly identical as we possibly can determine. If we measure the rates at which each cell processes the energy flux of our solution through its internal system and produces its products, we will find that each has its own unique temporal dimension for one, two, or more pathways of reaction and rates of product formation. They may be close, as those of two similar elevators moving together in space would be, but if we measure with enough specificity and resolution, we will find a difference. The difference is the independent dimension of time created within the structure-function of the cell referent frame. A simple, large-scale example would be the growth rate of any two identical flowers in the same soil and room. Subtle differences in the temporal dimensions of each cell become easily observable in large-scale behaviors. This is a *relativity effect* in biological systems.

The relativity effect of time dilation on biological systems was of course envisioned first by Einstein and is typically presented in the form of the twin paradox.[1] In this imaginary tale of twin brothers, one travels to a nearby star in a rocket that accelerates to a speed near that of light and finds upon his return that his twin has aged at an apparently accelerated rate relative to himself. This appears to many to be a flight of fancy, but the relative nature of the universe that Einstein revealed holds for all independent clocks in 4D referent frames: clocks of springs and sprockets, crystals and batteries, isotopes of radioactive elements, and cells and organisms. The first three are products, natural or synthetic, of the background field of matter and energy, whereas the last clock is created in the life field of cellular activity. Both frames of reference, the nonbiological and the biological, are populated by 4D referent systems creating an internal time flow that is affected uniquely by relative acceleration. Astronauts in Earth orbit have measured the relative rates of time of living systems at orbital acceleration and on the Earth and have found that biological clocks in acceleration move more slowly relative to ones at rest. Einstein's twin paradox is not a whimsical metaphor, but an illustration of a real phenomenon.

This is an essential point. We can imagine building a clock from almost anything; but there are only two natural temporal dimensions that exist for matter and life and thus are subject to relativistic effects: the time dimension in each particle of matter and any collection of matter, and the time dimension in each cell and any collection of cells. There is nothing that evolution has produced in between these two emergent systems. The third and final natural frame of reference, consciousness, emerged from the life field of cellular referent systems.

The Life Field

We may now begin to understand the concept of emergent evolution as it applies to life. Evolution is a process that transcends all levels of molecular organization and has operated since before the origin of life.

All life is cellular. The life field is the uncountable number of cells and their collective organizations that began over three billion years ago. At the highest level of classification, we give names to the properties of cellular systems in action. Properties may be defined in general as life (the name of the entire 4D field) or as cells (the name of each 4D unit of life), or be given more specific names, such as bacteria, fungi, plants, and animals. The most specific names we give to the entire behaving systems include red rose, oak tree, African termite, guppy, Spot the dog, and Melissa the girl. All the classification schemes in biology, from kingdoms, divisions, phyla, classes, orders, species, and subspecies to the pet names and names of individual people, are properties of living systems. And, as we have noted, each individual cell on the planet has the property of life.

Processes of living systems include the internal chemical pathways that maintain the system or produce a product and the behaviors of individual cells or organisms as they interact with one another and with the background environment. The general classifications of some internal processes include metabolism, respiration, digestion, and reproduction. Large-scale collective processes include growing, sporulating, crawling, walking, flying, eating, barking, and talking, and in the most general terms, living and dying. Products unique to life include all the gas, liquid, and solid molecules produced by single cells and all organisms.

The language of life pertains properly to cellular activities. We may employ this level of terminology with nonliving systems, either through poetic license or because of the illusion of animism. Thus, we may say that the river is running at a fast pace and digesting all materials in its path. Or we may give personal names to the planets and stars and believe that they are alive and have all the processes of life, including human emotion and intent. Even today, in our daily casual language, we speak of angry clouds, smiling suns, and sexy cars. We will continue to note the level of language use as we move toward the next frame of reference in nature.

The frame of reference approach to organic evolution, then, provides boundary lines for our operational definitions of terms that have application only when describing the properties, processes, or products of discrete referent systems and their 4D activity. Thus, we have operationally defined the term *emergence* to refer only to a frame of reference as it arises out of a background field. An emergent system or property or process, then, refers only to those things within each 4D frame of reference that do not exist in another referent frame. In this operational definition, all the state or phase changes or transitions that may be observed to arise either from matter and energy in action or from cells in action are not considered emergent properties or processes. The state transition of liquid water to steam, or the phase transition of swirling air currents to a vortex of a hurricane, or the swarm behavior of ants or bees arising from group interaction is not describing the emergence of a new 4D frame of reference. Strictly speaking, for science and medicine, we must remain aware of this distinction.

Finally, we may clearly see why life is usually defined by listing its key processes and products: metabolism, replication, division, and the production of a new cell. In biological relativity, we can define life as the 4D organic frame of reference. It is defined by its unit, the cell, and by the cells' individual 3D spatial arrangement and 1D internal temporal dimension. Upon this basic operational definition, which is just an extension of special and general relativity, we can project or map any of the names of properties (fungus, Fido, petunia, or Parker), layer upon them any of the names of processes (transduction, flying, or nesting), and identify any of the products (oxygen, dopamine, or bile). In doing this, we are classifying all structure and function relationships in living systems. Now, in the life frame of reference, we have a biology that studies anatomy (structure), physiology (function), and their interrelationships.

We have left behind the pre-life world of the protocell and with it our metaphor of the dance. Before we bring it to a close, however, we must note that with the emergence of a new organic frame of reference, the processes of evolution also became focused on the cell, its processes, and its products, heading toward more local regions of complexity and toward creating the next frame of reference. Thus, the dancers may change, the ballrooms may change, the choreography may change, the conductor and the pace he sets with his baton of relative time may change, but the evolutionary song remains the same. The cells now become the dancers; the timing of the dance is now in generations; the choreography is now written in genetic modifications that bring new metabolic pathways within the cell and new arrangements of cells in multicellular organisms—plants and animals. All these behaviors in evolutionary time, paced in generational moments of probabilistic modifications, at some critical threshold of order show new shapes and functions that we provide with classification names. Two conductors now exist in the world, one timing the background dance of biosphere evolution, and the other pacing the intracellular and between-cell dance of the new order of existence. Their destinies are intertwined, as the changes in the respective referent frame of each affects the other and they both travel along the background arrow of universal time.

The Life Effect

Life is a frame of reference, it is an emergent organization of organic processes, it is an irreducible system, and it is the most general name for the property of the entire field of cellular behavior. Therefore, we must explicitly state before moving on that in a seemingly paradoxical way, life has no inherent units of measure, no specific quantity, and absolutely no force of action back on the cell or background environment. There is no vital force of life, no *élan vital.* No cell has more life than another; no organism is less alive than another.

In order to make quantitative statements about cells, we must reduce our focus below the level of the living reference system and make measurements of individual biochemical reactions. Once we do this, however, the emergent system is no longer the referent system, and all statements of dimension are now made within the background environment of atoms, molecules, elements, and compounds. We may not measure the property of life by the relative dimensions of length, width, depth, or time as defined by the background system. For example, one cell may indeed have more energetic phosphate-containing compounds than another, and one organism may have more tissue types than another, but these are not measures of a force or quantity of life. We may also make statements about time, in the form of rate functions. One cell may catalyze a reaction 50 percent faster than another cell, but that does not mean that it has more life or a faster life. The tempo of life has meaning only for the whole system as it behaves.

However, the products and metabolites (e.g., novel enzymes, peptides, and fluids) created within the system of cellular life do have units of measure and quantity, and they absolutely do influence the larger biosphere. This, then, is what life does: In single cells, in plants, and in animals, the living cell reorganizes the substrate environment (matter and energy) via metabolic pathways to produce unique organic molecules. The truly overwhelming complexity and beauty of our biosphere can be felt when we reflect on the multitude of metabolic pathways within the diverse populations of cellular species.

Molecular oxygen (O_2) is but one, albeit rather important, example of the influence that a product of cellular function may have on the environment. The oxygen product of phosphorylation forever changed the conditions under which life evolved, and shifted the environment toward a vastly different future. In our biosphere, this led to the increase in atmospheric O_2 to its present concentration of 21 percent and provided a barrier against the harsh ultraviolet glare. Under the dominance of aerobic life, anaerobic cells were relegated to smaller niches by substrate compartmentalization. The nearly four-billion-year panorama of evolutionary processes has taken the primitive single cell and slowly increased its internal complexity by adding more structures and organelles (e.g., a nuclear membrane, the Golgi apparatus, lysosomes, and mitochondria), energy transfer reactions (e.g., in chlorophyll and synaptic zones), and specialized enzymes and large-scale functions (e.g., hormone release and sensory transduction).

This climb against the second law of thermodynamics toward negative entropy, confined to discrete systems, exquisitely refined the intracellular and local extracellular environments and maximized the efficient use of available energy. Simple cells became cooperative networks of multicellular organisms, which then evolved as the flora and fauna of the planet. All of these evolutionary changes may be understood as quantitative modifications to cells within the single 4D frame of reference of life. The biological world has undergone tremendous expansions of diverse life forms and equally dramatic extinctions. The current state of the biosphere and the life field includes five general kingdoms of living organisms: monera, protozoa, fungi, plants, and animals. Our focus from this point on will be directed toward the animal kingdom and the processes of evolution and development that created the only other novel frame of reference in the biological world.

The Progression of Life

Sometime around 600 million years ago, the fossil record indicates that a successful new class of multicellular organisms began to populate various aquatic niches. These organisms, animals, were characterized by cellular structures forming saclike areas that trapped large particles (potential nutrition) that flowed through in the watery currents (Figure 3-1). The cells of these early animals (e.g., hydra and sponges) had no rigid membrane structures (like those of plants). Additional characterizing features of the animal kingdom that continued to appear and modify in evolutionary time included more specialized cellular tissues and layers of tissues. More systems of cells (e.g., organs) that performed specific functions, such as ingestion, respiration, digestion, or reproduction, gradually came to be present in various degrees of complexity in new animals.

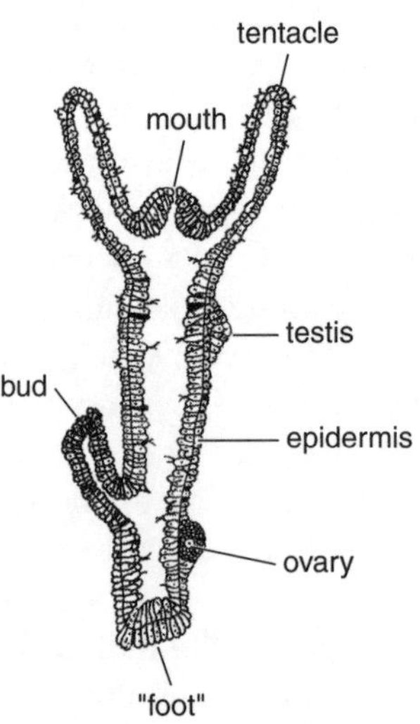

Figure 3-1 The hydra is one of the earliest animals to appear in evolution.

In early-appearing animals such as the hydra and the jellyfish, a new cell type was expressed from the genetic code: the nerve cell, which makes specialized cell-to-cell contacts with other nerve cells and with cells of other types. A small number of these nerve cells are found in the hydra and more in the jellyfish. The increase in the number and intricacy of connectivity of nerve cells kept evolutionary pace with the appearance of all other functional cellular systems. Thus, by the time the flatworms (e.g., planaria or tapeworms) evolved, a distinct system of nerve cells that formed a highly interconnected mass, a primordial brain, could be identified. And the nerve cell continued to function as an integral part of nearly every cellular system as these systems continued to modify under evolutionary processes. A most important function of animals, motility or movement, also came to be more and more under the influence of nerve cell activity.

In animals with many layers of cells, the extracellular milieu could not reach the inside cell layers. Thus, the microscopic solution between the cells, the extracellular environment (which is the internal or intercellular environment for the organism), had to contain a functional representation of the outside world, at least in terms of temperature range and the presence of inorganic and organic molecules in a solution that could support the existence of these isolated cells. Cellular systems evolved to create this representational environment inside the organism. The most complex plants have vascular systems that establish and maintain this type of environment deep inside dense cellular layers. In animals, this became even more important, as, by definition, they moved faster and further across more types of external conditions than any other organism.

Animals packed up the external milieu, wrapped it in protective coverings (shells, skeleton, or skin), and swam, crawled, walked, or flew away to new places. They had to regulate this internal world to an extremely fine degree, to keep all homeostatic functions intact as they roamed the Earth. Simultaneously, they had to react quickly to changes in the local external world in order to remain within their operating parameters of temperature, pressure, and metabolic demands. Reactive cells (nerve and muscle) endowed the multicellular organism with these astounding abilities. The evolution of animals is to a large degree the evolution of the nervous system. From jellyfish to centipedes, from lizards to bats, from dolphins to humans, the path of animal evolution is manifested by the creation of many specialized cells and cellular systems under adaptive control by the nervous system.

What, then, was the nervous system doing at each stage in evolution? And in what manner did the nervous system change, if at all, across the animal species in evolutionary time? Animals were able to move across different environments, ingest a variety of foods, and engage in successful sexual activity. The large-scale behaviors we describe with terms like ingestion or eating, moving or running, and reproducing or copulating are seen as driven, guided, and controlled by nervous system activity in its interaction with the external and internal worlds. Internal hunger drives searching, killing, and eating. Internal cold drives movement toward warmth. External smells, sounds, and movements from one animal drive courting and sexual activities. The nervous system appears to be acting to coordinate the activities of the animal to maximize its chance to exist until the next moment in time. How exactly does it perform this function? And does it operate in the same basic manner from animal to animal along the phylogenetic path?

In Part Three, "Dimensions of Consciousness," we address these questions and continue to present the model of emergent evolution in biological systems. We propose that nervous system activity generated unique products that evolutionary processes shaped over generations and across species. Moreover, evolutionary changes in nervous system structure and function (the morphology of nerve cells, functional parameters, cell-to-cell connectivity, and increased order of products) are expressed in the sets of reactions, the behavioral repertoires that each animal possesses.

Most important, we propose that, at an important point in our history, an animal's nervous system evolved that could maintain a sufficient order in its structure and function across a critical temporal threshold, thus generating a new biological organization: an emergent 4D frame of reference. We refer to this frame of reference as consciousness.

In keeping with the logical flow of our argument, we expect to be able to describe the properties, processes, and products of consciousness by examining the behavioral repertoires of those animals in which it operates. In the next chapter, we will follow the development of the nerve cell and the nervous system in the human. We will describe what special processes a nerve cell possesses, and how a system of nerve cells functions within the context of the entire developing organism. We will provide operational definitions for functions of the nervous system, and this will lead us to the unique processes and products out of which consciousness was forged in evolutionary time. These discussions will continue in Chapters 5, 6, and 7. We will start with the human nervous system, in part because it generates the consciousness frame of reference, but also because we will return to the subject of human development in later chapters.

Part Three

DIMENSIONS OF CONSCIOUSNESS

4

Development and Systems of Neurons

The human mammal, *Homo sapiens* or *wise man*, like all other multicellular animals, propagates the next generation by sexual reproduction. In the fertilization process, whether through intercourse or through *in vitro* insemination, an ovum and a sperm cell become a unicellular organism. A unique moment of human history is represented in the single cell, the zygote. In the fusion of two parental nuclei, genomes combine in a confluence of the three biological time scales: the long road of evolutionary modification to the DNA molecules from paternal and maternal family lines; the real-time process of novel chromosome creation in the act of conception; and the developmental procession of a newly propagated lifetime, whose initial moment, by definition, takes place at conception.

The number of cells making up the zygote increases exponentially. It is important to understand that all cells in each generation contain the same DNA, and thus have an equal potential to become virtually any type of specialized cell. The single factor that will determine the fate of each new healthy cell is its local external environment of chemicals and energies. This dynamic context determines the internal metabolic processes of each cell and what it will become in its mature existence.

In humans, the zygote cleaves into two daughter cells at about 30 hours after fertilization. A sphere of a dozen or more cells forms by 3 days, and by the end of week 1 there is an embryo composed of thousands of cells. In the third week of development, the embryo begins to divide into a distinctive three-layer or trilaminar structure. The three germ cell layers are called mesoderm, endoderm, and ectoderm. Cells of the mesoderm will produce connective tissues, striated muscle cells, blood vessels, blood cells, bone marrow cells, and the tissues of the excretory and reproductive organs; endoderm cells will divide and differentiate into epithelia of the respiratory system, glandular cells, and the pancreas and liver; and the ectoderm layer will produce outer epithelial tissues and the cells that make up the nervous system.

Early in the third week of human development, a thick band of cells appears along the midline of the embryo. This *primitive streak* begins at one end and elongates toward the other. The formation of this structure provides the landmark by which a three-dimensional (3D) morphological coordinate system for the growing embryo may be defined. The origin of this streak is at the caudal (rear or posterior) end, and its growth is toward the cranial (head or anterior) end. Thus, the right and left sides and the dorsal (top) and ventral (bottom) surfaces of the embryo may now be identified. The primitive streak is eventually replaced by a tubular column of cells called the *notochord*, which also migrates from the caudal region toward the expanding cranial end. The vertebral column eventually forms in the notochordal region. The mesodermal cells of the notochord become the defining bony structures of the midline axis: the cranium, the vertebrae, the ribs, and the sternum.

The central nervous system, which comprises the brain and spinal cord, arises out of the neuroectoderm, also called the *neural plate*, a region of cells that runs parallel and dorsal to the notochord. By the end of the third week, the entire length of the neural plate has folded into the *neural tube*, whose ends close to form a protected space inside the larger embryo. The interior space of the neural tube becomes the fluid-filled ventricular system of the brain and spinal cord central canal. The *neural crest cells*, situated along the outer length of the neural tube, give rise to most of the *peripheral nervous system*, which extends throughout the body. All the progenitors of the cells that make up the central nervous system—the neurons and glia cells—exist in the inner walls of the neural tube, a region called the ventricular zone. Thus, nerve and glia cells are intimately related, from their origins in primordial cells of the ventricular zone to their final destinies as intertwined functional systems within the brain and spinal cord.

The developing spinal cord becomes anatomically divided into a dorsal and a ventral region, and groups of nerve and glia cells called the *dorsal horn* nuclear groups and the *ventral horn* nuclei develop in the respective regions. The dorsal region will receive sensory information from the peripheral nervous system and send it toward the brain (*afferent* flow), and the ventral nuclei will transmit nerve impulses from the brain to all areas of the body (*efferent* flow). Clusters of neural crest cells that lie alongside the spinal cord differentiate to become the spinal ganglia (*dorsal root ganglia*) and the ganglia of the *sympathetic nervous system*. It is through these peripheral systems of cells that we experience the external and internal sensory worlds, send the information to our brains, and generate our behaviors and memories. All that we are, and can be, must relate to the basic patterns of afferent and efferent activities of the nervous system.

During the fourth developmental week, three primary brain vesicles form out of the neural tube: the *forebrain*, the *midbrain*, and the *hindbrain*. The forebrain further divides into two distinct regions, the *telencephalon* and the *diencephalon*, and the hindbrain partly divides into the *pons* and the *medulla*. Simultaneously, all other human body systems—respiratory, cardiovascular, musculoskeletal, endocrine, reproductive, and so on—are developing from the mesodermal and endodermal germ cells. In just 4 weeks of development, genetic expression and epigenetic influences have shaped the protected embryo into a basic three-dimensional design that reveals its future developmental course. Through massive waves of cell division, migration, and differentiation, the embryo has developed a definite rostral-caudal organization, in addition to dorsal, ventral, and midline axial orientations. Furthermore, after only 1 month of growth, the approximately 5-millimeter (mm)- (0.2-inch-) long embryo has minute but obvious arm and leg buds.

Local regions of specialized cells, their chemical products, and energy transfer reactions, on a scale of cubic micrometers, create extracellular environments or milieus that significantly influence cellular development. The exchange of materials and energies between local cells and the milieu affects all cellular metabolic pathways, including those of gene transcription. The environment of all cells in the growing embryo is a highly regulated, complex solution of inorganic and organic compounds, maintained in a very narrow range of acid-base balance (the pH value), supplying oxygen, glucose, and all other nutrients necessary to sustain metabolic function. The life-giving source of this delicately balanced bathing medium is the maternal blood supply. Initially this acts as an *embryotrophic* solution that reaches all cells by diffusion. As the sheer density of the mass of cells becomes prohibitive to a passive diffusion of the mother's sustaining nutrients, blood vessels begin to form (a process called *angiogenesis*), and by the third week of embryonic development a *cardiovascular* system is functioning and begins to actively participate in maintaining a relatively steady flow of all necessary energy sources to each and every cell. This is the first organ system to become operational in the embryo. At the end of the first month of embryonic development, we see a tiny living mass, formed by millions of cells, creating a wealth of local milieus in dynamic feedback with ever more specialized cell types.

The Nerve Cell Membrane

The interdependency between the extracellular and intracellular milieus is prominently evident in the life of the nerve cell. The nerve cell develops specialized structures and functions that differentiate it from all other cell types. The specialized neuronal membrane is defined, in part, by the large number of complex proteins that modify its phospholipid bilayer and create a highly reactive bioelectric field around the entire cell (Figure 4-1). The nerve cell's electromagnetic field converts local fluctuations (perturbations) in membrane charge into large, rapid, and recurrent waves of electrochemical activity that flow in only one direction and that reach the most distant portions of the membrane undiminished in intensity. A precise balance between the chemical composition of the extracellular and intracellular milieus, mediated across the neuronal membrane, must be sustained in order for the nerve cell to function properly.

As we discussed in Chapters 2 and 3, all cells have semipermeable membranes that create a nonequilibrium thermodynamic system. Furthermore, molecular concentration gradients that form across the membrane can give rise to momentary imbalances of charged ions on either side of it, thus creating a state of electric charge or voltage potential. The movement or flux of the charged particles through selective pores creates an electric current across the resistive membrane, as the ions follow the thermodynamic course toward an equilibrium state. Just as negatively charged electrons move along potential energy gradients to create a current in wires, resistors, and integrated circuits, so sodium or potassium ions create an electric current in biological systems. Their relative volumetric concentration across a living membrane and their ability to move through it determine the nature of the electrical property being measured. And in all cells the electrical state, or *membrane potential,* is measured as a relative negativity on the inside of the cell with respect to the outside environment. Thus, the convention is to state that a cell has a negative polarization of so many fractions of a volt. When the movement of ions through the membrane pores creates a change in the relative electric charge distribution, the cell is said to be *depolarized* if the intracellular side become less negative, and *hyperpolarized* if it gains more negative charge.

We must not lose sight of the fact that the development of knowledge, and thus our language, regarding the anatomical and electrical nature of bio-

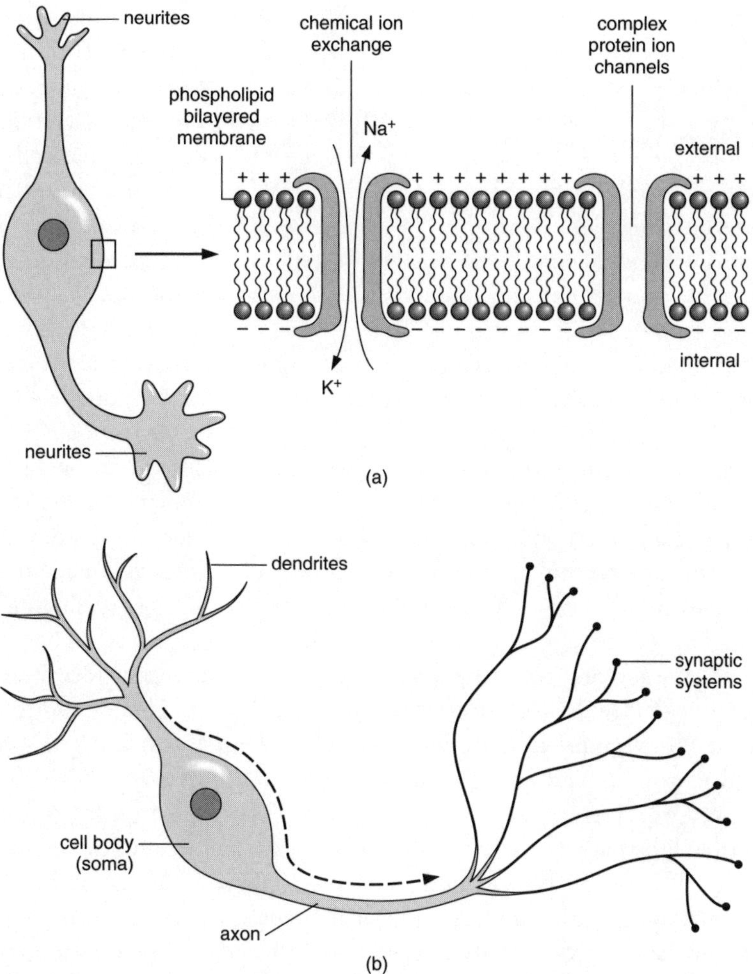

Figure 4-1 (*a*) Developing neuron with growth cone expansions called neurites. Microscopic view of the membrane shows the relative negative electrical charge along its interior surface created by ion exchange through protein channels. (*b*) Mature anatomy of a neuron illustrating the distinct polar arrangement of its structure. Arrow indicates the unidirectional flow of all electrical impulse waves.

logical tissues has a long and distinguished history that actually predates much of the terminology used in standard inorganic electronics. In groundbreaking work in the late 1800s and early 1900s, Sherrington, du Bois-Reymond, Katz, Bernstein, Eccles, Ramón y Cajal, Golgi, and others applied novel technologies to the examination of our biological existence.[1] The invention of the light microscope made it possible to view the cell on the scale of the millimeter [10^{-3} meter (m)] and micrometer (10^{-6} m). The introduction of the electron microscope in the 1940s opened up the Angstrom (10^{-8} m) or nanometer (10^{-9} m) scale of the natural world, making it possible for scientists to see such structures as the bilaminar cell membrane, intracellular organelles, and the synaptic system. The theory of the electromagnetic field and the development of devices to measure charge [volts (V)} and current [amperes (A)] brought to our perception important forces at work in cells and neurons on the scale of the millivolt and the microampere. The invention of the membrane *patch-clamp* technique in electrophysiology now permits analysis of bioelectric activity in a single protein channel measured at the picoampere (10^{-12} A) and picomole scale.[2]

These important developments in the past century have made it possible for us to produce models, hypotheses, and theories of neuron and brain function. No engineering schematic of electric circuits, no computer program written in any coding language, and no collection of integrated circuits can begin to rival the work of nature on the molecular scale of activity that produces the dynamic electric fields generated by all living cells, and particularly the highly responsive field possessed by neurons.

The underlying structural properties of nerve cells that form the basis of the bioelectric field are found at the micrometer and nanometer scale of nature in the unique distribution of membrane ion pores or channels, intracellular proteins, and energy-consuming ion transport pumps. *Ion channels* are large transmembrane (also called integral) proteins that form complex multiple loops across the lipid bilayer to create an opening that allows the passage of particular atoms under specific conditions. Many of these complex macromolecules undergo physical shape changes, or *conformational shifts*, in response to a variety of extracellular or intracellular influences that result in an opening or closing of the ion passages or pores. Channels that have such properties are called *gated*, while other channels appear to be *nongated* and consistently accommodate the flow of specific ions down their concentration gradients. The electrically polarized state of the nerve cell is primarily produced by the flow of sodium, potassium, chloride, and calcium ions through their respective gated and nongated channels.

The concentration gradient, defined by the partitioning of the ions on each side of the nerve cell membrane, creates the force for the movement of each ion species. Sodium, chloride, and calcium are more concentrated in the extracellular medium; thus, their unimpeded diffusion direction is toward the inside of the cell, where their concentrations are lower. Potassium, conversely, has an intracellular concentration nearly 10 times higher than its concentration outside the cell. The nerve cell membrane at its baseline state is significantly more permeable to the potassium ion, reflecting the distribution of gated and nongated ion channels and their pore states. Therefore, in the *steady-state* or *dynamic equilibrium* condition, the electrochemical drive forcing the positively charged potassium ions out of the cell leaves the intracellular side of the membrane with a relative negative charge (hyperpolarized). The presence of large intracellular proteins that carry a net negative (anionic) charge also contributes to this polarized membrane condition. The hyperpolarization inside the nerve cell membrane is typically between 60 and 80 millivolts (mV) negative potential difference with respect to the extracellular medium.

While potassium ion efflux determines the majority of the voltage difference at the steady-state condition, called the *resting membrane potential* (rmp), the sodium influx through its own set of channels limits the magnitude of the hyperpolarization by adding positive charges to the intracellular side of the membrane. However, because the membrane is far more resistant to the passage of sodium ions, the electrochemical drive for these ions is small compared to that for potassium. Therefore, the effect on the total potential difference at the resting membrane potential is likewise small. The other abundant ions, chloride and calcium, are concentrated in the extracellular solution and have low permeability across the membrane, and thus they also have small electrochemical diffusion forces. Additionally, the chloride ions' negative charge is electrically repulsed by the negative intracellular potential difference, further reducing the influx drive.

The resting membrane potential, then, is simply a product of a net excess of positive electric charges on the outside of the very thin and highly resistant membrane, and a net excess of negative electric charges along the inside of the membrane. This bioelectric field covers the entire cell, but it extends only about a micrometer on either side of the membrane and thus is generated by the diffusion of an extremely minute fraction of the ions present. Therefore, it would take a long time for a nerve cell to lose its resting membrane potential as a result of the passive diffusion of the principal ionic species to a final equilibrium state. But, as we soon discuss, many influences affecting the nerve cell create a highly dynamic situation in which the ionic flows are differentially increased and decreased in a wide variety of combinations at hundreds to thousands of locations on an individual cell membrane.

In order to maintain the resting membrane potential within a strict range of voltage values, all cells, including the neuron, expend metabolic energy to actively transport ions into and out of the cell. The principal ion transporter, called the *sodium pump*, is a large integral protein enzyme that uses *adenosine triphosphate* (ATP) as its energy source. Basically, the enzyme is a *sodium-potassium ATPase* that extrudes three sodium ions out of the cell while sequestering two potassium ions in the cell, at a cost of one molecule of ATP. Actively pumping ions against their respective diffusion gradients regains the resting levels of concentration differences for the ions as they are degraded during cell function. Note that the sodium pump ion-exchange ratio of three positive charges into two positive charges out of the cell per ATP molecule creates its own net negative potential difference for the cytoplasmic side of the membrane. The sodium pump is thus termed *electrogenic*, and its activity contributes to the hyperpolarized state of the cell.

The resting state is, of course, far from a state of tranquil quiescence; it may be more accurately described as a complex baseline or *homeostatic bioelectrical state*. Thus, the electrical potential of the nerve cell membrane and its dynamic response to intracellular and extracellular stimuli are shaped by the rich variety of ion channels and their unique functional properties. All along the membrane, millimeter by millimeter, gated ion channels are affected by a variety of influences that cause an opening or closing of their pores. This activity may alter the transmembrane flux of one or more ionic species and move the local membrane potential away from its baseline toward a more depolarized or hyperpolarized condition. And, in constant dynamic reaction, the collective processes of passive electrochemical diffusion and active ion transport act to reestablish the homeostatic bioelectric field. Many dozens of transmembrane glycoproteins have been identified as gated ion channels for sodium, potassium, chloride, or calcium. They may be classified by the type of stimulus that causes the conformational state change of the ion pore. The *voltage-gated* channels have intramembrane peptide sequences that appear to be sensitive to minute voltage changes in the membrane potential. *Chemically gated* channels shift conformational states when extracellular portions of the molecule, called receptor sites, bind with certain neuroactive compounds. *Ion-gated* channels open or close in response to changes in local intracellular ion concentrations. Other channels appear to be influenced by intracellular mechanical forces of adjacent proteins or by interaction with intracellular molecules bearing energetic phosphate bonds. Many channels have voltage-sensitive portions and also respond to changes in the concentration of cytoplasmic ions (e.g., calcium).

The Nerve Impulse

The young neurons of the neural crest and neural tube grow into their mature shapes by extending portions of their cell bodies, called cytoplasmic growth cones, out toward nearby and distant destinations. As these cellular extensions begin to interact with other cells, the neurons begin to take on a defining geometry. One or more growth cones from the central cell body (soma) become the branches of the cell (dendrites) that receive most of the connections from other neurons. Typically, at the polar opposite portion of the cell, a single growth cone becomes the primary pathway (axon) by which a neuron communicates with other cells (Figure 4-1*b*). The elemental dendritic, somatic, and axonal membrane segments thus mature under the constant influence of genetic, epigenetic, intracellular, and extracellular factors, wherein an ever-changing complement of gated and nongated ion channels and ion transporters are being produced by the cell and inserted through the membrane.

While all cells have a charged membrane that is populated by a variety of gated ion channels, and may have portions of their membrane depolarized or hyperpolarized by changes in ionic flux, only the nerve cell generates a *unidirectional*, traveling electrical potential along the entire extent of the axonal process. (Muscle cells also generate a traveling electrical impulse along their membranes and thus, like neurons, are classified as excitable cells. However, they do not have the polar arrangement of the neuron, and they do not extend growth cones to form dendritic and axonal segments of membrane.)

The mechanisms of development that determine the fine details of channel type, density per millimeter of membrane, and pattern of channels over the entire cell surface are not yet well understood, but we can describe a basic relationship between the elongated shape of the neuron and its electrical behavior. In general, the dendrites form a pole at one end of the nerve cell, where a complex arrangement of ion channels at hundreds to thousands of locations is receptive to neuroactive compounds coming from other nerve cells and the bathing fluid. The body of the cell will typically have a lesser amount of these specialized regions of dense channel aggregation. At the other pole, the axon segment will develop its own specialized pattern of ion channel distribution that produces a unique bioelectrical function in response to membrane depolarization in the dendritic and somatic regions: the *nerve impulse* or *action potential*. Thus the unique morphological polarity of the neuron gives it the characteristic functional properties that define it as a *nervous* or *excitable* cell.

As each young neuron modifies its membrane with ion channels and transporters, the bioelectric field forms and moves toward the mature steady state or resting membrane potential. Moreover, the membrane response of the dendritic and somatic regions becomes increasingly sensitive to local stimuli, thus heightening the reactive nature of the cell. At some point in this developmental progression, when a sufficient number, type, and distribution of ion channels and pumps are present and a critical amount of membrane tissue (in square millimeters) has its voltage potential depolarized beyond a threshold amount [in millivolts per second (mV·s)], for an adequate duration of time [in milliseconds (ms)], a young neuron will generate its very first nerve impulse or action potential, which will travel away from the point of membrane origin to the farthest extent of the axonal projections.

The nerve impulse is, in its basic description, a sequential progression of voltage-gated ion channel openings and closings that progress along the cell membrane from the start of the axonal segment (axon hillock) to each and every tip of its endings. As we have seen, the baseline membrane potential or voltage state is modulated when ion flow is altered by gated pore activity. Therefore, the biophysical structure of the nerve impulse rests upon ion influx and efflux through a unidirectional series of conformational state changes in distinct channel types. The nerve impulse is initiated when a sufficient portion of the cell membrane is depolarized to a critical voltage value of about 10 to 15 mV more positive than the resting membrane potential. When the transmembrane potential value is raised beyond this threshold, voltage-sensitive sodium channels open and the permeability of the local membrane to sodium ions is increased. As sodium ions diffuse along their concentration gradient into the cell, this movement of positive charge through the membrane further depolarizes the local region.

This sequence begins a self-perpetuating process of depolarization that quickly overcomes all homeostatic mechanisms of resting membrane potential restoration. In about 0.2 to 0.5 ms the sodium current (influx of ions) is at a maximum, and the voltage measure of the affected membrane potential has been elevated into the positive range by about 10 to 30 mV: the *reversal* potential state. Simultaneously, but at a slightly slower rate, voltage-sensitive potassium channels also open to increase the permeability of the membrane to this ion. During the *rising phase* of voltage shift, the sodium effect overwhelms the potassium influence, but when the *repolarizing* effect of potassium efflux reaches a point of dynamic equilibrium, the peak of the reversal voltage is reached. The subsequent *falling phase* of the voltage shift is also very rapid and involves the closing of sodium channels as the membrane potential moves toward a negatively polarized value. As the membrane voltage nears the baseline value, potassium channels are closing and the sodium pumps are expending metabolic energy to reestablish the concentration gradients for the two ions.

Once the initiating depolarization event occurs and the voltage state for a critical portion of cell membrane has risen and fallen, the nerve impulse proceeds along its characteristic course without any further need for a driving force. The rate and magnitude of the *voltage spike* are not affected by the initiating stimuli beyond what is needed to reach the threshold depolarization. Thus, the nerve impulse is an *all-or-nothing* event. The process is self-limiting at each small patch of membrane that is affected, and it is also self-propagating. From the region of origin, the impulse moves in one direction along the axonal membrane to the far, or distal, ends of the cell. As one portion of membrane is repolarizing, the next portion is depolarizing under the influence of the electrochemical field change brought about by the preceding voltage spike. The propagation of the nerve impulse becomes a *bioelectric wave phenomenon*, a wave that maintains the same magnitude and velocity throughout its course. The cell membrane behind the nerve impulse wave regains its resting potential and is then capable of propagating another action potential.

An impulse wave may travel over a centimeter of membrane length in a millisecond. The speed of wave propagation is limited in part by the electrical properties of the axon membrane. Most simply, the resistance to electrical wave movement is greater in small-diameter axons and less in large-diameter axons. Thus, impulse wave velocity varies greatly across nerve cell types.

While the movements of an electric charge along an axon share some common elements with those in an inorganic cable conducting electricity, there are important differences. The electron flow in a cable is based on the singular voltage potential gradient that exists from the positive end of the cable to the other, negative, end. When such a circuit is complete or closed, the electrons move along the cable, overcoming its inherent resistance and creating heat in the process. In contrast, the nerve impulse is a cumulative property of many sequential fluctuations of voltage potential across the membrane and is dependent upon the ionic concentrations of the solutions outside and inside the cell.

Moreover, many neural cells have axonal modifications that produce conducted nerve impulses at a speed up to 50 times faster than the basic membrane resistance properties could allow. Fast-conducting axons of these neurons are wrapped with thin membrane extensions from glial cells, called *myelin sheaths*. *Oligodendroglia* in the central nervous system and *Schwann* cells in the peripheral nervous system extend portions of their cytoplasm that tightly wrap around nerve cell axons. The effect of this peculiar arrangement, or cell system, is to isolate the axon membrane from the extracellular medium, except at regularly spaced segments along the extent of the processes. These small lengths of axon membrane (about 10 μm) that are exposed to the extracellular fluid, called *nodes of Ranvier*, are dense with sodium and potassium channels and sodium pumps. Under these conditions, the electrochemical field changes across a local membrane segment that are induced by the action potential may extend their depolarizing influence with far less resistance along the axon to the next exposed segment at approximately 1-mm intervals. This jumping of the impulse wave, a *saltatory conduction*, greatly increases nerve impulse velocity in small-diameter axons.

The velocity of nerve impulse propagation sets an absolute constraint on the time it takes for the wave to reach the distal extent of the axon projection that is specific for each nerve cell. There is also a maximum rate or frequency at which new action potentials may be initiated. The limiting factor in this process appears to be the time it takes for the repolarizing portion of the membrane to regain the ability to produce another voltage spike. This *absolute refractory period* lasts only a few milliseconds, and thus theoretically a cell could operate at an impulse frequency of 1,000 spikes per second. However, most neurons produce action potentials at rates in the range of less than 1 to over 200 per second. Nerve impulse activity, especially when maintained at a high rate, creates additional disturbances in the concentration gradients of the principal ions. In order to restore and maintain all ion gradients, neurons expend up to 50 percent of their metabolic energy in the form of ATP to drive the enzymatic ion transporters. This is the cost of maintaining a highly reactive bioelectric membrane that can generate a propagated wave of voltage force at rapid velocity and frequency.

Growing young nerve cells thus acquire the capacity to produce frequent, recurring nerve impulses in response to extracellular and intracellular stimuli as they migrate within the embryonic nervous system and extend neuritic processes. In this phase of maturation, the nerve impulse courses along the axonal process to the ends of the cell membrane. As this distal portion of the growth cone also enters its next developmental stage, each approaching voltage wave will initiate a sequence of events that leads to a discharge of molecules from specific regions of membrane into the extracellular space. This new functional property heralds another critical milestone in cell-to-cell interaction.

The Axon Terminal Region and Synaptic Zones

The developing axon, an elongating cytoplasmic cylinder, may produce from one to many hundreds of branching points at the extremes of its growth cone tip. Secondary and tertiary extensions may also protrude from each primary branch of the growth cone. The entire cell segment that includes all the endings may be referred to as the *axon terminal region* (Figure 4-2*a*). The region of axon termination is thus a 3D volume of coordinated bioelectric and biochemical activity. Through this region, a single nerve cell may have an effect on many other neurons simultaneously, and these, in turn, may send their cascade of axon branches on to other neural arrays. The magnification of a single nerve impulse by this branching effect leads to an exponential increase in the subtleties, and thus the complexities, of the interaction of nerve cells as unified arrays of synchronized volume elements.

The axon terminal region develops very differently in each neuron as it matures into its final position and functional role. In general, however, most axon terminal regions that reach their anatomical destinations and begin to form functional contacts with other cells have certain defining characteristics. First, as mentioned previously, the glia-neuron system of myelin sheathing is absent in the axon terminal regions, and so the axonal membrane of the neural cell is exposed to the surrounding medium. Next, in most axon terminal regions, the thin, nearly circular axon changes its shape near the end point of the cytoplasm. Depending upon the specific type of contact to be formed, the axon terminal regions can be identified by their small bulging regions of membrane (bulblike under light microscopic examination; hence the term *bouton*), but they also may form very massive and irregularly shaped cytoplasmic expansions (Figure 4-2*b*). These distinctive terminal portions of the neural cell function to create and maintain the points of contact between cells, the *synaptic zones*.

The secretory ability of the neuron localized to the synaptic zones is in many aspects not unlike that of all other cells that produce and release compounds under a variety of stimulus conditions. But in the neuron, the distance from the cell body to the axon terminal regions makes it necessary for the far regions of the cell to conduct some of the manufacturing and processing of the unique molecules involved in secretion. Depending upon the length of the axon, it can take many hours or days for key peptides and proteins to be transported from their site of production in the cell body to the terminal sites. Hundreds or thousands of small spherical structures [10 to 60 nanometers (nm) in diameter] called *synaptic vesicles* also fill each terminal region (Figure 4-2*c*). These complex protein spheres store and transport the molecules to be secreted, and may also contain other compounds and ions such as ATP and calcium.

One or more synaptic zones may exist in each axon terminal region and define the uniquely neuronal locations where the arrival of a nerve impulse wave initiates the secretory release of neuroactive molecules. At each site

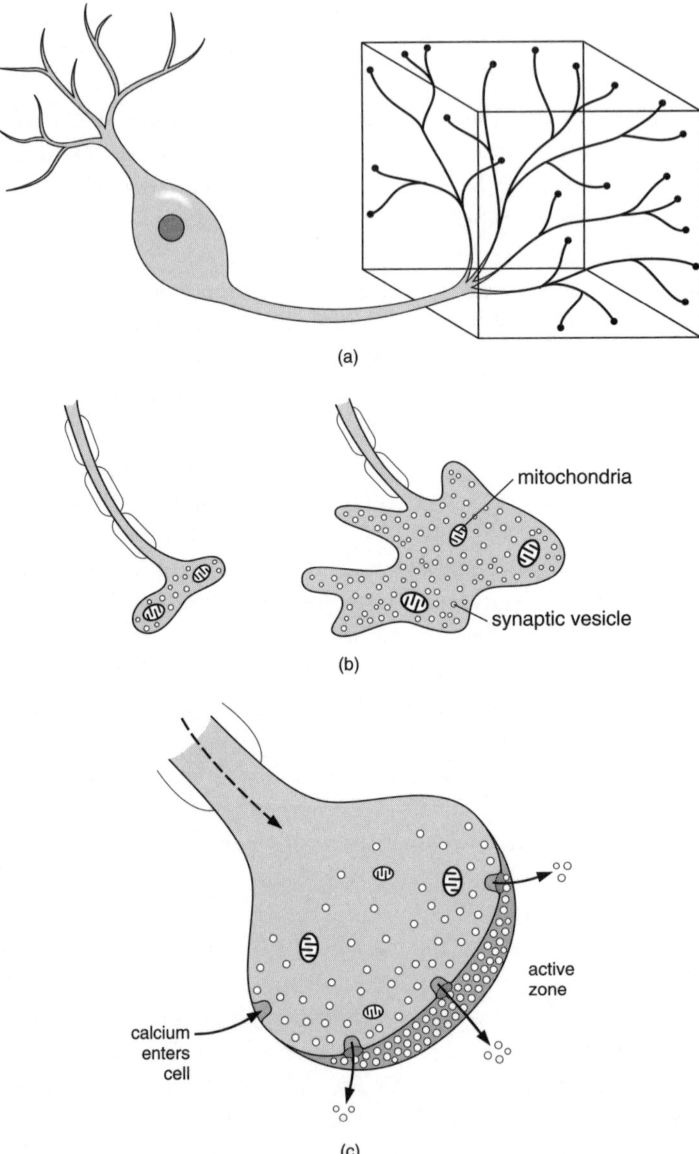

Figure 4-2 (*a*) Axon terminal region and synaptic zones of a nerve cell. The synaptic zones create 3D regions of tissues and solutions charged with electrochemical energy activity. (*b*) Presynaptic portions of axon terminal regions demonstrating the wide range in shape and size that exists in nervous systems. Each terminal is filled with mitochondria and spherical synaptic vesicles filled with neuroactive and other high-energy compounds. (*c*) Nerve impulse wave entering synaptic zone and release of chemical transmitter into a volume space near another cell.

of release, sometimes called the *active zone*, the cell membrane contains a high concentration of calcium channels and a fascinating gridlike arrangement of complex proteins that organize the synaptic vesicles that are poised to release their contents (Figure 4-2*c*). When the axon terminal region is depolarized by the nerve impulse, voltage-sensitive calcium channels allow the entry of calcium ions. In this millisecond event, coordinated sequences of calcium-dependent molecular changes ensue. The proteins of the synaptic vesicles, called *synapsins*, and the filamentous web of proteins and enzymes that compose the active zone undergo conformational changes that cause synaptic vesicles to fuse with the cell membrane grid and then open to allow the expulsion of their contents into the extracellular environment.

This rapid exocytotic release of bioactive compounds must end as suddenly as it begins if the entire *bioelectrical-to-biochemical* process of neural activity is to function at or near the rate of nerve impulse activity. A critical factor in the pulselike aspect of vesicular release is the calcium concentration at each synaptic zone. Thus, when the impulse wave causes calcium channels to open, the intracellular calcium concentration rises rapidly and significantly. It has been experimentally demonstrated that in the absence of a depolarizing event, the injection of calcium ions into an axon terminal region is sufficient to induce the synaptic release mechanisms. In order to halt this exocytotic process, the calcium concentration must fall below a critical threshold level. Calcium-ATPases, sodium-calcium exchange enzymes, and intracellular calcium-binding proteins all act to remove calcium ions from the active release zone less than a millisecond after the stimulated influx. In addition, the local metabolic machinery of the axon terminal region creates new synaptic vesicles to replace those used in the preceding secretory cycle, and fills them with the appropriate bioactive molecules.

The arrival of the depolarizing impulse wave and the calcium-dependent exocytotic event are not simultaneous; there is a delay of about 0.5 ms between the opening of the calcium channel and the secretion of vesicle content. Thus, the biophysical parameters of axon terminal region and synaptic zone function set an upper limit on the rate of secretory activity. And, of course, subtle changes in the concentration of calcium ions or the timing of influx or postinflux ion sequestration can affect the number of synaptic vesicles that fuse and open and thus may increase or decrease the number of molecules released per event. Many other normal and abnormal dynamic influences can also affect the function of the axon terminal region and synaptic zone, thus modulating the release of bioactive molecules. Such factors will be discussed as the functional roles of systems of neurons are elucidated.

Many, if not most or all, neurons create and release more than one bioactive substance. In fact, neurons may be named by the primary compound they release at synaptic zones. Other nomenclature schemes use shape, location, position in a network, or some other structural or functional property of the neuron. During development, many neuron types actually undergo a change in the synthesis and release of primary and secondary bioactive molecules. This alteration in biochemical phenotype can be under genetic control, but it also may occur under the influence of normal or abnormal stimuli in the local environment. These molecules, like any cell product secreted into the extracellular environment, are the primary agents of effect or action on other cells and thus on the organism.

In speaking of the bioactive molecules secreted by nerve cells, the terms *neurotransmitters* and *neuropeptides* are used to classify them. Neurotransmitters are typically amino acids or small molecules that cause an immediate change in the membrane potential of the receiving neuron, while neuropeptides are short or long chains of amino acids that usually affect the receiving neuron along a slower time course. The action of these substances on other cells is mediated by receptor proteins, and this may take place at general or very specific locations at which these receptor proteins exist and neuroactive compounds interact. Dozens of receptor types have been identified for nerve cells, and more will continue to be characterized. It is the properties of the receptor that determine how a specific neurotransmitter or neuropeptide affects that particular cell. Rapid shifts in membrane voltage may occur when a neurotransmitter binds to a receptor that controls an ion channel, causing the pore to open. Conversely, slow and longer-lasting changes in cell function may be produced when a neurotransmitter or neuropeptide binds to a receptor linked to intracellular enzymes and other proteins that alter the transcriptional and translational processes of the genome.

Decades of painstaking research has allowed us to identify a number of bioactive compounds synthesized in neurons and released at synaptic zones that produce changes in other cells.[3] The classic neurotransmitters include the *biogenic amines, acetylcholine, dopamine, norepinephrine, serotonin,* and *histamine*. Certain amino acids, such as *glutamate,* gamma-aminobutyric acid (*GABA*), and *glycine,* also function as key neurotransmitters. These molecules are known to bind to receptor proteins that modulate membrane ion channels, and thus can cause immediate (millisecond) changes in the depolarized state of the local membrane. It must be noted that the biogenic amines also bind to other types of receptors that initiate a metabolic cascade that leads to slower changes (seconds, minutes, hours, or days) in cell function.

The neuropeptides (e.g., *enkephalin* or *substance P*) are initially synthesized in the cell body and then are moved to axon terminal regions by axonal transport. They produce a variety of changes in cells with the appropriate receptors, but they are not known to have an immediate (millisecond) effect on ion channel functions. The important finding that a single nerve cell may synthesize and release both a biogenic amine or amino acid and one or more neuropeptides has added a layer of functional complexity to neuronal activity. Thus, a neuron may secrete a rapid-acting neurotransmitter and a longer-acting neuropeptide in response to each impulse wave. In the following sections and chapters, we continue to examine neurotransmitter function, as well as other neuronal effects on adjacent cells that do not appear to be purely mediated by impulse-wave-initiated synaptic vesicle release mechanisms.

Now we have a picture of the unique, singular neuron as a cell that is integrated into the surrounding environment and of its basic structural and functional properties. At this point in the embryonic development of the human neuron, we must explicitly shift from a discussion of the single nerve cell to a discussion of cell-to-cell interactions. In general, all cells interact with other cells. For example, large molecules extending out from cell membranes may affect nearby cells in a structural manner. The bioelectric field of a cell also may influence the development of other cells. And secreted cellular proteins, peptides, or other released molecules affect cells both locally and at a distance. Thus, where, when, and to what extent the primordial neural crest and neural tube cells project growth cones and form connections with other cells are, in a way, directed by the presence and products of other cells. Developmental interdependencies extend to all cell types and to all cell systems.

The Synaptic System in Neuron-to-Neuron Interaction

The generic bipolar neuron, aligned to represent the basic one-to-many array pattern of neuron-to-neuron interaction, is depicted in Figure 4-3*a*. The synaptic zones of the axon terminal regions are shown to lie near several locations, including the dendritic projections, cell body, initial portion of the axon, and the axon terminal region of adjacent cells. As embryonic development proceeds, these basic arrangements of nerve cells form throughout the organism in a wide variety of combinations and patterns.

To adopt a consistent terminology for discussing how neurons in a system influence one another, we must arbitrarily designate one cell as the point of origin of activity and then follow the subsequent sequence of biochemical and bioelectrical events. The temporal dimension of nerve cell–to–nerve cell function now becomes a critical variable. Following the sequence of connections depicted in Figure 4-3*a*, we note that a nerve impulse starting at neuron A will cause the release of neurotransmitters at

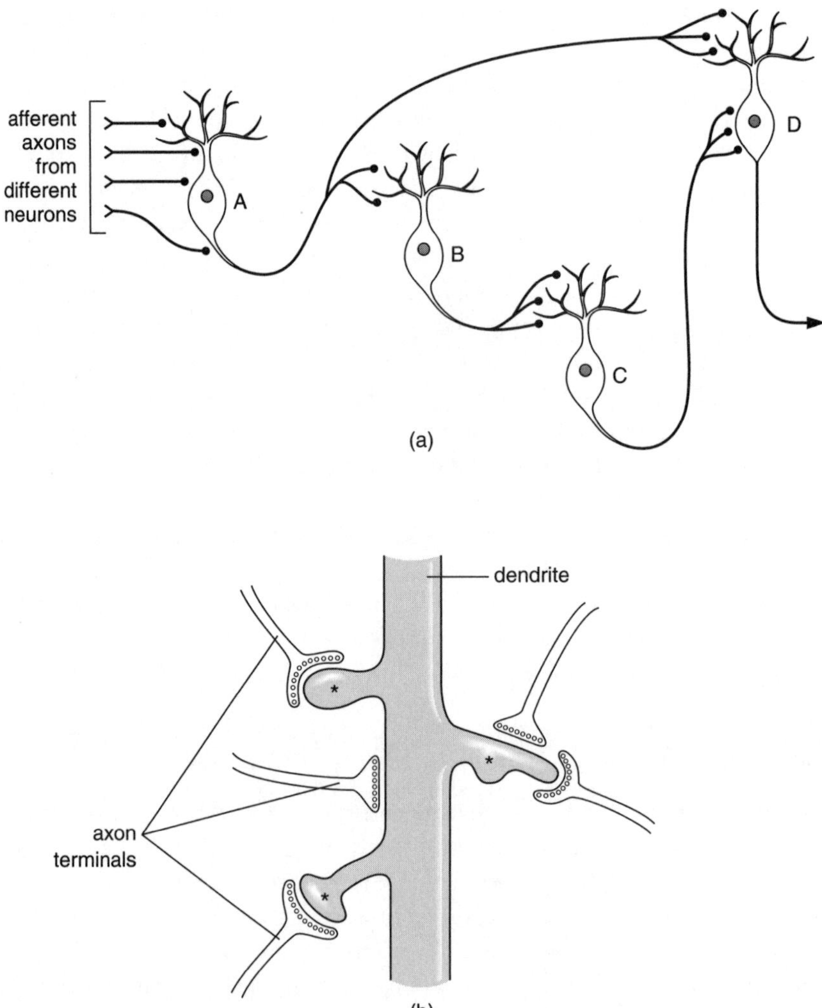

Figure 4-3 (*a*) Neuron-to-neuron synaptic systems. (*b*) Synaptic systems at high magnification on dendritic branch of a neuron. * = dendritic spines.

all synaptic zones within a volume of tissue space. On neuron B, the minute regions of dendritic membrane directly across from each synaptic zone of neuron A contain a dense collection of receptor proteins with which the released bioactive molecules will interact. Thus, in the relational description of this system, the synaptic zones of neuron A are referred to as the *presynaptic* components or elements, and the receptor zones of neuron B are called the *postsynaptic* elements. The term *synapse* is typically used to indicate the entire *synaptic system* and therefore refers to portions of two different cells. This basic terminology holds for all locations of synaptic elements, from the dendritic tree to the distal axon terminal regions. An illustrated electron micrograph (Figure 4-3*b*) shows several synaptic systems located at the dendritic tree and a schematic drawing of the key elements of a synaptic system. The distance between the presynaptic and postsynaptic cell membranes is on the order of 10 to 20 nm and is typically called the *synaptic gap* or *cleft*. The nanoworld of this important system is not fully understood, but it is clear that the synaptic system is a critical control point in neuron-to-neuron interactions.

A close-up of the dendritic portion of the B neuron shows a fine level of membrane specialization that exists on many types of neurons. A synapse may form along the shaft of the dendrite (axodendritic), but many smaller cytoplasmic extensions, called *spines*, may also form off the dendrite to create one or more synapses with other cells. Such *axospinous* synapses are nearly always found on dendritic branches, although exceptions do exist. Synaptic systems also form on the nerve cell body (axosomatic) and at the initial segment of the axon or at the most distal portions of the axon near the presynaptic zones (axo-axonic).

In the dynamic balance of neuronal influences produced by synaptic system activity, we must note that rapid depolarization of the cell membrane may occur in *excitatory* synaptic systems that cause the opening of sodium channels, but that hyperpolarization may also occur in *inhibitory* synaptic systems that cause the opening of chloride channels. In most cases, inhibitory synapses are located on the cell body or the initial and distal axonal segments. Thus, a neuron such as B may produce a nerve impulse in response to the moment-to-moment *spatiotemporal integration* of a multitude of minute hyperpolarizing and depolarizing ionic currents (*postsynaptic potentials*), each lasting up to 20 ms, caused by neuroactive molecules binding to millions of ion channel receptors. These cascading cumulative events may occur up to the maximal possible rate of action potential generation, which is highly constrained by the biophysical parameters of neurotransmitter release, receptor binding, ion channel dynamics, and bioelectric membrane properties. The threshold of depolarization that a neuron must undergo in each *temporal window of opportunity* to initiate a synaptically driven nerve impulse represents a complex set of postsynaptic ionic shifts over the portions of the cell membrane receiving neurotransmitter molecules.

We can imagine that a cell with thousands of synaptic systems formed with tens to hundreds of other neurons may be stimulated to initiate a nerve impulse in response to a wide variety of combinations of numbers and locations of synapses being activated, ratios of excitatory and inhibitory neurotransmitters being released, and the millisecond-to-millisecond timing of all this activity. This, then, is the beginning of the pulse or rhythm of the neuron-to-neuron interaction within the nervous system. The progression of our view of the developing nervous system will become more and more focused on the interactions between neurons; each cell propagates its own nerve impulses and releases bioactive molecules, but in increasingly complex networks of hundreds to millions or billions of synaptically linked arrays embedded in the living fabric of the cellular surround.

Neuron-to-Neuron Activity in the Life Field

The human embryo that we followed through the first month will continue to grow and develop along with the nervous system. Thus far, all the metabolic and neuronal functions that we have discussed fall within the four dimensions created by the life-field frame of reference. The unique nerve cell and its charged membrane represent a quantitative modification of the basic cell. Its presence in integrated systems of other cell types, in large part, marks the transition from the plant to the animal kingdom (along with the loss of a rigid membrane and ingestive methods of nutrition consumption). But, however spectacular, it remains a quantitative transition.

The changes in neuronal membrane potential brought about by ionic flux, nerve impulse cascade, propagation, regeneration, and exocytotic release of neuroactive compounds at the synaptic zones all occur within the biophysical parameters (entropic constraints) of the nonneural cells that provide the support for these high-energy nervous cells. The neuronal impulse wave that is initiated and propagated and the synaptic events that subsequently proceed also take place within a limited frequency range (events per millisecond). Indeed, nerve cell dynamics are rapid processes with respect to other large-scale cellular actions, but no new 4D space-time order that includes a novel temporal dimension is required for a full accounting of all functions.

What does occur in neuronal activity is an electrochemical discharge along complicated, dynamic nonequilibrium potential, kinetic, and thermal energy pathways. The effect on the next cell or cells receiving the released neuroactive molecules is not the propagation of an ordered 4D structure, as we defined for the referent system of the living cell. Postsynaptic cells that are affected by presynaptic neurotransmission may have their structure or function momentarily altered under this pulsed influence, but all such changes are ultimately described by the biochemical and biophysical energy exchange pathways that lie within each cell. Furthermore, any transmitted order, as indicated by propagated potential energy, has been severely degraded by the time released neuroactive molecules bind at postsynaptic receptor sites. The potential energy order in any neuron, a propagated 4D reference system, is maintained by the metabolic function of the cell and its supportive environment, and is fundamentally the same as in all other nonneuronal cells.

The temporal function or event that is created by the wave nature of the nerve impulse ends at the synaptic zones, although the synaptic vesicular release of substances as a function of the impulse wave frequency can be viewed as another timed event. In any event, there is nothing unique about this inexact quantized chemical pulse in terms of a 4D propagated system, and certainly not from the point of view of the postsynaptic receptors under neurotransmitter bombardment. Although it is a relatively rapid way to transfer specific forms of energy to widespread portions of the supporting system, nerve cell function is not different from the metabolic functions of any other cell, which also lead to a release of unique compounds into the extracellular environment, either at specific locations with respect to other cells or as general exocytotic mechanisms. Thus, as we discussed in the previous chapters, each cell has a multitude of temporal functions defined by each and every metabolic (entropic or energetic) process. Nearly all such propagated energy flows or exchanges, most of which are regenerative in nature like the membrane charge, take place inside the cell, but nevertheless they can result in the extracellular release of quantized amounts of compounds such as oxygen, peptides, hormones, or other complex proteins. And the temporal parameters of all cellular metabolic processes are altered by a variety of general and specific extracellular and intracellular stimuli, as expressed in positive or negative feedback influences on rates of biochemical actions.

Thus, while nerve cell function involves a highly charged transmembrane bioelectrical wave, traveling fast, far, and frequently with respect to all other cells, its operating parameters and the released products of metabolism lie within the 4D life field of biological order. Just as the protocell's operating parameters, and thus its existence, were entropically bound to the background flux of energies in the local biosphere, so the neuron's operating parameters and entire existence are likewise bound to the rise and fall of the local metabolic activity in the living multicellular organism.

The synaptic release of neurotransmitters by one neuron onto another will alter the probability that a nerve impulse will be generated in the receiving cell. However, nerve cells are not affected exclusively by other nerve cells. Many other influences may cause certain neurons to rapidly generate a nerve impulse, or in some cases may inhibit one. Nonneuronal stimuli, such as sensory energies, that may cause neurons to generate impulse waves provide a key driving force for the nervous system as it develops and functions *in utero* and after birth, and ultimately as it defines the limits of our experience of the world.

Sensory Neurons and the Stimulus World

We have now placed the functional nerve cell in the context of the complex developing organism. The many biochemical, electrical, and mechanical forces that impinge upon neural and other cells indeed affect their growth, maturation, connectivity, and survival. In addition to the bioactive molecules classified as neurotransmitters, neuromodulators, or neurohormones, there are many other energy sources, or stimuli, that influence the membrane potentials of neurons and initiate or inhibit the impulse wave activity. This begins the afferent flow of information from the external and internal stimulus worlds toward the brain. The basic processes of stimulus conversion and conduction capture the entire universe of what we may experience and know; they generate all our sensations, perceptions, emotions, thoughts, and memories. All our sensory realties are based equally upon these cellular functions, where the physics of matter and energy become the biology of nerve impulses and neurotransmission.

One term used to describe the conversion of one form of energy to another is *transduction*. The entire synaptic process of converting the nerve impulse wave to expelled bioactive neurotransmitter molecules may be seen as a transduction of electrical energy to chemical energy. Conversely, receptor proteins of the synaptic systems transduce the biochemical energies contained in the neurotransmitters into electrical potentials across the cell membrane. We now expand this view of transduction to understand how specialized cells react to a wide variety of stimuli that originate internal and external to the developing human—that is, how the nervous system begins to sense the world and send each transduced sample of the world to the brain.

The human nervous system contains an impressive array of *sensory receptors.* The term *receptor,* when used in this context, refers to a portion of a cell or one or more cells that function as a coordinated *sensory receptor unit* to convert a particular stimulus to a bioelectrical nerve response and transmit it toward the brain. A general scheme for classifying sensory receptors is to refer to the type of energy or stimulus that causes a neural response at the lowest level of energy relative to other stimuli that may be present. This scheme reflects the fact that specialized neural cells evolved in a manner that resulted in a highly selective response to a particular energy source or stimulus modality. The basic classifications include *mechanoreceptors, chemoreceptors, thermoreceptors,* and *photoreceptors.* Within the mechanoreceptor group are nerve cells that react to such mechanical forces as pressure changes in air waves; dilation or contraction of blood vessels or other tissue surfaces, such as those of the stomach or lung; stretching of muscle, tendon, fascia, or joint capsules; bending of hair cells; and a variety of pressure influences on skin tissues across the entire body surface. Chemoreceptors include cells on the nasal mucosa, cells on the tongue, and other cells positioned in large blood vessels and in the central nervous system. Also, many chemoreceptors react to bioactive compounds released by nearby damaged cells or by specialized cells of the immune system that expel substances under other stimulus conditions. Thermoreceptors respond to changes in the temperature (thermal energy) of the local environment. Photoreceptors are the cells in the retina that react to light waves of the electromagnetic spectrum. Many transducing cells of sensory units do not produce complete nerve impulses, but instead respond to the stimulus energy with graded electrical potentials called *receptor potentials.* In these systems, the first full action potential will be initiated in the nerve cell in functional contact with the transducing cell. As we can see, there are a wide variety of sensory units in the nervous system.

In the growing embryo, systems of neurons begin to form that can be viewed as having their starting point (cell A) at the interface with the internal or external environment. Then, following a stimulus transduction event, any subsequent cascade of neuron-to-neuron transmissions by synaptic systems may be viewed as a biochemical and bioelectrical method of energy transport between cells and across distances through the ever-increasing density of the cellular mass of the developing human form. All thresholds of stimulus and response for transduction and nerve impulse generation must be surpassed by the intensity of the stimulus, the number of cells

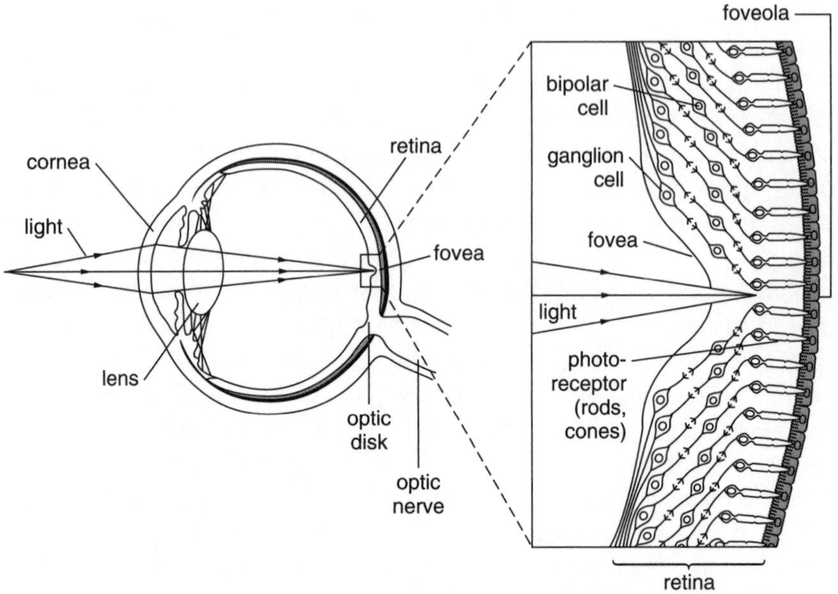

Figure 4-4 Human eye: retinal anatomy and optic nerve. (*After E. R. Kandel et al., Principles of Neural Science, 4th ed., McGraw-Hill, 2000, p. 508; reproduced by permission of The McGraw-Hill Companies*)

transmitting sensory signals to generate an action potential; and at each point along a neural pathway, each neuron must reach a threshold excitation/inhibition balance to generate its own action potential, moving the initial transduction event to its next location in the body and nervous system. From the external and internal stimulus worlds, we may catalog the sensory units that develop in concert with all other tissues and structures of the embryo (0 to 8 weeks) and the fetus (8 weeks to birth).

Formation of the human eye, indicated by a simple pair of grooves in the primordial forebrain, begins as early as embryonic week 5. The sensory unit, the retina, is a complex, multilayered structure that contains the receptors for photoenergy, the *rod* and *cone* cells, and several other types of neurons (Figure 4-4). The *ganglion cells* of the retina form the *optic nerve* that courses into the brain. The human retina has about 130 million receptor cells. Only about 5 to 7 million are cone cells, which react to photon wavelengths between 370 and 740 nm (violet to red), and these are most dense in the central portion (*fovea*) of the retina. The majority of the receptors are the rod cells, which generate potentials only when the illuminating photoenergy is at low intensity. The rod cells are not present in the foveal region of the retina and do not have a specific response to particular photon wavelengths. The human eye, the visual organ, will transduce only a minute fraction of the energy range in the electromagnetic spectrum. The ultraviolet and the infrared lie outside the two ends of the visible spectrum and cannot stimulate the rod or cone cells.

The human ear transduces air pressure waves from the external sensory world, as well as stimuli related to head position and acceleration through space. All these transduction events take place within the structure of the inner ear, which appears bilaterally in the fourth week of gestation. The middle ear and the external ear primarily serve to direct sound waves to the inner ear. The sensory cells that transduce pressure waves are called the *hair cells;* they exist as part of the *organ of Corti,* which resides in the *cochlea* (Figures 4-5, 4-6). Auditory waves traveling through the air are converted to fluid waves in the sealed cochlea that cause bending of the extended *stereocilia* (the hairs of the hair cells). This mechanical deflection induces depolarizing potentials in the cell membrane and leads to synaptic release of a neurotransmitter. Hair cells do not extend axons but form synaptic sys-

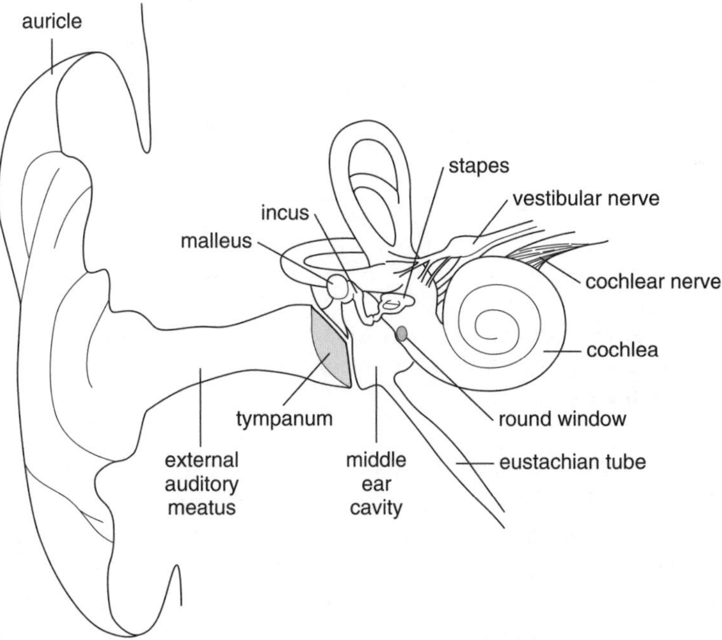

Figure 4-5 Human ear: inner ear anatomy and cochlear nerve. (*After E. R. Kandel et al., Principles of Neural Science, 4th ed., McGraw-Hill, 2000, p. 591; reproduced by permission of The McGraw-Hill Companies*)

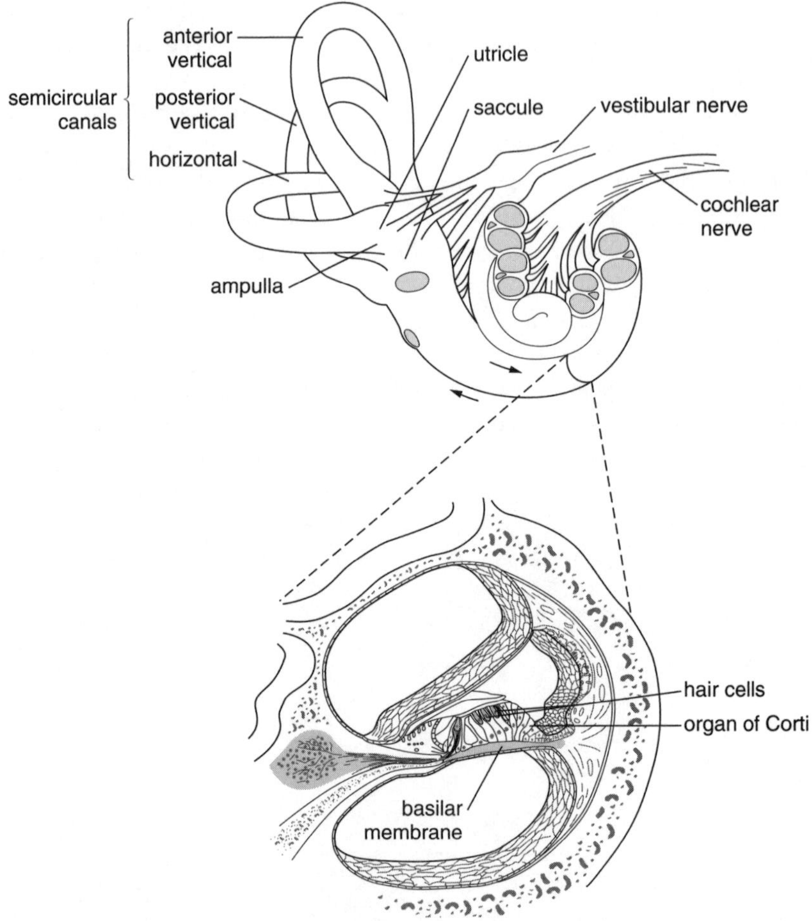

Figure 4-6 Human vestibular organ: semicircular canal system within inner ear. (*After E. R. Kandel et al., Principles of Neural Science, 4th ed., McGraw-Hill, 2000, p. 592; reproduced by permission of The McGraw-Hill Companies*)

tems at the base of the cell membrane. The postsynaptic component is the dendritic portion of ganglion cell neurons whose axons form the *auditory nerve*. The auditory nerve contains about 30,000 axons, reflecting approximately the same number of hair cells. The range of human hair cell response to sound waves, as measured by auditory testing, is from 20 hertz (Hz), or cycles per second, to 20,000 Hz. However, the range of highest sensitivity is only between 1,000 and 4,000 Hz. In this frequency range, an amazingly complex variety of different patterns, or variations in combined frequency and intensity parameters, can be differentiated. One such set of patterns, human speech, occurs typically between 100 and 5,000 Hz, and its intensity is usually below 60 decibels (dB).

The *vestibular* portion of the inner ear, like the cochlea, contains sensory hair cells that transduce mechanical force energy into neural impulse waves. The sensory units are found in an arrangement of cavities (the *vestibule*) formed in the very structure of the temporal bone adjacent to each cochlea. The *semicircular canals* create nearly orthogonal planes at right angles to each other (Figure 4-6), a fascinating biological reflection of the three spatial dimensions. The wave energies produced in the fluid-filled semicircular canals are transduced by the stereocilia of the hair cells into membrane depolarizations. This synaptic system, like that of the auditory organ, produces nerve impulse waves in the axons of the ganglion cells making up the *vestibular nerve*. Thus, virtually any rotational movement of the head in space will initiate a stimulus to some portion of the sensory cells, sending the transduced energies toward the brain in the afferent nerve fibers. The hair cell stereocilia of the utricle and saccule are embedded in a layer of thick gelatinous substance that contains a large number of calcium carbonate crystals, called *otoconia*. These sensory cells transduce the mechanical pressure on the cilia produced when the head changes direction with respect to the external inertial environment, including acceleration and deceleration changes. This stimulus energy is also sent toward the brain in the vestibular nerve.

The primary sensory function within the nasal cavity, *olfaction*, reacts to chemical stimuli in the external world. Early facial development of the human embryo is observed by the fourth week of gestation and includes paired nasal indentations. Only a few square centimeters in the uppermost chamber of the nasal passage contain sensory units of olfaction. Like the retina, cochlea, and vestibular organ, the olfactory organ is made up of a number of types of cells that transduce stimulus energy and transmit this event toward the brain (Figure 4-7). However, in this system, the primary sensory receptor cell is a bipolar neuron whose axon transmits the receptor potentials to the next neural connection. The vertical dendrite ends in a coating layer of mucus as a bulb-shaped projection (the *olfactory vesicle*) containing many long cilia. The cilia and perhaps protein complexes in the membrane of the dendritic projections act as general or specific receptors for a wide range of stimulus molecules. The interaction of adequate chemical stimuli with a sensory receptor induces a generator potential. The axons of the sensory neurons are myelinated by Schwann cells, and they pass through the *cribriform plate* of the *ethmoid bone* as the *olfactory nerve*. Each nerve from one side of the nasal cavity forms synaptic contacts with neurons of the *olfactory bulb* on the same side of the brain.

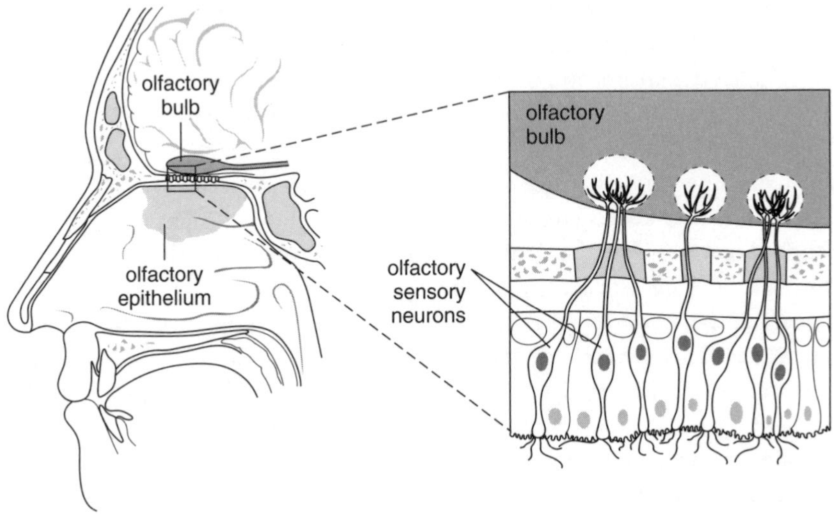

Figure 4-7 Human olfactory organ. (*After E. R. Kandel et al., Principles of Neural Science, 4th ed., McGraw-Hill, 2000, p. 626; reproduced by permission of The McGraw-Hill Companies*)

Special sensory cells on the tongue and pharynx transduce taste or gustatory stimuli: chemical products entering the oral cavity. The *taste organs* or *taste buds* consist primarily of two cell types, *receptor cells* and *supporting cells* (Figure 4-8). Taste buds develop in the *papillae* of the tongue, which begin to appear during week 8 of gestation. Each papilla may contain over 100 taste organs, and each organ contains many receptor and supporting cells. Most likely, molecules that bind to surface membrane receptor sites stimulate the sensory receptor cell. The exact nature of the taste receptor cell's particular affinity for a certain type of stimulus molecule is unknown. The sensory receptor cell produces graded electrical potentials and releases neurotransmitter molecules that stimulate the nerve endings forming synaptic systems with its basal membrane. Branches of three different *cranial nerves* (CNs) innervate the sensory receptor cells of the taste buds. The *facial* (CN VII), *glossopharyngeal* (CN IX), and *vagus* (CN X) nerves all innervate the taste buds with *pseudounipolar* neurons. A single fiber may make contact with several receptor cells, and a single receptor cell may make contact with several different fibers.

The final and most extensive transduction of external world stimulus energies is found in the organ that covers the entire body: the skin. The two layers of skin tissue, the *epidermis* and the *dermis* (derived from surface ectoderm and mesenchyme germ layers, respectively), are in development throughout the fetal period. There are many types of sensory cells in the

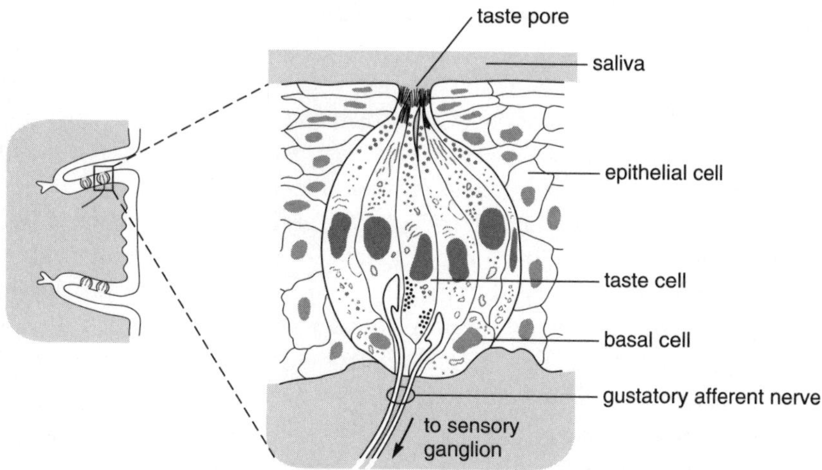

Figure 4-8 Human gustatory (taste) organ, showing receptor and supporting cells. (*After E. R. Kandel et al., Principles of Neural Science, 4th ed., McGraw-Hill, 2000, p. 638; reproduced by permission of The McGraw-Hill Companies*)

skin, and they transduce several forms of stimulus energies originating outside of the body (Figure 4-9). The mechanoreceptors of the skin include all sensory nerve endings that transduce pressure forces on the skin, including those of a high-frequency, vibratory quality. The thermoreceptors of the skin transduce changes in the temperature of the local environment. The neural crest cells that differentiate into dorsal root ganglion cells and transduce these cutaneous stimuli send one dendritelike process into the skin and another axonal process into the spinal cord.

The nerve endings in the skin subserving pressure and temperature transduction become encapsulated with connective tissue or epithelial cells that play a role in transmitting the stimulus energy to the neural membrane but do not perform the transduction event. Pressure forces or temperature changes induce generator potentials in the receptor nerve endings. These all-or-none nerve impulses are transmitted to the axonal process of the nerve cell, thus sending aspects of the stimulus event to the brain. The hair cells are an integral part of much of the body's skin. Hairs only begin to develop in the fetal period; they are visible at about week 20. Non-encapsulated, or so-called free, cutaneous nerve endings wrap around the hair shafts in the dermal layer of the skin. This arrangement provides an additional source of pressure stimuli transduction.

At the interface of the external and internal stimulus worlds, the skin contains a dense network of *free nerve endings* that appear to be chemoreceptors sensitive to bioactive compounds and other ions that are locally released as a result of tissue damage and other biological processes. Either external or internal forces may cause the release of bioactive molecules. Moreover, chemical solutions that are external to the skin but come into contact with the receptor nerve endings by diffusion through the epidermis may also cause a transduction event. These nerve endings may also respond, less specifically, to external pressure forces as mechanoreceptors.

From the most superficial layers of the epidermis to the deepest portions of the body core, a vast array of mechanoreceptors, thermoreceptors, and chemoreceptors appear in virtually every portion of the developing human embryo. The internal sensory world of the human organism is as actively transduced as is the external sensory environment. The number of neurons acting as receptor cells for the transduction of internal stimulus events far exceeds the number of receptor cells devoted exclusively to external energy source transduction. Blood vessels are lined with nerve endings that transduce expansion and contraction forces, and the concentrations of organic molecules such as glucose and oxygen stimulate receptors at several locations in the vascular system (e.g., the *carotid body*). *Fascial* tissue sheaths that line every body cavity, every muscle group, and each organ have receptor nerve endings that react to mechanical and chemical stimuli. Each smooth or striated *muscle cell* that stretches or contracts creates a transduction stimulus to a nerve ending, as does the movement of each *tendon* attached to a muscle group (*Golgi tendon organs*). Every *joint* in the body is encapsulated with tissues that contain nerve ending receptors that

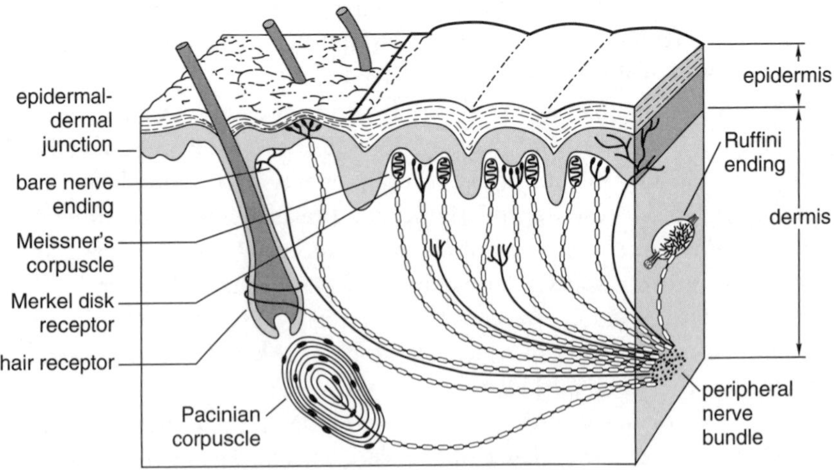

Figure 4-9 Sensory receptor cells in human skin. (*After E. R. Kandel et al., Principles of Neural Science, 4th ed., McGraw-Hill, 2000, p. 433; reproduced by permission of The McGraw-Hill Companies*)

transduce mechanical and chemical stimuli. The *periosteum* (fibrous covering on bone) is also densely innervated by sensory fibers, as is tooth pulp.

The *viscera* of the body—the lungs, heart, liver, gall bladder, pancreas, spleen, kidneys, ureters, urinary bladder, stomach, intestinal tract, and all reproductive organs—have varying amounts and types of sensory receptor nerve endings. The intestinal tract is densely populated with nerve endings that transduce pressure and chemical stimuli. Cardiac muscle tissue itself has few sensory fibers, but the covering tissue sack (the *pericardium*) contains an intricate network of receptors. The brain and spinal cord tissues do not have sensory receptor nerve endings, but the protective layers (the meninges) do possess them.

Thus, through the embryonic and fetal periods of development, sensory transduction cells populate each growing organ system and begin to convert one form of energy into a neural event of membrane current change. When each sensory neuron (or specialized transduction cell and neuron unit) reaches a critical functional threshold, the stimulus transduction event will begin to result in an impulse wave in a neuron whose axon enters into the spinal cord, part of the central nervous system. Thus, these transduction events, brought about by external or internal stimuli, also begin to influence the migration, synaptology, and survivability of neurons as they form functional collective systems integrated with each portion of the growing organism.

Regardless of the type of receptor cell or the form of stimulus energy being converted, each transduction event can be viewed, measured, and understood as a biochemical change in the membrane conductance of the receptor cell. Ultimately, all internal and external stimuli are sensed only as bioelectrical activity in small patches of cell membrane. The nature of the converting process varies greatly among the stimulus energy sources and within each sensory receptor group, but the outcome of each and every transduction in the nervous system is an increase or decrease in membrane potential. Each and every transduction in the nervous system that is of adequate stimulus intensity and duration will initiate a propagated wave of impulse activity that results in the activation of synaptic systems. The propagated impulse wave activity will vary among classes of sensory receptors and even within each class by the frequency with which a particular fiber will initiate generator potentials for a given type of stimulus or for certain qualities of a particular stimulus (e.g., intensity, duration, or a combination effect). The speed or velocity of the nerve impulses will also vary widely among and within receptor classes, depending upon nerve fiber diameter and myelination (usually between 0.5 and 120 m/s).

However, from the point of view of neuron B, C, or D (Figure 4-3*a*) receiving a synaptic contact from a sensory receptor neuron, the transduction of photoenergy, mechanical energy, or chemical energy is manifest only in 3D waves of impulse activity that enter synaptic zones and release neurotransmitters and/or neuromodulators in synaptic systems on dendritic spines, shafts, cell bodies, or axons. That is, the particular physical forces from the external or internal world that act on the organism do not directly affect any neural cell other than those specifically performing the transduction process. Except for the sensory receptors themselves, each neuron senses, or transduces, only biophysical stimuli from other neurons. (We note again that the local milieu of each neuron, including the ionic balance, pressure and temperature, bioactive molecules, and bioelectric currents, may affect the delicate multiplicity of shifts in membrane potentials that either increase or decrease the probability of an impulse potential's being generated. This local biomolecular volume effect either may exert its influence as an enduring *metabolic tone* affecting the overall membrane potential or, perhaps, may play a critical role as a dynamic variable at each stimulus moment affecting local synaptic activity.)

The afferent flow of transduced sensory stimuli from the receptor cell to the first synaptic contact in the spinal cord or brain is shown in Figure 4-10. The total picture, of course, includes the efferent outflow of the synaptic systems to skin, muscle, organ tissues, and so on. As we discuss earlier, the nervous system has been classified into a series of divisions based on evolutionary, developmental, structural, functional, and historical factors. Neural crest cells become the neurons and glia of the peripheral nervous system (PNS), which is further divided into the *somatic* and *autonomic* systems. The autonomic division is subdivided into the *sympathetic* and *parasympathetic* systems. The somatic system includes all neural processes that result in actions of the musculoskeletal system, from simple reflex responses to complex behavior. The autonomic system classically refers to the neural functions that regulate all internal organs. The neurons that convey transduced stimuli from the retina, cochlea and vestibular organ, and olfactory receptors are not of neural crest origin. The cell bodies of the somatic sensory receptors aggregate in clusters (ganglia) that organize parallel to the dorsal (posterior) spinal cord. The axonal processes of these cells enter the spinal cord to form synaptic contacts with cells of neural tube origin [the central nervous system (CNS)]. These afferent synaptic contacts thus form a PNS-to-CNS transition. Collectively, the axonal bundles and their tissue coverings create rootlike structures—thus the term *dorsal root ganglia*.

The sensory receptors of most modalities found in the skin, skeletal muscle, joints, and other portions of the body form the somatic or spinal division of the peripheral nervous system. The autonomic sensory receptors include all fibers transducing stimuli from the internal organs, glands, smooth muscle, and blood vessels; hence the common use of the name *visceral* nervous system. The cell bodies of the sympathetic division, sensory receptors are also in the dorsal ganglia, but these neural groups are found only in the thoracic and lumbar segments (the *thoracolumbar* division) of the spinal cord. The parasympathetic neurons transmitting sensory stimuli can be found in brainstem clusters and in the caudal or sacral portion of the spinal cord. The parasympathetic nervous system is thus also called the *craniosacral* division.

We began this discussion by examining the range of stimuli that the human nervous system will transduce in addition to the neuron-to-neuron

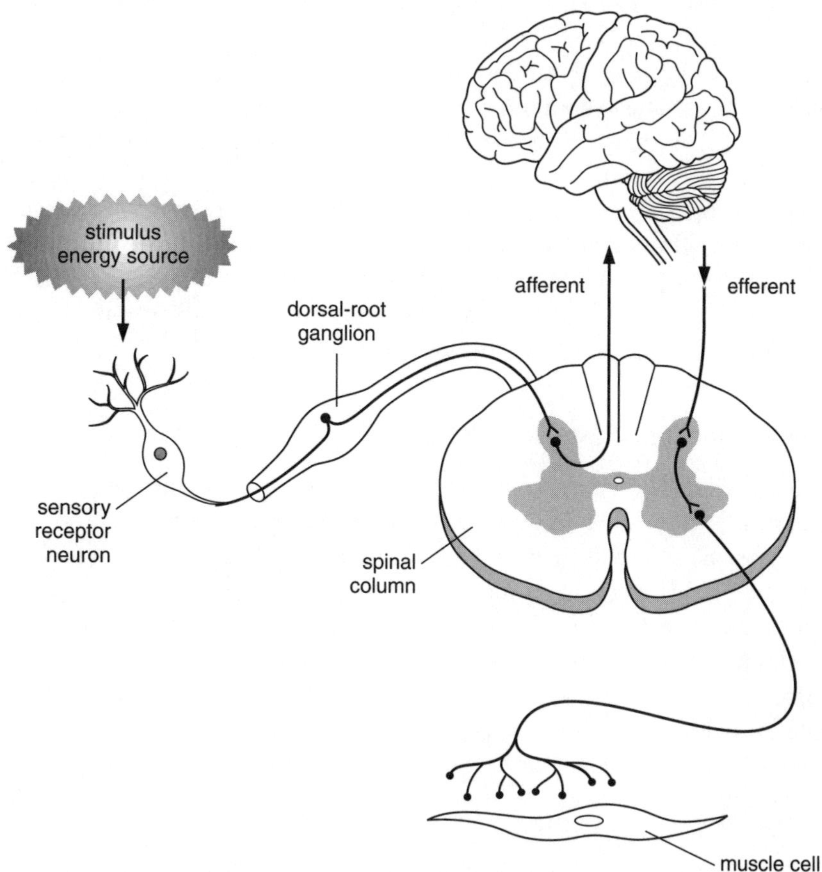

Figure 4-10 Diagram of afferent flow of sensory information to the brain and efferent output from the brain to effector (e.g., muscle) cells.

transduction process conducted in synaptic systems. Even in the womb, as embryonic limb buds develop into the bones, muscles, and joints of the fingers and toes, as the early circulatory system brings oxygen and nutrients to ever more dense and complex internal organ systems, and as newly differentiated skin cells begin to build the layers of dermal and epidermal covering, the energy forces of the external and internal worlds exert an influence. While the retina develops behind closed eyelids and the ears, nose, and mouth await the full stimulation that postnatal life will bring, photoenergy and sound energy are present in diminished form, and pressure, temperature, and chemical stimuli abound. Through the embryonic and fetal periods, more and more cells differentiate into specialized status, begin a specific function, and live or die. The number of cells that die may actually outnumber those that survive in most systems.

As the size, density, and complexity of the fetus increase, the nervous system keeps pace. The particular classes of stimulus energies that can be transduced by the receptor cells will be transduced, but only if their physical effects are above a minimal threshold of intensity or duration and, conversely, only if these effects are below a maximum threshold of intensity or duration. The mammalian nervous system may sense only a very narrow spectrum of the electromagnetic and mechanical universe. Those energy sources for which no receptor cell exists and those that reside outside the receptive range of a given class of cell types will not be transduced, will not be sensed, and will not be transmitted through neural systems—critical constraints that limit our sensory existence.

Space, Time, and Systems of Nerve Cells

What does the nervous system, at least the described peripheral system of nervous tissues, *do*? We know that cells derived from the neural crest form receptors to transduce a number of stimulus sources of the external and internal worlds, that they propagate nerve impulses toward their synaptic zones, and that they form synaptic systems with other neurons in the spinal cord and brain. We know, then, that this energy transduction is a driving force for the nervous system. It is a complex, multimodal force that helps mold the developing nervous system to its unique environment, creating a dynamic structural and functional shape that cannot be fully predicted in the genetic code.

The nervous system activity must also have an effect on the development of every other cellular system, to the extent allowed by genetic-coded plasticity. Just as nonneuronal cells that release bioactive compounds as an output (e.g., hormones) have an action on many other cell types, so do neurons that release bioactive molecules. The output, or action, neurons are called the *effector* cells; in some manner, they convey transduced stimulus energy to other organ systems. Between the sensory receptor cells and the effector cells there may be between zero and billions of neural cells. These *interneurons* (using the most general definition) exist in the peripheral and central nervous systems, but predominate in the brain structures.

In this discussion of the nervous system below the brain, we have noted that the dorsal horns or columns of the spinal cord contain neurons that form the first synaptic contact with the neurons transmitting action potentials produced by sensory cell stimulation. These *first-order* neurons may send axons toward the brain (rostral), to lower segments of the spinal cord (caudal), to the same side of the spinal cord (homolateral), across the midline to the other side (contralateral), or to both sides of the cord (bilateral) to form synaptic contacts with other neurons. Other first-order neurons, also functioning as effector cells, send axons out of the spinal cord to form synaptic contacts with nonneural cells (e.g., muscle cells). The various neural loops, or circuits (note the generally used electronic terms), beginning at the sensory receptor and ending with the effector neuron may involve one synaptic link (a *monosynaptic reflex loop*) or may involve several stages of synaptic processes (e.g., *neocortical* network processes). The designation of neurons as second-order, third-order, and so on thus denotes where the particular nerve cell lies in the direct path between the first sensory transducing neural element and the final output nerve cell. This designation does not indicate the tremendous synaptic interplay between dozens to millions of other interneurons that may affect the ultimate impulse wave output in a particular synaptically driven pathway. As we know, a single neuron may receive the synaptic output of hundreds of other cells. So, in tracing a loop or circuit, we may count the number of direct point-to-point contacts between a sensory event and an ultimate, effector cell-mediated output back onto a nonneural cell.

For the life frame of reference, we described the language change that was needed in order to characterize or define single-cell functions that cannot be reduced to the background biophysical frame of reference: the emergent properties or functions, such as metabolism, respiration, exocytosis, pinocytosis, and reproduction. When we looked at multicellular life, new words to describe the processes of systems of cells were required. We say that flowers bloom, fish swim, and cats meow. These multicellular processes or behaviors are not emergent, by our operational definition, but describe the collective actions of many single cells.

We now have examined the single nerve cell in the context of the developing human and have noted some of its defining structures and functions with respect to the many other cell lineages. In our efforts to initiate a descriptive analysis of the embryonic nervous system, we had to adopt a sequential, A-to-B approach: neuron-to-neuron connection by synaptic system activity, and stimulus energy source-to-receptor cell transduction event. Now that we have introduced the concept of the output or effector neuron, another change in the language is necessary if we are to adequately describe these loops or circuit systems of neurons and the effect they collectively have not only on other neural circuits, but on all other cellular systems of the human organism and on the world of living and nonliving things.

Each neuron, like each and every cell in the life field, functions or behaves as a cell. Therefore, each nerve cell circuit, from a two-neuron loop to the multibillion-cell entirety of brain function, behaves, in general, like any other system of cells. Like each nonneuronal single cell or multicellular system that can be described by its unique structure, function, and products, the specialized nerve cell and systems of neurons have unique behaviors and products that integrate them into the overall existence of the entire organism.

It is our human behavior to provide definitions for functions or operations of the collective cellular activity. For example, within complex multicellular animal life, which includes humans, we can say that the circulatory system carries nutrients and oxygen to all cells so that they may continue to live in the dense environment of tissues and organs. It also carries away the products of life, cellular metabolites such as CO_2 that cannot be allowed to accumulate, and performs many other functions necessary to the survival of the animal. Thus, we describe the behavior of this system composed of many cell types by saying that it transports, it exchanges, it feeds, or it removes. The digestive system can be said to filter, extract, absorb, and secrete. Like these descriptions of the circulatory and digestive systems, descriptions of nervous system behavior encompass not only the functions of the principal tissue type, in this case the neuron, but also those of all other cell types (e.g., neuroglia) that are integral to the overall system function.

Nervous system processes can be classified into two simple organizing schemes: *between-system* functions or behavior and *within-system* behavior. A between-system classification is required for a complete description of nervous system behavior because neural cells are a critical component of nearly every functional, systems-level organization of tissues and organs in all animals. The nervous system-to-nonneural system behavior is mediated by the effector neurons mentioned previously. At some stage in a short or long chain of synaptically linked neurons, an axonal synaptic zone may innervate a nonneural cell and effect an action, or output function. Muscle cells of the musculoskeletal system, from eyelids to vocal cords to toes, form neuromuscular junctions with axons of effector neurons. The synaptic release of acetylcholine, as the primary fast-acting neurotransmitter, causes a muscle cell to contract, and thus, at the system-level observation, an action (from a single muscle cell contraction to a blink, laugh, or curl) is performed. Special cardiac muscle cells form synaptic systems with neurons of the vagus nerve, whose neurotransmitter release, also acetylcholine, causes the heart cells to lower their rate of intrinsic rhythmic contractions. Conversely, synaptic contacts with effector neurons of the sympathetic nervous system release norepinephrine onto cardiac cell receptor molecules, resulting in an increased contractile rate. Glandular cells (e.g., salivary, sweat, pituitary, or adrenal) are stimulated or inhibited in their function of cell product secretion by synaptic activity from effector nerve cells. We can catalog almost every function or behavior of the human body and locate a direct nervous system effector influence that causes a between-system behavior: the dilated iris, a cough, stomach acid release, ejaculation, or a pirouette.

These behaviors reflect the coordinated action of an incredible number of cells, many under significant nervous system influence. What, then, guides the nervous system in its effect on the other organ systems of the body? What determines the location and timing of effector nerve cell impulse wave activity? For specific examples, we could ask how jellyfish decide to move left, right, up, or down; how termites build mounds with gardens and nurseries; how chimps choose leaders and mates; or how people invent and understand calculus. The answer is that animal behavior, from the simplest muscle twitch to the unfathomable complexity of human imagination, expressed in effector-mediated activity, invariably involves a critical amount of within-system neural function. Many within-system neural processes have easily observable (and thus classifiable) between-system outputs through the musculoskeletal, digestive, circulatory, or some other nonneural functional system. Other behaviors, however, such as wanting, caring, loving, hating, or contemplating, are not as easily observed in effector cell-driven outcomes. But in a general sense we still consider these descriptive verbs to reflect behaviors, and as such they must be produced within the nervous system. In broad strokes, we have just defined the within-system behavior of the nervous system.

Following stimulus transduction through receptor cells, within the neuron-to-neuron transmission of synaptic activity and before the effector synaptic contacts with other cellular systems, the nervous system itself performs functions. The terminology to describe these within-system functions is varied and includes words like *compare, extract, weigh, add, subtract, multiply, divide, calculate, integrate, compute, encode, depict, represent, decide, understand, predict,* and *remember*. In its most basic function or behavior, the neuron-to-neuron, within-system transmission of the transduced internal and external environments serves to *bind in time* the stimuli present within the organism and in the nearby external world.

We can see that a single-cell organism has its entire outer membrane in contact with the local external world, transducing all stimuli to the extent of its capabilities. The internal consequences of external influences, changes in metabolic rates or products, or genomic transcriptional modulation will reflect an interplay of all the stimuli converging on the cell. A single-cell life form senses the world and reacts to it in a manner that maximizes its potential to exist to the next moment; this is a homeostatic function or behavior (as we discussed in Chapters 2 and 3). If we constructed a hypothetical *freeze-frame portrait* of all the metabolic pathway states (indeed, intracellular systems) and the unique structural configuration of the cell, we could derive knowledge about the local external world and the various energy forces that have an influence on the cell. Thus, we could say that the momentary structural-functional state of the intracellular environment is a reflection or representation of or *complex code* for the extracellular stimulus moment. All transduced energies are bound in a *temporal metabolic moment* spanning the spatial extent of the single cell's internal world. [We can actually see that it is even more complicated than this, for within each single cell of any evolutionary maturity, there are systems (organelles) that will react to a specific type of stimulation. Thus, a product of an organelle will act as a unique internal stimulus source at a distant part of the internal world—all in a single cell!]

However, as multicellular life developed in evolutionary time, the external world of background energy forces and their fluctuations could not reach each cell membrane directly. The effect of stimulus transduction, or some aspect of it, had to be transmitted from a cell positioned at the interface of the organism with the background environment to those cells not so exposed. Looking back upon the phylogenetic pathway, we see the specialization of cells within ever more densely tissue-layered plants and animals. Most of the specialized cellular systems that we partition and name by various structure-function criteria serve to transmit or transport some aspect of the external environment to deeper layers of the organism. Indeed, if we were to freeze-frame a metabolic moment of a small piece of artery and examine its contents, we could derive a representation of the outside stimulus world (e.g., temperature, oxygen tension, food energy types and availability, and even time of day).

Each system within a complex organism thus developed to help create and maintain a viable metabolic environment that would keep all cells functioning within their parameters—the interdependent, collective process of homeostasis. The time function, or operational rhythm, that each cellular system possesses was also shaped in evolutionary time and varies from organism to organism and from system to system. Again, the fossil record and tree of life show not only the great breadth of cellular systems that developed in multicellular plants and animals, but also the limits to size, complexity, and operational parameters that our changing biosphere has imposed. Across the multicellular species, oxygen and nutrients are extracted and transported within specific temporal parameters to keep all other cells alive. These operations are performed more quickly for some plants and animals than for others. Aspects of all other external forces that may determine the survival of the organism, whether mechanical, thermal, photo, or chemical, are transduced and transmitted in different manners and at different rates within and between species by all specialized cellular systems. In this general functional description of the evolution of cellular systems, nervous systems are not qualitatively different; the general function of the nervous system must in some way also help to maintain the overall homeostatic condition of the organism.

This is why we said that the basic within-system function or behavior of the nervous system was to *bind in time* the stimuli present within the organism and in the nearby external world. From the small number of nerve cells in the flatworm to the billions of neurons in the human, all neural circuits or networks bring together aspects of transduced stimuli from various locations—all at the rhythm of action potential propagation, and at the specificity and resolution provided by the types, distributions, and densities of receptor cells. Thus in the human fetus, driven (and limited) by the pulse of moment-to-moment sensory stimuli transduction, the synaptic system activity within a set of interneurons may in some way reflect not only a pressure change on a patch of skin, but simultaneously a temperature change deep in the dermal layers. Also, a set of neurons may bind in time highly different mechanical forces affecting sensory cells from different sides of the body.

These simple word descriptions belie the functional dominance that within-system neural behaviors have imposed upon the world. This binding in temporal moments of synaptic system operation of aspects of the external and internal worlds that may exist meters apart and may span several energy forms provides the fundamental basis for all complex animal behaviors, including those that are most difficult to ascribe to neural processes. The pulse of the nervous system, set by the transduction and transmission parameters and varying across sensory receptor systems and species, determines the rate at which these temporal bindings of spatial and sensory aspects may occur.

The outcome of these functions, whether they are transmitted to another interneuronal binding moment or expressed through effector cells, thus is also limited to the rhythm of the system. From a homeostatic standpoint, the within-system behavior of the nervous system provides a rapid way to bring together one or more vital aspects of the external and internal milieus that certainly could not otherwise have a direct influence on the incredibly dense body of cells the nervous system serves. The effector cell-mediated outcomes of these binding moments in nervous system activity bring to the other cellular systems all the comparative, weighed, integrated, or calculated actions that are needed to regulate, control, or guide the fetus through intrauterine development and, eventually, the young infant through the life span. The nervous system's function is quantitatively different from that of other cellular systems in the ways in which its transmissions of transduced stimuli are conducted through an interaction of synaptic systems. Only the nervous system binds such a wide variety of stimuli from every possible location in or on the body, and it does so more rapidly and at a higher resolution than other cellular systems. Thus, the primary difference is the quantitative or *computational interaction* within the systems of neurons.

Below the Brain: A Finger in a Pool of Mud

We have limited this chapter to the general developmental and functional aspects of the human nervous system below the brain. The sensory receptor cells of the somatic and autonomic divisions of the peripheral nervous system and all the special sensory fibers of the optic, olfactory, gustatory, auditory, and vestibular nerves transmit the stimulus universe to the central nervous system. In the spinal cord and brain, networks of neurons conduct most of the within-system functions of calculation, integration, and computation. Output effectors are activated from spinal cord networks in short loops to influence reflex and regulatory functions within the musculoskeletal, respiratory, cardiovascular, digestive, and endocrine systems. Brain effector outputs influence many of the spinal cord networks as they produce their efferent waves of neural activity that activate somatic and visceral systems. Before we move to the brain and its development, structure, and function, and the production of consciousness, we will look at one example of the nervous system in action that may serve to integrate many of the concepts outlined in this chapter.

For this example, we will advance along the developmental timeline of the human fetus and imagine that a baby girl has been born and is now growing and maturing in the world, separated from the mother's protective womb. As we watch the young infant at play, we will not be surprised to see her become attracted to a pool of glistening mud and proceed to dip her index finger into it. We focus on the tip of her finger and acknowledge the astounding number of nerve fibers coursing from all the sensory receptors in the layers of skin tissues, hair cells, blood vessels, and membranous sheaths surrounding tendons, joints, muscle, and bone. And in effector cell reply, we note all the axons bringing action impulses from the brain and spinal cord to the muscle fibers, blood vessels, hair cells, and sweat and sebaceous glands.

As the infant pushes the tip of her finger into the pool of mud, a local explosion of activity ensues with the millisecond-to-millisecond transduction of the changes in the external and internal worlds of a few cubic centimeters of one of the body's most distant outposts. The temperature of the mud, if different from that of the ambient air, is converted to a series of neural impulses in thousands of afferent axons. The viscosity of the water and dirt suspension serves as a source of mechanical stimulation as the nail and skin are pushed against it. (Is it watery or pasty?) The movement of the mud, enveloping her finger as it descends into the pool, stimulates a succession of different sensory cells and nerve endings in the skin and on the hair cells that reside only on the dorsal side. (Is it slippery or sticky?) All of these forces, through moment-to-moment transduction events, produce a massive barrage of neural impulse waves that somewhere, somehow, contain information about or a representation of the temperature and density of the suspension.

The delicate little fingertip is now submerged. If the average thermal energy of the mud is significantly greater or less than that of the finger, an energy exchange begins that can cause local blood vessels to expand or contract, small muscles around hair cells to contract, and sweat glands to begin secretion activity—a homeostatic process. Below the brain, the neural circuits subserving these behaviors would be of the short-loop class that reacts quickly to stimulus energy afferent flow. The homeostatic knowledge or decision-making machinery that determines what to do when the local temperature in the fingertip changes is built into the structure-function of the nervous system. It is a design feature forged during billions of years of evolution. And, it is basically the same response that would occur in the digit of a raccoon or leopard.

If the temperature difference were too dramatic, a very short neural circuit from the sensory receptor to the spinal cord and back to skeletal muscle cells might be stimulated, resulting in the rapid withdrawal of the finger from the pool. The same reaction might occur if the fingertip happened to strike a sliver of glass within the thick solution. The situation becomes much more complicated when we acknowledge that brain effector systems (descending in the ventral tracts of the spinal cord) can modulate some of these reactions to some finite extent. Such complex variables as hunger or attraction could produce a shift in the threshold of pain tolerated by the infant if there was a piece of food or a glittering object to be obtained. This represents a partial override of one basic homeostatic mechanism by another, the result of a millisecond battle fought primarily in the brain. Perhaps this is a factor that will differentiate the raccoon, the leopard, and the human.

The coordination of musculoskeletal activity that allows the kneeling or sitting infant to extend her finger and push it into the mud involves multiple simultaneous assessments of overall body position and the balance between the left and right arms, legs, hands, and fingers. This seemingly flowing and flawless progression of a delicate hand and finger toward and through the surface of the pool is in fact a massive sequence of parallel events, transduced and transmitted within the nervous system and between cellular systems at a millisecond rate of operation. Thousands of starts, stops, errors, adjustments, and resets thus define the internal reality underlying this external illusion of seamless motion and purpose across many seconds of time. Here, now, we may begin to understand the relationship between the Muybridge illusion of motion at the flicker-fusion threshold for a series of pictures and the illusion of ongoing behavior as a fusion of underlying neurobiological processes. In both instances, the illusion is generated in the mind of the observer.

If the fingertip is held still at a certain depth in the mud, other interesting processes may occur. The heat exchange between the body and the mud may begin to equilibrate; when there is no longer a relative temperature difference, the external surrounding mud may no longer be sensed as a source of thermal energy stimulus. As the microscopic swirling of the muddy solution slows to below a particular threshold of mechanical energy per square millimeter of skin surface per millisecond, the mud may no longer be detectable as a mechanical energy source.

When the finger is moved along a path in the mud, a new set of stimulus transductions related to the force of motion, thermal changes as new areas of mud come in contact with the skin, and so on will be initiated—as a result of a simple line in the mud made by an infant finger. Actually, this produces an incredible series of transduction, transmission, integration, and effector events involving nearly every major class of sensory receptor, autonomic and somatic pathways, short reflex arcs, and long circuits to the brain. Billions of cells in networks of connectivity are reacting to the onset of stimuli, velocity changes, and equilibrium effects on transduction cell activity in the tiny fingertip. The utter complexity of this seemingly simple act becomes even more imposing when we realize that other sensory systems—e.g., the visual, auditory, olfactory, and gustatory systems—were not even involved in the account. (The mud-covered finger in the mouth event at least once in an infant's life is a certainty in the quantum universe.) Extrapolating the transduction, transmission, and feedback effector activity in this small region of a finger to the entire human infant or adult in his or her moment-to-moment existence provides a sense of the magnitude of the operations that our nervous system conducts in concert with all the other biological systems of the body. For the most part, we ignored the enigmatic human brain functions related to motivation, mood, meaning, or memory in this example. We will, of necessity, be addressing all these processes in the next chapter.

Information, Computation, Representation, and Complexity

Before we continue with the development and function of the human nervous system, we must again take a moment to come to terms with our terms. We introduced the class of words that became necessary in order to describe the emergent behaviors of cells, the functional units of the life field. All the metabolic and reproductive processes of each individual cell and the larger-scale properties and behaviors of systems of cells required words that denoted the 4D quality of a cell or cells across moments of time. For one specialized cell, the neuron, we introduced the properties of an action potential or nerve impulse and synaptic transmission. Each term describes a modification of other basic cellular functions. The collective activity of nerve cells in systems required additional words to describe what appears to be happening between the stimulus transduction and the effector action. *Something* happens within the systems of nerve cells that can cause subtle or dramatic changes in internal (regulatory) processes or in various somatic muscular systems. The terms *information, computation, rep-*

resentation, and related words were introduced when we began to describe these neuron-to-neuron and collective nervous system activities.

From our human viewpoint, it appears that the nervous system, by binding in time various distant and disparate stimulus energy events, is internally reflecting or representing the external and internal worlds in its nerve impulse and neurotransmission activities. The terminology we invoke to further describe this basic process of representing is that of mathematical operations. Thus, we say that the nervous system performs summations, calculations, integrations, or computations within its neuron-to-neuron network activity. Depending upon which part of the nervous system we examine, we may infer either that a representation is being computed (e.g., from initial sensory transduction transmissions) or that a computation is being performed on a representation (e.g., by interneuronal networks in brain nuclei). Finally, the representations derived by the computational processes of neuronal systems must be based upon some type of substrate data, or information contained in basic neuronal activity.

The code, or the basic information upon which the nervous system computes representations, appears to be contained in the singular and collective nerve impulse, the frequencies of impulses, and the relative rates of impulse conduction.[4] In addition, many aspects of synaptic system activity may also contain a basic code to fuel the computational engine—e.g., the relative timing and location of synaptic system activity on a single or group of neurons and the types and amounts of bioactive molecules released per nerve impulse. At this point in our presentation, all information generated (as aspects of nerve impulses or synaptic activity), computations performed (as a change in the information as it proceeds through a system of nerves), and representations created (as the collective information at some location, at some moment, in some portion of the nervous system) by the systems of neurons described thus far remain within the dimensional parameters of cellular systems, and thus within the referent system of life. No new biological system possessing a unique order and temporal dimension, with respect to the time functions of general cell metabolic activity or of specialized nerve cell impulse generation activity, has been uncovered. The within-system neural processes, binding in time informational aspects of the stimulus world, are indeed an amazing evolutionary modification, but they appear at this point to function well within the rise and fall of stimulus energies and cellular metabolism.

The descriptive words we have used to define the collective behaviors of neural systems may of course be applied to many other types of systems across many scales of measurement. Information, in its most basic usage, may be related directly to a change in the entropic state of a system, either biological or nonbiological. Thus, information, like entropy, is a reflection of the order or disorder in a defined system.[5] When entropy or uncertainty is reduced and order is increased, information is said to be created, attained, or at least theoretically attainable. The seminal underpinnings of modern information theory may be found in the works of Shannon and Weaver, Wiener, and others.[6] In this basic and general definition, we may say that information is present in any system in which entropy and order change, from quantum states to biological events, to the electronic circuits of computer systems, to neural networks.

Related to information theory, the development of modern computational theory by Turing, von Neumann, McCulloch and Pitts, and others predicted and subsequently demonstrated the utility of harnessing, if you will, the information contained in a series of basic state transitions (e.g., 0/1, negative/positive, off/on, etc.).[7] Both simple and complex mathematical problems could be solved if enough binary events were purposefully strung together by any device set up to follow a basic, repetitive set of rules or operations. Theoretically, the time it took to step through each set of binary data points was irrelevant. A computation was accomplished when the device completed a mathematical operation, however simple or complex. An abacus and a slide rule, in effect, are basic computing devices that can work in binary code, but that also may operate at other levels of numerical representation (e.g., base 10). These devices can work only at the speed and efficiency of their human operators.

Practically speaking, the advent of the integrated circuit, which now supports trillions of binary operations per second, has made our time the digital age, a computational age. So, like entropy, order, and information, computation may be used in reference to many different types of systems on many scales of operation. However, it basically is defined as a mathematical operation performed by any device or system following its own set of operational parameters, and that includes the nervous system. We can say that a single neuron (or, for that matter, a single dendritic spine) is performing a spatiotemporal integration of all synaptic and other influences per stimulus moment, and that this operation either does or does not result in the generation of an action potential. This is an example of how we impose our notion of a computation on a nerve cell function. We may expand this conceptual process to the moment-to-moment input of many synaptic zones to many neurons and the resultant output of the pattern of nerve impulses from the neuron set. Computation by a single cell and computation by a neural network may or may not follow the same set of operational rules.

Representation is also a generalizable concept, and it also depends on how we partition various systems, their momentary states, and the changes in those states. If we make a series of hypothetical freeze-frame assessments of the structural and functional states of a single cell while we vary the oxygen tension in the bathing solution, we may find that a set of measurable parameters correlates with (partially reflects) or represents the concentration of oxygen molecules outside of the cell. The intracellular state is not the same thing as the oxygen concentration, but it can be seen as a representation of it—that is, if we make the mathematical comparison that projects one data set onto the other. We will avoid delving into the philosophical tangentials that immediately come to mind (e.g., isn't a dollar a representation of ten dimes?). We will just note that, again, it is our human organization of biological functions that places representations of the external and internal stimulus worlds into the properties and the behaviors of nervous systems. Therefore, if stimulus transduction and transmission contains information about the world, then it appears logical to infer that within some set of neurons at a given moment in stimulus processing, there is a representation, a correlate, of some aspects of the stimulus world. At a more general level of logic, it could be said that we *just know* that the nervous system represents the world, at least the external world, as one might exclaim, "I just close my eyes and I can see the room I'm in and the street where I grew up!" This proposition could be absolutely correct, or it could be erroneous on an important fundamental level of knowledge. (Again, we will avoid a discourse on epistemology at this juncture.) Information, computation, and representation are all interrelated and perhaps indispensable in discussions of nervous system activity.

At this time, in the search for knowledge and understanding of the biological universe—its operations manual, its secrets—we do not know what information a single neuron derives from its environment. We do not know what the absolute basic code of information transmission in the nervous system is. We do not know the full set of computational rules that operate in a single neuron or a network of neurons. We do not know exactly if, where, and how the nervous system represents the external and internal stimulus environments. We can model some components of neural behavior in electromechanical circuits and mathematical equations, together expressed in computer simulations, but these are our constructs. We can build a mechanical finger that moves and makes a line in a pool of mud, but we still do not know the mathematical operations, the algorithms, of the nervous system. We may even write computer programs that calculate a bewildering number of possible moves in a game of chess and related probabilities of successful end games, but we have not encoded the operation of the nervous system. For example, the staged events of human-computer chess competitions only serve to underscore the illusion of knowledge that we tend to project onto inanimate objects.[8] No chess master has a 100 percent success rate for all games played against human opponents. Why, then, do we attribute humanlike abilities to a software program when a human displays the normal tendency to fail in a competition where it is employed? In fact, most players of chess are readily beaten by relatively simple software programs. Does this fact necessarily mean that computers running chess game software are more intelligent than most people? Hype, hope, and illusion must be understood and respectfully separated from insight if we are to make progress in our efforts to reveal the neural computational code.

Is the information contained within a bundle of axons conducting nerve impulses transmitted to a receiving network of neurons in the central nervous system entirely by a code generated collectively at the synaptic contacts? And does the network then perform its functional operations entirely by synaptic excitation/inhibition transduction events? We do not know. It must be remembered that it is only recently that we even began to understand and conceive of the nervous system as the substrate of computation and behavior. We are limited, and humbled, in our understanding of the basics of neural function when we begin to speak of such things. We will return again and again to our limitations in knowledge in the following chapters. This is not necessarily a sad state of affairs, as the nervous system is the most complex biological system known. It is more of an indication of how much more we have to discover; how much more beauty and excitement nature holds for the interested.

The human embryo was selected as the model system for this chapter to enable us to describe the special properties of the nerve cell and its development into integrated systems that subserve all human behaviors. This was done, in part, because the human is the only animal that studies other nervous systems and writes papers about them. Such activity appears to be among the most complex expressions of the nervous system that we know. And, while this chapter is primarily limited to the nervous system below the brain, most of the basic structural and functional components of the nervous system have been introduced. We know that the nerve cells participate in stimulus transduction and transmit this complex information to spinal cord or brain nuclei. In the spinal cord (and brain), small to enormously large networks of neurons, glia, and other cells perform complex computations, and effector outputs are activated. But is the human nervous system the most complex?

To prepare for the discussion of brain development, the birth of a human infant, and the emergence of consciousness, it is pertinent to again examine this much overworked word: *complexity*. How do we know which nervous system is the most complex? Are not the behaviors that humans engage in more complex than those of other animals? If this is true, what makes it so? If this is false, is there no significant difference between the structure and function of the human nervous system and those of some other animals, or other primates? In general, complexity is a relative term. Something is more or less complex or intricate only in relation to another item.

The judgment of complexity is centered on the interrelationships among parts of a whole, but it typically is a judgment nevertheless. Increased complexity may refer to a larger number of things contained in one item or system compared to another. One maze may have more pathways than another, and thus contain more choice options for someone who tries to solve them both. One cell may contain certain DNA in its genome and produce a particular protein that protects it during harsh environmental conditions that kill other cells without the protein. Is the cell with different DNA, a different protein, and a different response to external stimuli more complex? If one nervous system contains more synaptic systems than another, it could be said to be more complex in that there may be additional informational, computational, or representational functions or capacities. But this is not always so clear, as in some cases a larger number of neurons or synapses may not necessarily lead to more intricate operations or behavioral consequences.

Discussions of what variable qualities or quantities one is referring to when one applies the term *complexity* and what systems are more complex than others range far and wide, without absolute agreement. Complexity could be correlated with entropy, order, information, or the possible states or conditions that a system might attain. The total number of mathematical equations needed to provide a complete description of a system might be another measure of complexity. In cell biology, it thus appears that the term *complexity* is primarily used to infer or suggest either that one cell or multicellular system has more functions, processes, or behaviors than another, or that the cell or system has particular properties that differ in a manner that gives it a greater probability of survival than a similar cell or cellular system.

In the hypothetical protocellular world presented earlier, evolutionary changes to the internal structures and functions that led to the maintenance of an internal order with respect to the background flux were regarded as increasing complexity on a quantitative scale. At the critical flicker-fusion threshold of collective internal function, the living cell emerged as a new order of organic complexity; this was a qualitative, 4D change. From that moment on, biological evolution brought paths of quantitative modifications and additions to cells and cellular systems that in many cases resulted in a more intricate and successful species.

This generational time-scale interplay between cells and the environment—that is, the evolution of life—also produced many complex organisms that did not survive in a changing world and others, perhaps less complex, that developed an enduring relationship with their local biophysical contexts. Thus, evolution as an engine of complexity is constrained by local environmental conditions. It is our premise, or model, that while we can identify these quantitative changes across the species in all systems of cells, including the nervous system, it is only in the nervous system that we can identify a qualitative change that we commonly refer to as consciousness.

We may ask, in an extreme comparison, if a starfish and an eagle differ in complexity. From an evolutionary perspective, each animal certainly possesses enough complexity to survive in its respective environmental niche. Moreover, we note that each multicellular animal has differently modified cellular systems that function for its particular environment, in this example aquatic or land and air. And each animal has a nervous system that senses the external and internal environments, transduces and transmits stimulus information, and initiates a behavioral repertoire.

From the perspective of relative behavior, we may say that the eagle seems more complex in that it moves faster, travels farther, and has more flexible behavior. If we look at the internal structures, we note that the eagle has more cells that form more intricate systems (e.g., respiratory, circulatory, digestive, reproductive, and musculoskeletal systems) and that it has a larger nervous system to control these systems. If we look at the nervous system of each animal, we note that the eagle has more nerve cells and that they form larger, more interconnected networks of interneurons (the eagle has a bigger brain). The eagle thus may be viewed as more complex than the starfish on the basis of some cellular systems and its behavioral flexibility or *plasticity*; it has a more complex functional capability endowed by the structure and function of the nervous system.

While one may argue that the starfish has all the behaviors that it needs in order to function maximally in its environment, it can also be argued that the eagle's environment (external and internal) presents a more varied set of stimulus forces, and so the eagle requires a larger repertoire of behavioral responses if it is to survive. But, for all of the eagle's apparent greater complexity, the sum total of the differences between the starfish and the eagle, as wrought in evolutionary time along very different pathways, may be seen as quantitative modifications. Each individual cell of the starfish and eagle is essentially the same, operating in the life field. Are there behaviors that the collective activity of all the cells that we call eagle generates over the animal's lifespan that are qualitatively different from the behaviors generated by the collective activity of all the cells that we call starfish?

On the generational time scale, both the eagle and the starfish are born, undergo development, behave to the extent they can, perhaps reproduce, and die. Can we adequately describe all the moment-to-moment behaviors of one animal with the same terms used for the other? Or is the mother eagle's feeding of her young so vastly more complex than anything that a starfish can do that it must be a new order of existence, a qualitative shift in the behavior of organized cellular systems? Is something new happening in the nervous system of the eagle as it soars above the treetops and then dives to snatch a fish from a river that could never be experienced by a starfish as it encounters its own prey? Is there an emergent order of functionality, such as feelings, cognition, sense of self, or some other state of being, that is a true measure of the greater complexity in the eagle?

Of course, it is exactly this line of questioning that we are addressing throughout this book. The answer to these questions have not been definitively formulated in any type of quantitative, mathematical, or scientific terms. At first, it may seem easy to assume that there must be some qualitative difference between a starfish and an eagle. However, when we take the time to start with the single cell, understand the development of cellular systems within an organism, and integrate the structure and function of the systems of nerve cells in the animal, it becomes a more difficult task. And when we begin to compare two animals that are closer together on the mammalian branch of the family tree—say a mouse and a dog or, in the primate branch, a chimp and an orangutan, or a chimp and a human, for that matter—issues of complexity and qualitative differences become more demanding, more frustrating, and even more contentious.

When we observe the evolutionary process and try our best to classify the fossilized extinct and surviving forms of single and multicellular life, we make complexity judgments based on unique cellular systems expressed through the genetic code. We are still in the process of making an evolutionary map based on the behavioral repertoires of each animal, the cellular substrate of which is nervous system activity. When we make an observation that one animal has a behavior (a multisystem collective process driven by nervous system computational activity) that is not present in another, must we always assume that a radical, qualitative phenomenon in the nervous system of the animal possessing that behavior underlies that difference? Or, is it more correct to assume that the same operational system of neural network computational activity—the substrate repetitive machinery—is processing a different set of information from external and internal stimulus transduction, forming a different set of representations, and thus driving a different set of effector outputs? Perhaps it is processing more information, more computational operations, and more representations, but qualitatively it is in the same class.

Can we apply these quantitative changes as a *complexity index* for the vast range of behaviors observed in nature, or at least for animals within the same environmental niche? Even with these constraints, complexity assessment is not so easy. A bear and a beaver, two mammals, may live near the same stream, but one builds dams and the other does not. The genetic expressions of behavior are different, but is one animal more complex than the other? In what animal or animals has a qualitative, emergent, neural operation evolved to produce behavior that is *not* comparable to the entire set of all other animal behaviors? If this has happened, was it due to a change in the information, the computation, the representation, or something else? Where do we draw the line, if a line is to be drawn? Is a human finger making a line in a pool of mud a more complex act than a chimp making the same line? These are nagging questions that will not go away.

Anthropomorphic Lexicology

The specialized academic and general societal discourse about these topics has always been advanced by new terminology arising from arduously attained knowledge about our biophysical existence. The latest additions to the dictionary on the neuroscience of behavior include such words as *network, nonlinear, computational, combinatorial, parallel processing, reentrant pathways*, and *chaotic systems*, among many others.[9] However, when the level of description reaches the systemwide output stage, the *computational solutions* that are expressed by an organism through some type of sequential effector activity collectively referred to as behavior, the definitional language becomes more difficult. To say that a flower *basks* in the sunshine, that a termite *valiantly defends* its home, or that a stallion *boldly befriends* a mare may cause problems. We will always enhance and add life to our spoken and written descriptive phrases in our daily routine of talking with friends and family (or to pets) or when we write poetry or tell a bedtime story to a child. But when we wish to systematically define any type of behavior, from that of the single neuron to that of the fly, to that of the human, within the context of biophysical constraints, we must be very careful with our descriptive terms and operational definitions.

We have noted changes in terminology when it became necessary to do so. Up to this point, we have purposely avoided using certain terms, and we have placed many words in italics to alert the reader to a particular usage. This approach has absolutely restricted the use of many wonderfully demonstrative words, phrases, metaphors, allusions, and analogies. However, at the potential cost of momentary literary enjoyment, this is the only way to remain consistent with the major theme of this work. Thus, by carefully maintaining a certain level of descriptive terminology and providing a reference set of definitions, we can be more consistent and coherent as we proceed to an operational definition of consciousness.

We will continue to impose limits and constraints upon the overall conceptual (philosophical) foundation of the model, as we feel this more accurately reflects the biophysical constraints within which we exist. When we describe the electrochemical or mechanical processes that operate around or in a single cell, including the nerve cell, we use words and phrases that reflect the level or scale of behavior within the biophysical substrate frame of reference (ionic concentration, charge, current, or potential). That terminology is sufficient to relate the knowledge. Only when we examine the emergent system of the cell, the life unit, relative to other cells or to the background system are we compelled to invoke a different set of nouns and verbs. The descriptive language of metabolism, nerve impulse, neurotransmission, and stimulus transduction is sufficient to impart this scale of processes. The criteria of necessary and sufficient in the application of terms are vital if we are to present a model that, indeed, draws lines across which we argue that emergent, qualitative, four-dimensional systems became operational in the evolutionary time scale. These criteria are monumentally vital if we are to propose that in nervous system activity we may actually identify the emergence of consciousness as the only emergent biological system other than life.

One way to view this is to say that we have taken care not to use larger-scale terms for smaller-scale phenomena. We did not use the language of the life field for individual biophysical events or processes: The potassium ions did not *gallop* or *scurry* into and out of cells; the nerve membrane depolarization events did not *fly* or *rush* down the axon. The descriptive terms *move, flow,* or even *cascade* were sufficient. It was not necessary to invoke more lively verbs, adjectives, or adverbs. When we described the processes of individual cells or multicellular systems, we used the language of life: The cell differentiated or metabolized; the growth cone expanded and migrated;

the heart began to beat. For larger-scale activity, these terms are necessary only in that they can convey a complex process in a single word. They are a device, a chunking method, a collapsing convention that permits a reasonable rate of communication. (This type of linguistic necessity is itself a reflection of a limitation, a constraint in our ability to communicate.) But we did not need to say that a cell *grabbed* a molecule or that a growth cone *searched* for its *awaiting* target cell. That scale of language is not necessary. It may be sufficient, but it is not constrained to only that level of behavior.

Our point of view, in human consciousness, permits us to watch and study all scales of organized space-time and to describe what we see and learn with words and definitions. Where to draw the lines and how to determine what term is necessary and sufficient is a dynamic process, and not always a simple or obvious one. When we apply the largest-scale terms that exist, those of complex human behavior (including emotions and all the qualia of philosophical categorizations), to any smaller-scale or other system phenomena, we are projecting a property of human consciousness on that process or activity. We are imposing an anthropomorphic lexicology.

But, again, where do we draw the line? We may agree that a rock cannot *swelter* in the heat and that a caterpillar cannot *dream* of becoming a butterfly. But we will find much less unanimity if we propose that a cocker spaniel cannot be *embarrassed* to urinate on a busy city street or that a gorilla cannot *dread* the coming of old age or *contemplate* the moon and stars. Is this just anthropomorphic lexicology, or do dogs get embarrassed and nonhuman primates contemplate? Which nervous system, other than the human, produces all the thoughts and emotions for which we have such words? Is anthropomorphic lexicology an invalid concept? Does each and every animal (leaving out inanimate matter and plants for the moment) produce each and every computational product that a human does? Or do only mammals, or only big mammals, or only primates, or only big primates have a nervous system that functions like that of the human? Where we find the qualitative change in behavior is where it becomes necessary to apply our self-descriptive lexicology. It is also where we can begin to look for the biophysical modifications that altered nervous system processes and generated the behavior. If that threshold to consciousness has an identifiable behavioral expression, then we can draw the line. If this can be accomplished, it may have utility in the science and medicine of nervous system function.

The model of biological relativity proposes that we will find the threshold of consciousness in the human nervous system and its behavioral expression. This is why we used the human embryo to introduce nerve cell and nerve system development. After we complete this part of the developmental story, which we will do in the next chapter, we will then take the time to look across the animal kingdom for evidence of consciousness. With our behavioral model of human consciousness in hand, we will apply it to other animals and make complexity judgments about which levels of terminology are both necessary and sufficient to describe their expressed computational products, their behaviors.

Toward the Brain

The ascending afferent tracts of the spinal cord and the afferent fibers of the optic, auditory, vestibular, olfactory, and gustatory nerves transmit all the transduced sensory stimuli toward the brain. The entirety of human sensation, experience, and action is derived from these basic informational sources. From the viewpoint of the brain, massive bioelectrical wavefronts of nerve impulses enter into a succession of highly interconnected groupings of interneurons, the nuclei, and are repeatedly converted or transduced into a mixed biochemical, bioelectrical, and biomechanical code in and around billions of synaptic systems. At each brain nucleus, the neural networks perform their computational operations on this information and produce representations of the transduced sensory worlds. It is deep within the isolated environment of the brain tissues that the individual sensory modalities will become more and more intermingled, the right and left will be fully merged, and representations of the external and internal stimulus worlds collide.

The information carried along the afferent pathways heading toward the brain is substantially limited in its scope, reliability, and resolution. Our receptor cells cannot transduce many potential stimuli, and at certain minimal and maximal thresholds, other stimuli are not detected. The temporal dimension of the sensory worlds—that is, the flux of stimulus energies—is encoded in the nerve impulse wave frequencies, but this transduction of time by the receptor cells is limited by the biophysics of the individual sensory transduction process, action potential generation, and axonal conduction. If too many stimulus events occur within a certain time frame, the full magnitude of the event may not be detected, and a partial (erroneous) computational solution may be produced. For example, we cannot see the discrete spokes of a spinning wheel after it reaches a critical rotational rate. The nervous system cannot process the information contained in the event, and we perceive an illusion of a static mass.

We are thus *locked in* or highly constrained with respect to the larger spatiotemporal field of potential stimulus events in the external and internal worlds. Moreover, the potential maximum amount of information that could be transduced and encoded is further degraded by the inexact functions, the noise, of the substrate biological and biochemical systems. All cellular functions that depend upon metabolic and mechanical processes, including transduction, transmission, and neurotransmitter release, have their own fluctuations, as they are large-scale operations built upon many individual substrate molecular events. Therefore, the information in the afferent fibers does not consist entirely of the sensory stimuli that can potentially be transduced. These constraints on the scope and reliability of sensory transduction set limits on the resolution, or detail, that can be represented in any transduction event.

At the brain, massive neural activity brings the transduced sensory stimuli of the world into networks of cells. The information encoded in each individual nerve fiber, however, is essentially a 2D code for each stimulus event. That is, information about the existence, persistence, or magnitude of a stimulus may be contained in the frequency of nerve impulses in a single axon. But information about the relationships of a stimulus with others, the 3D landscape of the external or internal world, is beyond the capabilities of a single axon. Stimulus energy is transformed into a depolarization of the neuronal membrane, and a nerve impulse wave may be generated, but these waves are generated one at a time. The synaptic transmission of bioelectrical transduction to biochemical exocytosis is also a 2D code, a singular and serial spatial event. However, somewhere in the neural network processes, somewhere in the 3D arrays of cell-to-cell interconnectivity and volumes of tissues containing synaptic zones, the dimensions of space and time are computed and represented. The pulse or rhythm of informational activity in the waves of afferent impulse conduction is a function of the temporal parameters of the background stimulus worlds and of the cellular parameters of membrane conductance. Thus, we may say that the stimulus worlds are encoded by the nervous system in collective moments of transduction; a *transduction moment* or *point representation* is therefore operationally defined as a momentary state of all nervous system activity, which changes on a millisecond time scale and which represents the maximum amount of information about the external and internal stimulus worlds. It is a finite set of biophysical conditions. It is the freeze-frame or snapshot analogy applied to a cross-sectional moment of the entire afferent wavefront entering the brain; it is a *flicker of representation*, a peak state, that rises and falls with the temporal fluctuations of the substrate neural impulse and synaptic system activity. All the information, the order, the entropic state, is time-locked to the pulse of the underlying nerve cell activity.

No new temporal dimension, independent of the background flux, is created in this wave of individual fiber information.

From the first young nerve cell to generate an action potential to the first sensory cell to transduce an energy source, the human embryo, then the fetus, develops billions and billions of cells that generate and process an ever-increasing barrage of transduction events. Afferent and efferent pathways transmit the neural code to either enter ever more intricate computational fields of the central nervous system or effect an action in the internal or external environment—moment-to-moment point representations of basic sensory information or derived output solutions. The nervous system becomes alive with activity; it begins to sense the world around and within and ultimately to understand and wonder. We will continue the developmental story of the human nervous system in the next chapter. There we will see the brain constructing the final dimensions of space and time from the flux of substrate neural information in the human infant exposed to the new stimulus worlds. There we will see where our sense of the 4D reality is born. However, we must present this model using the language of information, computation, representation, and complexity, with all the appropriate humility and respect for our embryonic state of knowledge.

5
The Brain and Sensory Information

We are now equipped with a view of the specialized morphologies and behaviors of the developing nerve cell within the larger context of the growing human body. The transduction and transmission of the external and internal stimulus worlds sets the stage for our exploration of the information flow through the central nervous system. From here on, as we employ the language of information, computation, and representation to operationalize consciousness, it is even more important to remain aware of the interrelated nature of form and function in our nervous system.

The primordia of the brain structures are observed at the cranial end of the neural tube, where the primary vesicles are formed during embryonic weeks 4 and 5. Along the caudal-to-rostral axis, the neuroectoderm of the hindbrain, midbrain, and forebrain begins to generate millions upon millions of young nerve and glia cells in waves that migrate from their respective ventricular zones to form a wide array of cellular aggregations. Thousands, then millions, then billions of axonal growth cones extend out from brain nerve cell bodies to interconnect the cells of the brain. Other young brain cells extend growth cones out of the local regions to form axon terminal regions and synaptic zones with more distant neurons in the spinal cord. Simultaneously, the primordial axons from the spinal cord neurons begin to enter brain regions and create synaptic contacts.

As the embryonic brain is forming its unique cellular arrangements, the sensory worlds begin to impinge upon its development. Imagine the first nerve impulse wave along an afferent tract to the brain bringing mechanical pressure information from a patch of skin or stomach tissue, or the onset of optic nerve activity transmitting diffuse photic energy that has infiltrated the intrauterine world, transduced by a tiny collection of rod and cone cells.

At first there are just hints and fragments, then partial patterns, and finally the tsunamilike onslaught of the totality of stimulus energies as they are transduced in the moment-to-moment sensory cell activity that is transmitted in pulses of impulse waves to a brain that is ever more ready to receive and react to them.

Brain Nuclei, Cortical Regions, and Axon Tracts

The adult human brain is depicted in Figure 5-1. We will refer to this figure often as we follow the development of the specialized regions of the brain and the flow of sensory information through its networks.

In the terminology used to describe the peripheral nervous system, aggregations of nerve cell bodies, supporting cells, and their connective tissue

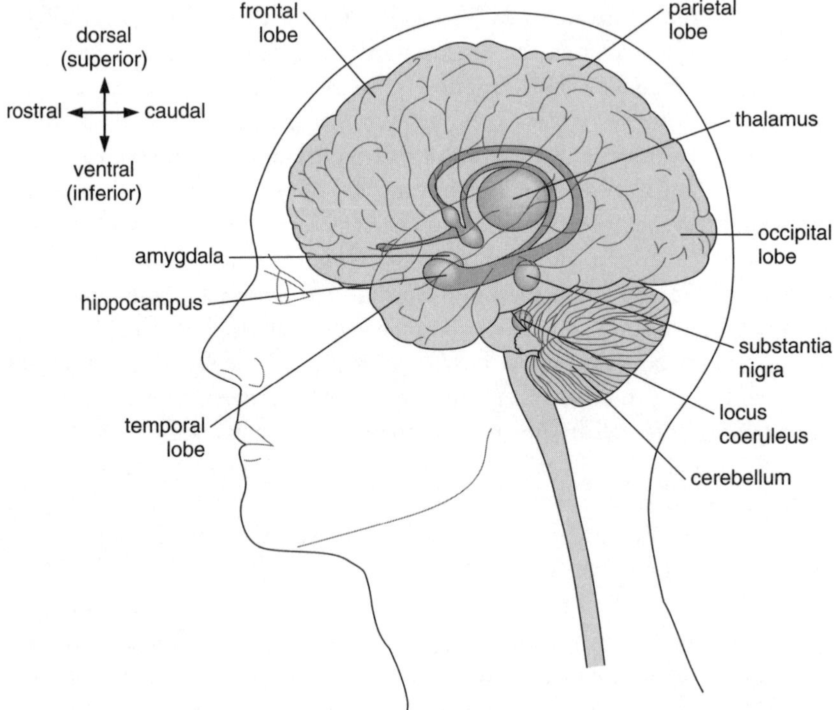

Figure 5-1 The adult human brain, showing axes of orientation, primary brain lobes, and key nuclei deep to the cerebral cortex.

coverings are referred to as *ganglia*, and the axon fiber bundles that bring information to and from these ganglia are referred to as *nerves*. In the central nervous system (the spinal cord and brain), nerve cells and surrounding cell clusters are called *nuclei*, and axon fiber groups are referred to as *tracts*. In the surface or cortex regions of the brain, such as the cerebral or cerebellar cortex, neurons and glial cells form distinct layers, or *lamina*. Each nuclear cell group or laminated region has its own specific collection of nerve cell types (defined by morphology or by the neurotransmitters and neuropeptides expressed) and numbers, arrangements of afferent axon terminal regions, synaptic connectivity (the various excitatory and inhibitory systems), and efferent projections to other nuclei or cortical regions. Thus, no two brain regions are exactly alike, although basic similarities in patterns of cellular arrangement and connections may be observed.

The descriptive analysis of brain structure based on particular cellular arrangements and axonal projections, called cytoarchitecture, has a significant history and has produced several different methods for delineating subtle distinctions in the boundaries of brain regions. That discussion is well beyond the scope of this current presentation, but we must comment that there was no official road map to follow when scientists began to explore the developmental and phylogenetic patterns of brain formation. And of course the laborious effort to add a functional overlay to the structural map, in terms of the information or representation present at each unique brain area, has proved to be an even more daunting task. Finally, from a single neuron to a nuclear group of interconnected neurons, measuring the changes in a particular bit of information as it is processed or computed by the neural machinery defines the ultimate quest to elucidate the computational nature of the nervous system. What information is located within a particular brain region at a particular moment? What biomathematical transformation is performed within that region, and how is it done? What representations are contained in the axon tracts leaving that region, and how are they coded in the spike train of nerve impulse activity?

Basic neuroanatomical, electrophysiological, and biochemical study; analysis of changes in neuron and neural system behavior over developmental and phylogenetic time scales; and examination of how use or experience affects the ongoing operation of neural networks all add to our collective knowledge of how the brain functions to produce behavior. Slowly we gather small insights into how a brain nucleus or network portion functions to modify or transform the information brought to it by afferent fibers. We collect evidence of the level of order or complexity of representation present in a particular brain region from electrophysiological recordings of a single cell or cell group activity in nonhuman experimental situations or from humans undergoing neurosurgical procedures. For example, there are neurons deep in the brain that alter their nerve impulse rate in response to sound stimuli applied to a peripheral hair cell, and this implies that they play a role in sound processing. Behavioral analysis of nonhumans and of humans with developmental disturbances in brain formation, disease, or traumatic effects on brain function also provides knowledge of how each region of the brain contributes to the processing of sensory stimuli. For instance, patients with damage to the left side of the brain often demonstrate an inability to control or sense portions of the right side of the body. This basic observation led to an understanding of the way the nervous fibers cross the midline on their paths to and from the brain.

We can trace waves of nerve impulses as they ascend the neuraxis toward and finally through the forebrain and cerebral cortex, and in this way define functional maps of the representation of the sensory world within each brain nucleus. Comparing the changes in the functional map from one brain nucleus to another gives us insight into the computational operations performed on sensory information as it flows through a particular brain network. Thus, if neurons in one region of the brain generate spike trains when any shape is presented in the visual field, but the cells in an adjacent region respond only to shapes of a particular size, it may be inferred that biocomputational activity brought a refinement of sorts to the selectivity of this network. In our investigations of brain function, we may then ask questions such as: Where does the nervous system compute and store the letter A? Where is the first place in the brain that the word FIRE is constructed from the discrete written or spoken letters? Where in the brain is a pencil represented as a structure with shape, dimension, color, name, and operational definition? Where is the face of a beloved relative created and stored? Where is the temporal dimension, the passing of the present into the past and the predicted future, generated? Where do hope, hate, and love exist in the brain? Where does the brain compute the totality of the sensory worlds in action, the moment-to-moment reality of consciousness?

As each nuclear group in the brain develops its own unique configuration, the afferent drive sources (whether from first-order neurons or several synaptic contacts downstream from initial energy transduction events) exert an influence through the particular synaptic patterns that are formed and the bioelectrical and biochemical activity patterns that are projected through these synaptic systems. Thus, as we discussed for the peripheral nervous system, brain nuclei form under the interrelated influences of genetic expression parameters; the background environment, which includes the adhesion, growth, and survival molecules; and the functional interaction provided by the innervating afferent projections. This activity molds or shapes the initial nuclear group and continues to modify its morphological and operational existence to the limits allowed by genetic plasticity over the lifetimes of the cells (abnormal extremes notwithstanding). The connectivity of afferent sources with the neurons of the brain region, the connectivity of the various neural cells within defined nuclei, and the connectivity of the efferent axon tracts with the next nuclei or other target cells are continuously being modified and reorganized to various degrees, from the first synapse formed during embryogenesis to the final nerve impulse generated at the end of life.

A generalized schematic of a basic brainlike nucleus, focusing on a few of the key developmental structural factors, is depicted in Figure 5-2. One afferent input (A1) consists of bundles of axonal growth cones that form synaptic zones with a nuclear cell group (N1). A second afferent fiber tract (A2) brings information from another nucleus and forms its synaptic zones on a separate set of neurons (N2). In this simple design, the A1 and A2 afferent fibers terminate on dendritic spines of their respective target neurons. The N2 neurons extend their axons toward the N1 cell bodies and form axosomatic synaptic contacts within the nucleus. The axons of the N1 cells collect into a bundle and leave the local nucleus to form synaptic zones with another brain nucleus, a spinal cord cell group, or both. The neurons that project their axons away from the local cell group (the N1 neurons in this case) are typically called projection or principal neurons. The nerve cells that

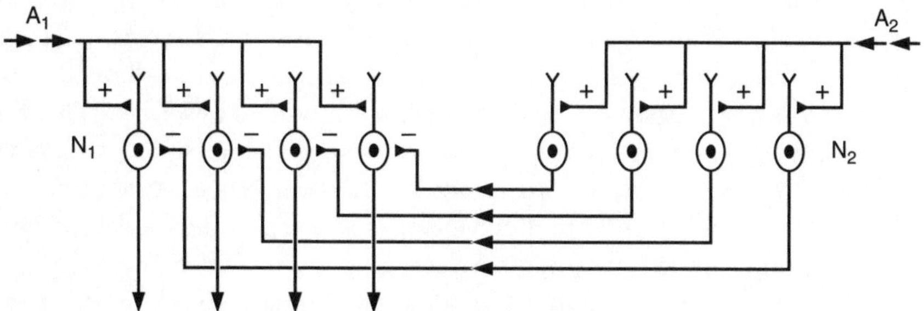

Figure 5-2 Schematic of a nerve cell-to-nerve cell network illustrating a basic organization in brain nuclei. Afferent projections (A) to groups of neurons (N) are noted as excitatory (+) or inhibitory (–) in their overall stimulatory influence.

form synaptic contacts within the local nuclear mass (the N2 neurons) may be referred to as local neurons or (in a more specific use of the term than we are employing in our terminology) interneurons.

The developmental sequence for this simple nuclear group of cells (a neural network) involves cell migration to specific intranuclear positions and the death of many cells during this process as a critical mass is attained. The migration of axonal growth cones into the forming target zone of cells takes place in a complex timing sequence that differs among brain regions and afferent sources. As the neurons in the target nucleus extend dendritic branches, the young axon terminal zones may form synaptic contacts and initiate the development of the highly plastic synaptic spine extrusions. The dynamic formation of synaptic systems also involves an early overabundance and gradual degeneration to achieve a stable configuration; the pruning is partly by genetic design and partly activity-dependent. Thus, as developmental time passes, the nuclear mass of cells—neural, glial, and other nonneural types—is shaped in terms of cell types, numbers of each type, and the source, number, and type of synaptic zones formed. The predetermined general size, shape, and connectivity are modified by the unique metabolic conditions present in the particular embryo or fetus and by the neural activity entering into the newly formed neural fields following sensory transduction events external and internal to the young human. The continual development of the simple nucleus in Figure 5-2, like that of all brain nuclei, will also involve the activity of neuroglia cells that form myelin sheaths around many of the axons in each fiber tract, as well as the formation and degeneration of synaptic contacts.

These activities continue after the fetus becomes a child and well into adulthood. Thus, important factors concerning the input of information into a nucleus, such as the speed of nerve impulse conduction (a myelination effect) and the pattern of synaptic influence (the number and location of contacts), will vary—one may say mature—over many years, perhaps even over a lifetime in some regions of the brain. The rate of cell death will differ across brain regions and will of course be modified by each organism's unique life experiences, such as trauma and illness. The possibility that new neurons are generated following childbirth is under investigation, but the evidence from most animal studies has not provided a strong model for new cell replacement in the mature brain, save for a few well-known exceptions.

The flow of neural activity through a developing network of cells partially depends on excitatory and inhibitory influences that shift the resting membrane potential toward or away from generating a nerve impulse in the axon. We see that the A1 synaptic zones (Figure 5-2) are designated as excitatory (+) in nature, as are those of the A2 field (as noted in Chapter 4, most axospinous synapses in the brain are likely to involve an excitatory neurotransmitter such as glutamate). As this nucleus develops, a critical number of functional synaptic systems will form in the A1 projection onto the N1 cells, and when a sufficient number of synaptic zones are activated, a nerve impulse may be generated in one or more of these neurons. However, the N2 cells are shown to form inhibitory (–) axosomatic contacts with the N1 group (most likely using GABA as a primary neurotransmitter).

When the A2 projection becomes mature enough to depolarize N2 neurons and initiate action potentials, the N2 cell will act to reduce the probability that an N1 neuron will generate a nerve impulse. The timing of differential afferent activity thus becomes a critical component in the function of this nucleus. This reflects the primary within-system neural function of binding in time sensory information from different portions of the organism. Nerve impulses generated in N1 cells exit the nucleus in the projection tract as patterns of spatial and temporal bioelectrical activity. The human brain contains an incredible number of variations on this basic theme of nuclear structure and function, but this general example serves as a model for some of the important developmental considerations that we must keep in mind as we look at the manner in which the brain begins to receive and process afferent sensory information.

Critical Postulates Regarding Neural Activity, Order, and Information

We may now present an important set of hypotheses regarding the interrelationship of brain nuclear structure and biophysical function. These constructs form the basis for the model of biological relativity as it relates to the generation of consciousness in neural activity.

Recall that we proposed that the protocell, and then the living cell, is a thermodynamically semiclosed system of a particular three-dimensional (3D) structure that created an organization or order of energy states within its structure for a critical duration. The degree of order attained in each protocell or cell was dependent upon a complex function involving the background biophysical energy sources and reflected parameters of the transduction and internal transmission of these energies. The order attained was thus wholly dependent upon the energy sources available, and it increased and decreased along a multifactorial curve related to the energy flux of the biophysical environment. The protocell lost a critical amount of internal order during periods of minimal background energy and thus could not sustain its existence. The living cell maintained a critical threshold order

(3D) for a sufficient time (1D) with respect to the background flux to permit its ongoing existence. The first living cell embodied a thermodynamic disconnect in its negative entropic order from the background frame of reference and propagated its own unique 4D existence.

Now, in an analogous manner, we propose that the waves of neural activity in the afferent fiber tracts entering brain nuclei may be conceptualized as a new background energy source, provided by the existence of the life field and the evolution of nervous systems. As we noted in the previous chapter, information or representations of the sensory worlds are contained within these active axonal arrays. Thus, in our basic example (Figure 5-2), the A1 afferent fibers, their axon terminal regions, and the synaptic zones possess an order or informational content that has a maximal and minimal existence plotted along a complex curve whose temporal axis is determined by the biophysics of neural transmission and transduction. The 3D structure of the brain nucleus, which includes the afferent terminal fibers and the synaptic systems they form and is shaped in development by genetic and epigenetic influences, defines a region with bounding limits through which the background neural activity flows, bringing additional order and thus information for a brief, momentary duration.

An entire brain nucleus, or defined networks within it, may therefore be viewed as a special volume of tissue (perhaps the most complex volume of tissue in the universe): a cellular-based living structure that functions as a thermodynamically semiclosed system. Within a constrained frequency range and maximal order limitations, a complex wavefront of electrochemical energies (the afferent nerve impulse wave and synaptic zone activities) adds momentary charge, force, and information to the tissue volume. We thus propose that brain nuclei, cortical regions, and portions of nuclei as defined neural networks may be conceptualized as cell-like 3D structures that produce a unique order in the background neural activity as it pulses through the constrained multicellular fields.

Thus, the entropic order, the information or representation possessed by a particular afferent nerve impulse wave, reflects a maximal state (and a quantifiable biophysical force) that declines along a curve after it enters a brain nuclear region and transfers its bioelectric energy to the tissue volume as it is converted into biochemical synaptic zone activity. The brain tissue charged by this ordered energy performs its computational operations (defined by its unique inherent cellular arrangements and connectivity), and the final output products (the computational solutions or transformed information) are encoded in the volumes of tissue containing arrays of axonal projection tracts. The efferent tracts, like the input tracts, possess a wavefront of nerve impulse charge in the 3D fiber array and contain order or information that is a complex function of the original afferent information.

In a manner of speaking, the flow of sensory information from brain region to brain region keeps a representation of the internal or external world alive, albeit transformed. As a representation of a moment of sensory transduction gets projected through brain nuclei, it is immediately followed by additional moments of sensory transduction. The farther along the neuraxis that a particular wavefront of sensory representation goes, the older it gets relative to the ongoing sensory transduction processes. The modified representations reaching the most rostral extent of brain cortex may form the *now* in that region, but they are the past relative to the representations in more caudal nuclear regions. It is in particular regions of the brain that portions of sensory representations that have been kept alive across several synaptic zones will bind with representations of a different transduction moment. It is also in this binding of past and present sensory moments that consciousness as a frame of reference will be formed.

In our basic neural network figure, we can see how the way in which the information contained in A1 afferent sources activates the neural field can be modified by varying the amount and timing of activity in the A2 afferent fibers. The efferent output of the N1 nerve cells may thereby contain a wide range of informational content that is a function of the A1-A2 interaction through the computational engine of the brain region. If we make this neural region more complex by adding additional layers of cells, more connections between the cells of the nucleus, or additional afferent sources, it soon becomes beyond our ability to understand just how the collective information entering the region at each transmission-transduction moment is being transformed by its flow through the tissue field. We can look at the efferent output and try to back-engineer the system to determine the computational operations generated during each information flux, but this approach has limitations and quickly becomes mathematically and conceptually overwhelming. We do not completely understand the underlying biophysical calculations of even the smallest of brain nuclei. Likewise, we do not completely understand the way in which the simplest bacterium orders the energy flux through its system to achieve its ongoing living existence.

If we now begin to view the information contained in neural activity as the background energy flux and to view the brain nuclei, or specialized volumes of brain tissue, as cell-like structures that have evolved to further provide order, create more information, and enhance representations, then we may begin to look for the evolutionary modifications that produced a neural structure whose function produces an informational or representational computation of the 4D nature of our stimulus worlds—an emergent 4D referent system from neural activity that we call consciousness. To best view where and how the brain begins to reconstruct the 4D sensory worlds, we will follow the path that each sensory modality takes through selected brain regions. Along this road, we will see the wide variety of brain nuclei and cortical areas that exist to bind in time sensory representations and reconstruct the dimensions of our 4D existence. At each nuclear region, we will look at a freeze-frame moment of neural activity flux and attempt to determine the representational order present in the afferent synaptic zones and what modification is computed and then transmitted in the primary efferent output.

Below the Cerebral Cortex

We will now examine the basic, somewhat simplified, flow of sensory information through the brain nuclear regions before the projections to the cerebral cortex and other forebrain regions. Important recurrent themes in brain design, such as laterality, crossed pathways, and topographic projections and maps, can be noted in almost every sensory projection.

The Visual System

The visual field is defined as the 3D outside world from which photoenergy sources emit stimuli toward the retinas of the eyes (Figure 5-3). For each concave retina, there exists a visual field with limits set by the size, shape, and range of movement of each retina. A central area of the visual fields can reach both the left and the right retina; this is the binocular field. The structure of the visual world, in the form of patterns of light, color, objects, perspective, and motion contained in waves of photoenergy, is transduced by the rod and cone cells and initially processed by the many cell layers of each retina. The approximately 125 million cone and rod cells in each retina transduce light energy stimuli and transmit them to only about 1 million ganglion cells. The retinal ganglion cells from both eyes collectively form the optic nerves [cranial nerve (CN) II] that carry all the basic information possible about the visual worlds toward the brain in waves of nerve impulse activity. The dramatic reduction in the number of neurons that carry the entire visual representation to the brain reflects the concept of the receptive field. Basically, each ganglion cell's nerve impulse activity is driven by a collection or patch of rods and cones in the retina.

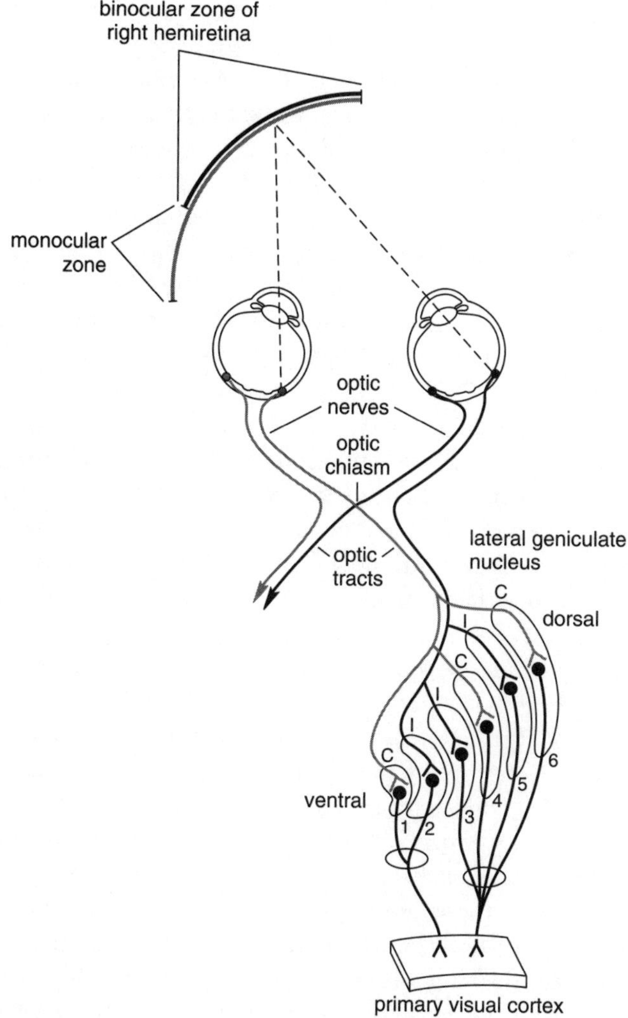

Figure 5-3 The human visual system, showing the external visual field transduced by the rod and cone cells of the retinas and transmitted to the brain. C = contralateral input. I = ipsilateral input. (*After E. R. Kandel et al., Principles of Neural Science, 4th ed., McGraw-Hill, 2000, p. 529; reproduced by permission of The McGraw-Hill Companies*)

Different regions of the retina have different receptive fields, with the central fovea having a ratio of nearly one cone to one ganglion cell, whereas at the periphery of the retina, the activity of many rod cells is reflected in one ganglion cell.

The myelinated axon bundles of the optic nerves converge at a midline location called the optic chiasm. Here the optic nerve fibers from the medial or nasal portions of each retina cross the midline to enter the brain on the contralateral side (Figure 5-3), while the fibers carrying visual information from the lateral or temporal aspects of the retina project into the brain on the same or ipsilateral side. Thus, the first part of each of the optic tracts (so called now that these axons are entering brain nuclei) contains fibers from both retinas. By examining the curved structure of the retina and the way that light from the visual field reaches the rods and cones, we can see that the information or visual field representation in each optic tract is derived from the contralateral visual field but includes the binocular portion of the field. The primary targets of the optic tracts in the primate and the human are shown in Figure 5-3. The lateral geniculate nuclei (LGN) of the thalamic group of nuclei receive a large number of optic tract axons. An LGN exists on each side of the brain, and so is bilateral, and, as we will see for most of the brain nuclei, it has a truly fascinating structure and function. The six layers of neural cell bodies are separated by layers of dendrites and axons that protrude from the parent cells. The primary subdivisions of the LGN are the ventral large cell layers, 1 and 2 (magnocellular laminae), and the dorsal small cell layers, 3, 4, 5, and 6 (parvicellular laminae).

The afferent flow of visual information through the bilateral nuclei begins with the interface of the optic tract synaptic zones and the LGN neural layers. The optic tract axons that originate from the contralateral ganglion cells form synaptic contact with the neurons in layers 1, 4, and 6, while the ipsilateral axonal fibers create synaptic zones in layers 2, 3, and 5. The mapping or topographic projection of the retina onto the LGN through the 3D organization of the afferent synaptic zones is remarkable and demonstrates the basic principle that the 3D structural organization of the axon array and the arrangement of the final synaptic zones within the target brain nucleus are as important as the pattern of nerve impulse activity that rides through this volume formation. It is our premise that discrete central nervous system regions function as a unified tissue volume that orders and modifies the electrochemical energy flux that flows through them. The synaptic contacts are a part of this computational machinery, but the importance of the overall structural organization of the individual nuclei or network cannot be ignored. The retinotopic arrangement is such that each point of the contralateral visual field is represented by a particular synaptic field in one of the LGN cell layers. This map maintains its topography across all six cell layers. The afferent source provides the stimulus energy that drives the LGN in its computational activities. The efferent outputs from the ventral layers project to many subcortical regions of the brain. The ascending efferent tracts proceed to the visual cerebral cortex. A feedback afferent source from the cerebral cortex, as well as afferent fibers from brainstem nuclei, also drives the operation of the LGN.

The modifications to the visual information contained in the activated optic nerve fibers as it pulses through the synaptic fields in the LGN are not completely understood. Individual neurons of the LGN appear to generate or inhibit action potentials in response to visual field stimuli with the same *receptive field* properties, as do retinal ganglion neurons. Thus, some cells are tuned by their network connectivity to respond maximally to a particular concentric spot of light in the center of a receptive field or to its removal. Other cells are stimulated or inhibited when the periphery or surround of the field is illuminated or its illumination is removed. The various combinations of excitation and inhibition of ganglion and LGN neurons following stimulus presentation determine their *center-surround* response properties. The cone cells selectively transduce photons in certain wavelength ranges, and this basic color information is detected in ganglion and predominantly ventral LGN neurons. Another class of ganglion and thus LGN neurons appears to respond to movements of edges (contrast points) across a receptive field.

We do not have evidence that the representation of the visual world at this point in brain processing reaches an internal order of resolution or complexity high enough to include specific shapes, depth perception, or combined properties of shape, color, and motion. It appears to be more of a point-to-point mapping of the ganglion cell array onto the layers of LGN cells. However, the ultimate computational functions of the LGN are not known at this time. As with most of the thalamic nuclei, it is common to see the LGN classified as a *relay nucleus*, indicating that it appears to play an intermediate role. We do not find evidence of a dramatic change in the way intranuclear neurons respond to sensory stimuli compared to neurons at earlier points in the sensory pathway, nor does the efferent output of this nucleus lead to an effector system where we can observe a behavioral reaction.

The other primary target nuclei of optic tract fibers include the superior colliculus and pretectal regions. These midbrain structures appear to utilize the basic visual field information contained in the optic tract fibers to effect the motor functions of eye, head, and neck movement (superior colliculus) and the various reflex actions of the pupils in response to light intensity fluctuations (pretectal nuclei). We see here another nervous system design feature: Reflex or rapid motor actions are produced within a sensory modality without the involvement of the higher brain regions.

Although there are fibers running from the largest and most recent evolutionary addition to the brain, the cerebral cortex, to the superior colliculus, these *corticotectal* fibers originate predominantly from the visual regions of the cerebral cortex (Figure 5-1). The evolutionary explanations for the direct subcortical pathways are obvious: Insects and nonmammals do not possess a cerebral cortex, and all animals must make rapid effector actions (presumably to enhance the homeostasis of the organism) with minimal time devoted to neural computational processes. We will continue to note that a great majority of observable behavior is initiated without significant cerebral cortex influence.

The Auditory System

Sound waves enter each ear as a mechanical force that leads the eardrum or tympanic membrane to vibrate. This energy is transmitted into the fluid-filled cochlea through the action of the middle ear ossicle bones on the oval window. Hair cells in the organ of Corti are stimulated by the force of the fluid wave. Different hair cells respond maximally to certain frequency ranges, based upon their position along the linear basilar membrane. Thus, a sound frequency topography exists along the hair cell distribution. The auditory or cochlear nerve (part of CN VIII) is made up of the central axon projections of the spiral ganglion bipolar cells. The hair cells form synaptic connections with the shorter projections of the bipolar cells, and thus provide the driving force for the nerve impulse waves moving toward the central nervous system. On each side of the pontine region of the hindbrain, the bilateral cochlear nuclei receive the afferent fibers of the ipsilateral auditory nerve (Figure 5-4). The cochlear nuclei are segmented into several sections on the basis of the wide variety of nerve cell types, the synaptic connectivity, and functional properties. The important consideration here is that the topography of the frequency spectrum among the hair cells as they are arranged along the extent of the linear basilar membrane in the organ of Corti is essentially replicated in each of the nuclear divisions. The multiple, repeating *tonotopic* maps are created by the organized afferent projections, which form orderly synaptic zone arrays in each portion of the cochlear nuclei. It appears that within each nuclear division, neurons responding to the higher-frequency sound stimuli are located in the dorsal portion, while ventral neurons are stimulated by the lower-frequency range.

The efferent fiber tracts leaving the cochlear nuclei travel many paths. An important aspect of the auditory pathways from each cochlear nucleus is that they are all bilateral in their projections. One primary projection is to the superior olivary complex, a group of small nuclei on each side of the

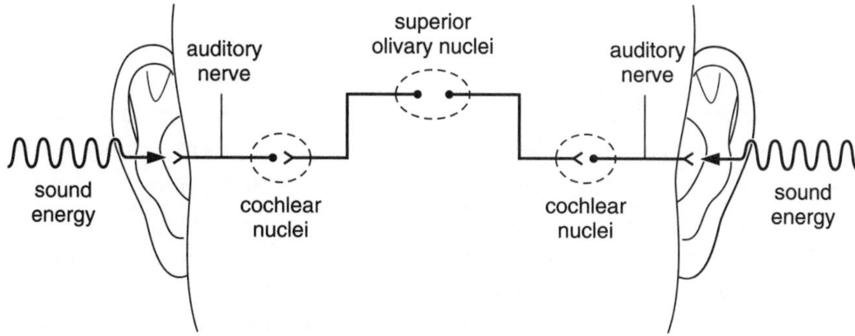

Figure 5-4 Brainstem portion of the human auditory system. The cochlear nuclei receive sound information from the auditory nerves. The superior olivary nuclei receive afferent input from the left and right cochlear nuclei.

brainstem (Figure 5-4). In the medial and lateral nuclei of this complex, neurons receive afferent fibers from both cochlear nuclei. This creates a bilateral tonotopic organization. As the afferent neural activity flows through these nuclei, there appears to be a computational function involving the relative difference between the time a particular sound reaches each ear (medial nucleus), the phase of the wave (e.g., the crest or the valley of a traveling sound wave), and the relative difference between the intensity of a particular sound as it reaches each ear (lateral nucleus). The biological computation of *binaural disparity* in the time, phase, or intensity of specific sound stimuli produces a new level of representation of the sensory world of sound. The efferent output fibers of these nuclei may contain the first information about the three-dimensional coordinates (the depth or volume of sound space) for the location of a sound source in the external environment. Although each derived moment-to-moment map of sound location produced by disparity computation can still be mapped onto a 2D plane (as a simple triangulation of three points in space), it provides the biological basis by which depth or volume may be derived from nerve impulse wave activity. That is, if the brain can effectively keep track of a series of 2D triangulated sound location maps over a period of time, the depth of the sound space can be determined by stacking the maps and connecting the common sound location points across the maps.

Thus far, we have been aware of the bilateral, symmetric nature of multicellular animals and that the nervous system develops afferent sensory nerves that tend to project toward the brain with only one side of the body represented in the information. While many projections do cross the midline to ascend on the contralateral side, they are primarily processed separately from the ipsilateral fiber projections. We noted this in the LGN of the visual system, where no convergence of the same regions from both retinas occurs. The binaural convergence of two afferent auditory representations within a single tonotopically organized neural group marks the first time that we will discuss an important event in nervous system activity, *disparity computation.*

We will keep this section brief, as this topic will demand our attention again and again as we approach the threshold of consciousness. Basically, within the nuclei of the superior olivary complex, the nervous system binds in time two similar but nonidentical representations of the external sound environment. Each afferent tract contains a transduction moment or point representation of the two-dimensional frequency spectrum derived from hair cell activity on its respective side of the body. There is no information about the 360-degree world of sound sources in each afferent wavefront. When the synaptic zones of the two afferent tracts energize the same nuclear tissue volume—when representation meets representation—a biological integration produces an output function encoded in a structured axonal array that may contain information about the three-dimensional sound wave environment external to the organism. A computational reconstruction of dimension within defined brain volumes has occurred.

It does not take the entire brain to perform this binding and integrative operation. At this brainstem level of processing, the output information may be a crude map of basic sound locations and may lack more complex properties of the auditory world (including language aspects). But we must see it as a vital functional operation and a deep insight into the evolutionary process. Nervous systems that can bring together two sufficient 2D representations of the sensory environment may derive information about the third dimension of that particular sensory stimulus. In the disparity computation, $3D = f\,(2D_{left}, 2D_{right})$, where f represents the biomathematical integration of timing, phase, or intensity differences. A more accurate representation of the sensory world is produced, and more dimensions of the 4D world are reconstructed within brain computation. The highest degree of implementation of this operational principle is to be seen in the cerebral cortex.

The efferent output of the superior olivary complex merges with both ipsilateral and contralateral fibers from the cochlear nuclei to form the bilateral fiber tract called the *lateral lemniscus*. These fibers enter the nuclei of the lateral lemniscus on their respective sides of the brainstem region called the pons, and again form tonotopic maps with their synaptic zones.

Neurons of these nuclei send efferent outputs across the midline to the contralateral nucleus. The bilateral tracts emerge from these nuclei and ascend to bilateral nuclei called the inferior colliculi at the midbrain level of the neuraxis. The same afferent input pattern exists in these nuclei, forming a well-structured map of the momentary bilateral auditory environment. The output tracts of the inferior colliculi form a minor crossing projection to the contralateral nucleus and a major projection to the ipsilateral medial geniculate nucleus (MGN) of the thalamus.

As we observed in the LGN, there are no crossing tracts between the MGN. The MGN has a distinct structural organization with three primary divisions: medial, dorsal, and ventral. As in the LGN, afferent fibers from the inferior colliculus form synaptic zones with individual layers or laminae of MGN neurons. The intervening dendritic and axonal zones are not as structurally distinct as in the LGN, and therefore the laminae of the MGN are not as visually prominent in tissue preparations. The MGN contains the bilateral tonotopic functional organization as in the lower auditory nuclei. The efferent tract emerging from the ventral division (and one portion of the medial division) projects ipsilaterally to the primary auditory region of the cerebral cortex, which, in turn, sends reciprocal fibers back to the ventral MGN. Other divisions of the MGN also send axon tracts to the auditory cortex, but these projections end in the region surrounding the primary auditory region, called the secondary auditory cortex.

The nuclear groups of the auditory system are also regularly called relay nuclei. This again indicates that our research efforts have not identified a significant computational transformation of information within these cell masses. It may be that neurons become progressively more restricted in the range of tonal frequencies that elicit nerve impulses, and thus their *tuning curves* become narrow. But it is within this brainstem system that a new order of information is generated by the processing of bilateral afferent projections within a common neural region.

The Vestibular System

Specialized hair cells of the ampullas, utricle, and saccule transduce fluid-wave mechanical energy in the semicircular canals. Movement of the head or velocity changes in the body create motion in the fluid by causing a shift in one of the orthogonal vectors relative to the local inertial field. The vestibular nerve (part of CN VIII) is composed of bipolar neurons whose cell bodies make up the scarpa ganglia. The peripheral projections of these cells form synaptic contacts with the hair cells, and the central projections form the axon bundle. The vestibular nerve on each side of the brain enters the pons and forms synaptic zones with the four vestibular nuclei: inferior, superior, lateral, and medial. Some fibers of each nerve do not enter these nuclei, but rather travel to the ipsilateral cerebellum (a complex region of the brain that plays a major role in our ability to move in a smooth and highly controlled manner). The four vestibular nuclei receive fibers conveying motion information from different canals or from the saccule or utricle. The pattern of innervation has no specific topographic organization like that seen in the visual or auditory systems, but there are differential inputs to each of the four nuclei that have functional importance with respect to the direction of motion and the control of the motor system exerted by this system. The vestibular nuclei also receive a significant afferent input from the cerebellum, but they do not receive descending fibers from the cerebral cortex.

Efferent output fibers from the vestibular nuclei travel to the cerebellum and to the cranial nerve nuclei (III, IV, VI) that control extraocular muscles and descend to spinal cord motor neurons via the vestibulospinal tract and the medial longitudinal fasciculus (MLF). The ascending vestibulothalamic tract carries fibers to the bilateral ventral posterolateral (VPL) and posteroinferior (VPI) nuclei of the thalamus. The vestibular nuclei of each side of the brain send fibers to the contralateral nuclei. And most ascending and descending efferent tracts contain both crossed and uncrossed fibers.

The computational nature of the vestibular nuclei appears to be involved in the subcortical control of eye movements and postural motor functions of the spinal cord. The vestibular information that reaches the thalamic nuclei, and thus is transmitted in some form to the cerebral cortex, is not well understood. Thus, we do not have knowledge about significant transformations of the basic information of rotational vector or acceleration that the vestibular nerve sends toward the brain nuclei.

The Olfactory System

The olfactory receptors in the nasal epithelium are stimulated by a wide range of molecules that enter the nasal passages. The bipolar receptor cells send their unmyelinated central axons through the cribriform plate of the ethmoid bone to enter the ipsilateral olfactory bulb as the olfactory nerve (CN I). It is important to note that unlike the neurons in other sensory systems, the bipolar olfactory receptor neuron has a limited lifespan of about a month. The basal cells of the olfactory epithelium are proliferative and generate new neurons to replace the old ones. Hence, in this phylogenetically ancient sensory system, new axons are continually migrating along the olfactory nerve and forming new synaptic connections in the olfactory bulb. The olfactory bulbs are bilateral structures that lie on the ventral surface of the medial frontal cerebral cortex and are the only brain nuclei directly innervated by the olfactory nerves. The bulbs have a laminar structure, but they have a less complex intranuclear arrangement than that seen in the LGN or MGN. The afferent olfactory fibers make contact only with the dendrites of the large *mitral* cells and the smaller *tufted* cells in the anterior portion of the bulb to form a layer of spherical synaptic zones called *glomeruli*. There is a significant convergence of the large number of olfactory nerve fibers to a much smaller number of mitral and tufted cells. The topographic nature of the projection of the nasal receptors onto the mitral and tufted cells is not known to be as specific as that found in other sensory systems, but it appears to exist. A topographical organization would provide a coordinate structure to guide the migrating axons of newly generated sensory receptors to the same location where the prior axons terminated. The axons of the mitral and tufted cells of each glomerulus form the olfactory tract that projects into other brain regions. The two olfactory bulbs are interconnected by a small group of neurons that sit caudal to the bulbs, the anterior olfactory nuclei. The dendrites of these neurons receive input from the mitral cells and send their axons to the contralateral nucleus by way of the anterior commissure. The olfactory tracts do not directly innervate the thalamic nuclei, another indication of their early functional status in the brain system. Instead, the vast majority of the afferent fibers synapse in a distinct region of the brain called the piriform cortex and in certain nuclei of the amygdaloid complex.

While there is evidence that olfactory bulb neural computations serve to encode spatial, temporal, concentration, and other qualities of chemical stimulus transduction, the exact nature of this process is unknown. Moreover, there is no fully accepted theory of the chemical-receptor interaction that describes the basis of our rich experience of olfactory information. We do know, however, that the bipolar sensory receptors are stimulated by certain types of molecules and not by others. The informational specificity of the *odor map* reaching the glomeruli of the bulbs per transduction moment is also influenced by contralateral input and by additional afferent input from some brain regions.

The Gustatory System

The sensory receptor cells of the tongue and pharynx produce graded electrical potentials in response to appropriate chemical stimuli. These cells are innervated by the bilateral, paired branches of three cranial nerves (CN VII, IX, and X) to form the gustatory nerve. A single fiber may form contacts with several receptor cells, and a single receptor cell may form contacts with several different fibers. The anterior two-thirds of the tongue is innervated by a branch of the facial nerve (CN VII), the posterior one-third of the tongue is contacted by branches of the glossopharyngeal nerve (CN IX), and a small region near the epiglottis is innervated by a branch of the vagus nerve (CN X).

A basic classification system for gustatory stimuli contains the four categories sweet, salty, bitter, and sour. A typical topological rendering of the tongue with respect to the taste stimuli that elicit the maximal response shows that the tip is most sensitive to sweet, the anterior lateral edges to salty, the posterior lateral edges to sour, and the posterior tongue to bitter stimuli. This is a relative response map, as sensory receptors on each portion of the tongue may respond to every class of stimuli. Also, recordings from gustatory nerve fibers show that the discharge rate frequency may correlate with the intensity of a taste stimulus. The brain nucleus that receives fibers from all three portions of the gustatory nerve is called the solitary nucleus and exists on each side of the brainstem region called the medulla. The afferent fibers primarily terminate in the rostral portion of this nucleus, which may be called the gustatory nucleus. The topographic organization of taste stimuli or receptor locations in this nucleus is not well understood. From this nucleus, output fibers ascend to the ipsilateral ventral posteromedial (VPM) nucleus of the thalamus. The functional changes in the representation of the taste world from receptor cell to solitary nucleus to thalamic nucleus are unknown at this time, but it does not appear that neurons of the target thalamic nucleus have a high specificity of response to any discrete quality of chemical taste.

The Somatosensory and Viscerosensory Systems

The chemical, mechanical, and thermal sensory receptors of most modalities found in the skin, skeletal muscle, joints, and other portions of the body form the somatic or spinal division of the peripheral nervous system. The autonomic sensory receptors include all fibers transducing stimuli from the internal organs, glands, smooth muscle, and blood vessels; hence the common use of the name *visceral* nervous system (or *viscerosensory* system). The sensory representations of the face, the nasal and oral mucosa, the anterior two-thirds of the tongue, the tooth pulp and gingival membranes, the muscles of mastication, the jaw, the eardrum (tympanic membrane), and the membrane covering the brain (dura mater) are all generated by branches of the trigeminal nerve (CN V). Dorsal root fibers enter the spinal cord carrying information from all types of somatic and visceral receptors (excluding the trigeminal fiber projections). Sensory representation patterns based on receptor types, such as thermal, pressure, joint capsule, and so on, are found in the fiber tracts that ascend toward the brain nuclei. The major ascending spinal fiber tracts include the posterior or dorsal white columns, the anterior spinothalamic tract, the lateral spinothalamic tract, and the trigeminothalamic tract.

POSTERIOR OR DORSAL WHITE COLUMNS On each side of the posterior spinal cord, large, paired, myelinated fiber tracts called the gracile and cuneate *fasciculi* (singular, *fasciculus*) ascend into the brain. These tracts are uncrossed or ipsilateral fibers that primarily convey sensory information from pressure receptors and from joint receptors transducing information related to position and movement. At each spinal level, more fibers enter through the dorsal roots and add to these fiber tracts, making them much wider in the rostral spinal cord. These afferent tracts form synaptic zones in the ipsilateral gracile and cuneate nuclei in the medulla. A somatotopic organization representing relative body location of sensory transduction is formed by the afferent terminal fields in these nuclei. The efferent output fibers of the two nuclei on each side of the medulla cross the midline and ascend on the contralateral side as the medial lemniscus. These large tracts maintain the somatotopic map of the contralateral body in the three-dimensional arrangement of the fibers. The medial lemniscal tracts terminate in the ventral VPL nucleus of the thalamus. These afferent synaptic zones in the bilateral VPL nuclei create the somatotopic representation of the contralateral body. The VPL output fibers terminate in the cerebral cortex.

ANTERIOR SPINOTHALAMIC TRACT These bilateral fiber tracts are composed of sensory fibers that cross the midline in the anterior white commissure and then ascend toward the brain. The sensory receptors that contribute to this tract transduce a specific range of pressure stimuli on the skin and are called the *light touch* receptors; they are found primarily on hairless or glabrous skin. These afferent fibers travel to the VPL nuclei and synapse in a somatotopic organization.

LATERAL SPINOTHALAMIC TRACT Thermoreceptors and free nerve endings in all regions of the skin provide the sensory stimulus drive to the fibers of these bilateral tracts. The axons of the lateral spinothalamic tract also cross in the anterior white commissure and then ascend on the contralateral side. These afferent tracts also synapse somatotopically in the VPL nuclei of the thalamus.

TRIGEMINOTHALAMIC TRACT The bilateral sensory branches of the trigeminal nerve (CN V) that innervate regions of the face, eye, tongue, oral cavity, and other areas are unipolar neurons whose cell bodies reside in the trigeminal ganglia. The three branches of this sensory nerve, the ophthalmic, maxillary, and mandibular divisions, are named for their relative fields of innervation. The central processes of these nerve cells enter the brain at the level of the pons and form synaptic zones in the sensory nucleus of CN V. A somatotopic organization is formed in the axonal projections from the endpoints in the face, eye, tongue, and other areas to the trigeminal ganglia and is maintained as the afferent fibers enter the brain nucleus. Each efferent output tract of the trigeminal sensory nucleus in the pons region crosses the midline and ascends on the contralateral side, although some fibers course ipsilaterally to the thalamus. This tract enters the VPM nucleus of the thalamus. Here again, a somatotopic map is created within the structure and synaptic function of this nucleus.

The computational activity in the VPL and VPM as these multiple sensory maps are flowing through the nuclei before traveling as output axons to the neocortex may involve some initial merging of sensory stimuli from different receptor types for an identical place on the body. Thus, the transformed somatosensory representations reaching the cerebral cortex would not have as distinct maps for each and every receptor type as those found in the afferent information reaching the thalamic nuclei. We note again that in the VPL, only one side of the body and its internal structures is represented in the informational flow.

The Thalamus and Thalamocortical Tracts

The thalamus is a vital brain region of the diencephalon, which also includes the epithalamus, hypothalamus, and subthalamus. The primary sensory relay nuclei contained within the structure of the thalamus include the LGN, MGN, VPL, VPM, and VPI (Figure 5-5). All these regions send projections to the ipsilateral cerebral cortex. Many thalamic nuclei do not receive direct sensory information from the ascending tracts, but have reciprocal connections to specific regions of the cerebral cortex, while other nuclei primarily (and in some cases exclusively) maintain subcortical afferent and efferent connections. The thalamic nuclei not only serve to integrate and coordinate sensory information to and from the cerebral cortex, but they function as primary integration sites of motor efferents from the cerebellum and other brain regions involved in movement (e.g., the striatum). The thalamus may thus provide a coordinating function between the high-order sensory processing of the cerebral cortex and the subcortical motor systems.

Toward the Cerebral Cortex

The many brainstem nuclei that we have described as playing a role in the ascending flow of sensory information toward the thalamus and cortical

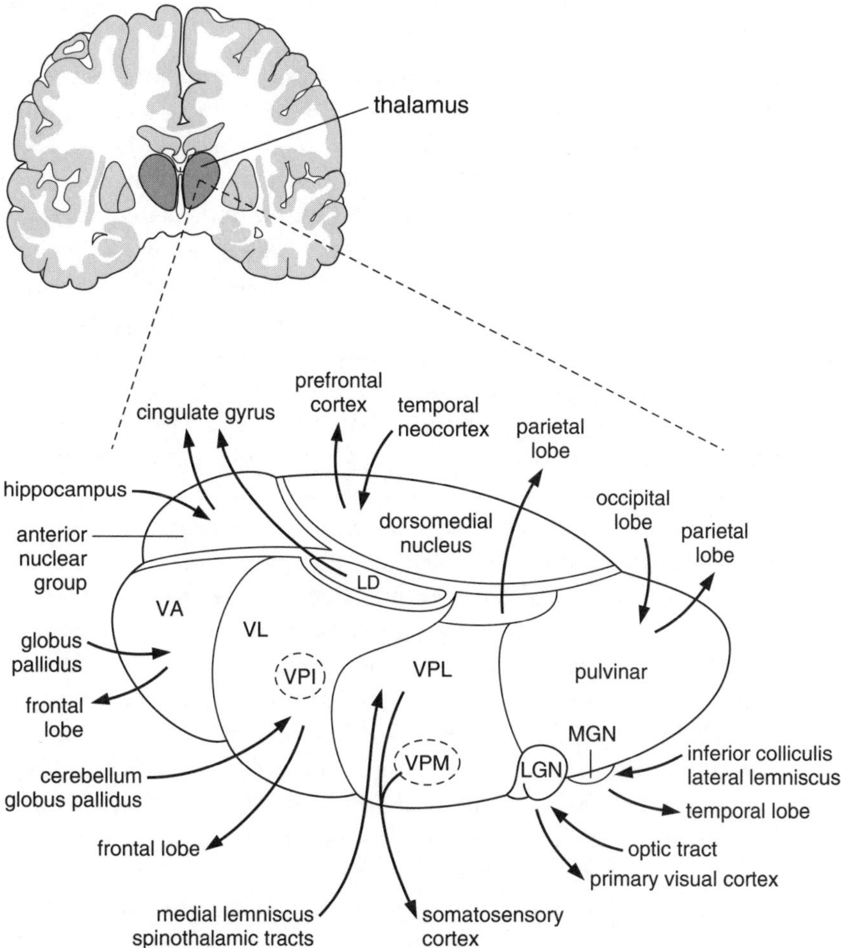

Figure 5-5 Many nuclei of the thalamus receive the vast majority of all sensory information and send it to the cerebral cortex. Only olfactory sensory information reaches the cerebral cortex without passing through the thalamus.

regions also operate as part of effector output systems that initiate motor and internal regulatory actions. These systems operate in animals that do not have a cerebral cortex, and they do so quite well. Much, if not most, behavior is initiated and regulated by the sensory input-to-effector output neural circuits that form between the peripheral nervous system and the brainstem nuclei. Rapid musculoskeletal movements, cardiovascular changes, respiratory function, and other homeostatic processes are conducted without strict dependence upon the higher cortical influence. Evolutionary modification brought forth the additional neural clusters and cell layers of the cortical regions, but the whole of the animal kingdom engaged in complex and productive behavior long before these structures came into being.

In mammals with a cerebral cortex, the sensory information processed by the brainstem and subcortical nuclei must be kept alive—its order must be maintained—so that it can be presented to the cortical fields. Thus, while the efferent output of the subcortical nuclei send information down the neuraxis (the descending tracts) to bring about immediate changes in behavior or internal regulatory functions, the efferent axons also include ascending tracts that contain sensory representations for each sequential stimulus processing moment. As the nucleus transduces, transforms, and transmits a moment of ordered flux in neural activity, it is functioning like a cell to create an informational product. It is making available over a long time frame an encoded sensory representation that will have an influence on another part of the nervous system, just as a cellular product may have an influence on other cells or the background environment.

These products that the nuclei of the brainstem send toward the cerebral cortex are relatively simple, unimodal fragments of the sensory world. The representational order within such a freeze-frame moment of subcortical nuclear network computational activity does not appear to increase dramatically across stages of processing, except for the binaural calculation of the spatial location of a sound source. This one example, devised early in mammalian systems, perhaps foreshadows a path of evolutionary modification in the nervous system that led to a threshold representational order that we call consciousness. We must, at this time, maintain our focus on the ascent of sensory information to the cerebral cortex, but it is important to note that these nuclei do function as computational engines for all subcortical initiated and modified behavior. In subsequent chapters, we will return to questions of evolution, phylogeny, and the effector systems that determine the entire behavioral repertoire of each animal and human.

Finally, we must again address the timing function of the nucleus-to-nucleus progression of sensory information and how it partitions the sensory representations. A sensory representation, as ordered neural activity, enters a nuclear region, is again transduced through synaptic zone function, is transmitted through the cellular field, and is encoded in the output effector axonal array. Regardless of the degree of transformation that is performed, some portion of the sensory representation is maintained to enter another nuclear region. For example, while a representation of the auditory world is present in the medial geniculate nucleus at a particular time t, another representation of sound stimuli that was transduced at a time $t+1$ following the one farther along the neuraxis is simultaneously present in the inferior colliculus. This timing function of information partitioning continues on a millisecond time scale as the nervous system senses the external and internal stimulus worlds.

As we have proposed, the nuclei may be seen as cell-like structures that serve to maintain an order of information contained within the biophysical afferent input as it flows through the bounded tissue field. Thus, each information pulse contained in afferent synaptic zones moves through a nuclear region, only to be followed by another. The rise and fall of information or order that corresponds to the pulses of afferent neural activity may be seen as the background energy flux that drives the biocomputational activities in the cell-like regions of complex neural tissues. We must keep in mind this process of energy, order, and information flowing along a temporal wavelike function between discrete networks of brain tissue as we follow the sensory representations into the cerebral cortex.

The Cerebral Cortex or Neocortex

At this point in our examination of the moment-to-moment flow of sensory information contained in neural activity through the brain nuclei, we see that the various sensory stimuli are being processed in a parallel manner, with little integration between the individual modalities. The full dimensionality and complexity of the entire sensory world thus remains scattered among many regions of representation. If we were to analyze the information contained in a selection of freeze-frame flickers of representation, we would see a fragmented, piecemeal sensory universe. No letter A, no word FIRE, no pencil, no face, no temporal dimension, and no emotion can be identified in the brainstem nuclear representations. It is the cerebral cortex and its neural fields that bring a novel order of representation of the sensory worlds, resolving their full dimensional nature and integrating the component modalities to reflect the rich, dense complexity of our existence.

The telencephalic portion of the forebrain gives rise to the corpus striatum, amygdala, hippocampus, and cerebral cortex. Prior to the evolutionary modifications that gave rise to the cerebral cortex, the other nuclei of the telencephalon existed as the outermost structure of the brain, that is, the literal cortex of that particular brain, and thus they retain anatomical names that identify them as cortical regions. The most recent addition to cortical structures, the new cortex or neocortex, marks the final large-scale evolutionary modification of the mammalian nervous system.

All cortical nuclei develop together in the rostral region of the neural tube and are most notable by the two cerebral vesicles that appear during embryonic weeks 5 to 7. The cerebral vesicles represent the primordia of the two cerebral hemispheres, the neocortices that dominate the adult brain structure. The proliferative cell layers that surround the fluid-filled lateral ventricles, the ventricular zone, generate many billions of young neurons and glial cells that give structure to the cerebral cortex (recall that a large majority of the 100 billion or so neurons in the human body reside in the neocortex, and that this number does not include the many glial cells).

The Cortical Structure

The basic neural cell layers and axon fiber arrangement found in most mammalian neocortices are shown in Figure 5-6. In intermittent waves emerging from the ventricular zone, the postmitotic young neurons and glial cells migrate to their final positions. The first layers form near the ventricles, and subsequent layers are superimposed in an orderly sequence. Specialized cells called the radial glial cells create a fascinating scaffoldlike arrangement upon which the young nerve cells migrate out from the ventricular zone toward their final position in the cortical mantle. Pasko Rakic's seminal studies of cortical development included the finding that the radial glial cells extend cytoplasmic processes across the entire width of the cortical layers, and that neurons move along these radiations before halting and taking up permanent residence.[1]

Thousands, then millions, then tens of billions of migrating axonal growth cones, with their own specialized rates of travel and timing of entry or exit from a cortical layer or region, form afferent or efferent synaptic zones under the guidance of a rich complexity of chemical, mechanical, and electrical influences. Large and small pyramidal neurons begin to fill the internal layers of the neocortex; they are found most prominently in layers II to V, less so in layer VI. Other cell types, generally termed nonpyramidal neurons, are found in various numbers in layers II to VI, but are most dense

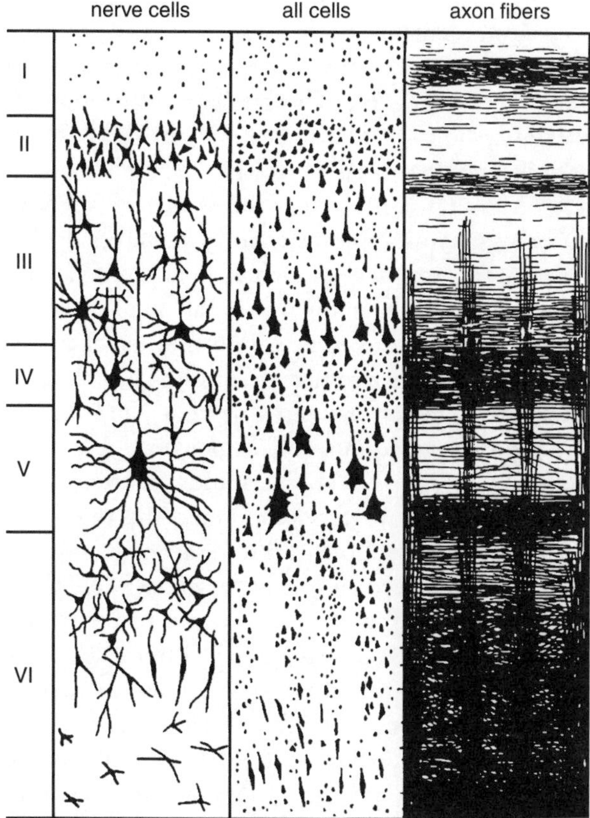

Figure 5-6 Structural arrangement of the human neocortex. Variations on the basic six-layered pattern are found across regions of the neocortex. Thalamic axons bringing sensory information primarily form synaptic systems with neurons in layer IV.

in layer IV. The nonpyramidal cells make up the vast majority of the inhibitory (mostly GABAergic) neurons of the cortex. One primary exception is the stellate cells, which are excitatory nonpyramidal neurons. Layer I, the molecular layer, contains dendritic projections and axonal fibers.

The basic six-layer neocortex is in place by the sixth month of fetal development. Migrating growth cones from pyramidal cells cross the midline to make synaptic contact with cells of the contralateral neocortex, thus forming the commissure systems. The anterior and hippocampal commissures begin to form during the third month of development, and the massive corpus callosum appears shortly thereafter and continues to grow throughout the fetal period until it includes several hundred million axons.

As in all other regions of the developing nervous system, an overabundance of cells and synaptic contacts are produced, and a process of selective degeneration, pruning, or shaping as a result of genetic design and activity-dependent influences is ongoing. The gradual myelination of axons proceeds in an interesting caudal-to-rostral direction of maturational development and continues to take place in the frontal neocortex into the second decade of life. Of course, the process of formation, modification, and degeneration of synaptic zones is continuous across the lifespan of the nervous system. Late in fetal development, a final proliferative phase brings about the folding patterns seen in higher primate brains. The warping of the cortical sheet is necessary if it is to fit within the cranial confines. The patterns of cortical convolutions are named according to the surface convex fold (gyrus) and the deep concave recess (sulcus), and the entire cerebral cortex may be grossly divided into four regions or lobes: frontal, parietal, temporal, and occipital (Figure 5-1). The adult neocortex has a surface area of about 2,200 square centimeters (cm^2), and the thickness of the six-layered structure ranges from 1.5 to 4.5 millimeters (mm).

A great variety of neocortical regions have been identified by cytoarchitectonic differences in the number, type, and arrangement of cells down the vertical six-layer axis. Functional differences, as we will continue to note, also may be found to correlate with structural variation. The basic patterns of afferent and efferent connectivity for most neocortical regions are as follows: Afferent input from thalamic nuclei (LGN, MGN, VPL, VPM), bringing specific sensory information, form very dense synaptic zones with nonpyramidal cells in layer IV. Association fibers from other neocortical areas and commissural afferents synapse in layers II and III. Efferent axons from layers II and III thus travel to other neocortical areas (association fibers), layer IV pyramidal neurons project axons to the thalamic nuclei, and large pyramidal cells of layer V project fibers to the subcortical nuclei and spinal cord (projection fibers). The commissural fibers arise from pyramidal neurons of layer IV. The reciprocal nature of corticocortical and thalamocortical connectivity permeates virtually every neocortical region.

Many axon fiber tracts from nonthalamic subcortical nuclei innervate the entire neocortex. The older designation "ascending reticular activating system" (ARAS) served to describe the direction of axon projection, the location of the cells of origin, and the overall functional effect. A more precise understanding of the nonsensory innervation of the neocortex by these subcortical regions must take into account their individual characteristics.

The primary divisions of this system include distinct cell groups that use one of the small molecule neurotransmitters called monoamines as their principal bioactive substance. The four primary cell groups are the cholinergic neurons in a region of the basal forebrain (using acetylcholine as the neurotransmitter), the noradrenergic cells in a brainstem nucleus called the locus ceruleus, the serotoninergic neurons of the raphe nuclei, and the dopaminergic neurons in small clusters of cells in the midline brainstem. Collectively, these monoaminergic nuclei (ignoring for this discussion the peptide neurotransmitters that are also produced) send axons to almost all the forebrain nuclei and to some regions of the brainstem and spinal cord. They each exhibit a distinct pattern of selective innervation across the regions of the cerebral cortex, and even within the layers of the cortical columns.

Differential activity from these afferent sources produces a multiplicity of neural effects and thus provides for a highly flexible, modulatory system that can influence the sensory processing activity of the neocortex and the entire forebrain. The cholinergic and noradrenergic systems may modulate a general state of alertness or arousal, as they are most active during high-arousal moments. Excitatory stimulation may serve to enhance modular computational activity, while selective inhibitory influences may serve to bring metabolic and informational focus to an adjacent uninhibited region of active sensory activity. The large-scale effects of biological rhythms, such as sleep and wake cycles, may be modulated by these neural systems.

The Cortical Module

A remarkable recurring pattern of anatomic structure and physiological function is embedded throughout the entire expanse of the neocortex in the form of cortical columns or modules. The full understanding of this modular genetic design feature may herald one of the greatest achievements in neurobiology.

When the six-layered cortical plate is viewed from the top down, as depicted in Figure 5-7, a rough pattern of repeating cylindrical connectivity may be observed. These columns or modules were first given a formal description by the anatomist Lorente de No in 1933.[2] Each columnar region extends across the six cortical layers, and its volume is determined by the local axonal connectivity between nearby projection neurons and interneurons. The resultant cylindrical volume of tissue, interconnected by corticocortical fibers and filled with millions of synaptic zones, is about 200 to 500 micrometers (μm) in diameter.

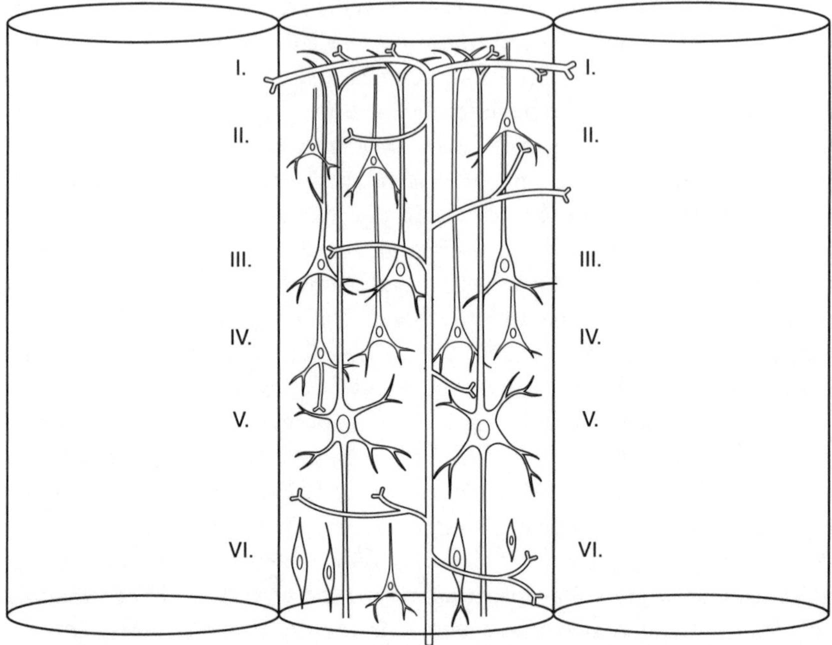

Figure 5-7 The cortical module, a columnar field of neurons, synaptic zones, and other cells that appears to form a basic, repeating structure through the neocortex. Each roughly cylindrical column extends across all six layers of the neocortex and may have a diameter of between 200 and 500 μm. These modules may function as biocomputational units in sensory processing.

Most astounding was the breakthrough discovery that in some regions of the neocortex, there is a well-defined correlation between the structural dimensions of a cortical column and its functional sensory properties. Much of the initial electrophysiological evidence for this structure-function relationship was provided by Mountcastle (1957)and colleagues.[3] Detailed studies of this modularity in the neocortical processing of visual sensory information were conducted by the preeminent team of Hubel and Wiesel, beginning in 1959.[4] Szentágothai hypothesized that the cortical module functioned as the "elemental integrative unit" (1967).[5] Study of the cortical module may ultimately provide deep insight into the manner by which sensory information is transformed as it passes through these tissue volumes. That is, these structures may carry out basic biocomputational functions by virtue of their inherent design. Thus, in the model of biological relativity, we propose that neocortical modules function as the cell-like structures through which the afferent waves of sensory information ebb and flow, and undergo transformation in the process. We will be referring to this concept as we trace the paths of sensory representations through neocortical regions, in a specific instance generating consciousness.

The developing human neocortex forms synaptic zones with the migrating thalamocortical axons as they bring the first fragmented sensory representations of the stimulus worlds. Feedforward afferent synaptic connections are made from neocortical module to neocortical module and from region to region, and feedback efferent projections form circuit loops with the thalamic nuclei and other nuclei of the forebrain, midbrain, hindbrain, and spinal cord. As the human fetus nears birth, the massive and convoluted neocortex is ready to process the full complement of sensory information to come. From its first breath, the young infant begins to experience a reality derived from the sensory representations of the external and internal worlds, a reality constructed in and constrained by the modular neocortical computational fields. We will now trace the flow of sensory information through this amazing living structure and present a model for the generation of an emergent biological order.

The Primary Sensory Neocortex

The specific sensory information emerging from the thalamus reaches the neocortex in regions of the occipital and parietal lobes called the *primary sensory areas* (Figure 5-8*a*). (Some fibers reach adjacent regions processing the same sensory modality that are called the secondary sensory cortex.) The olfactory bulbs, as the exception, project their sensory information directly to the temporal lobe region and the amygdaloid complex. The neocortex has no other way to directly sense the external and internal worlds. All the basic sensory information that provides 5 driving force for the neocortical computational machinery is contained in the successive structured waves of afferent nerve impulse activity.

The Visual Cortex

The LGN on each side of the brain sends the representation of one-half of the visual field to the primary visual cortex through a wide band of topographically arranged axon fibers called optic radiations. The primary visual cortex (also called the striate cortex) lies in the calcarine sulcus and on the cuneate and lingual gyri of the occipital lobe. We will primarily refer to the

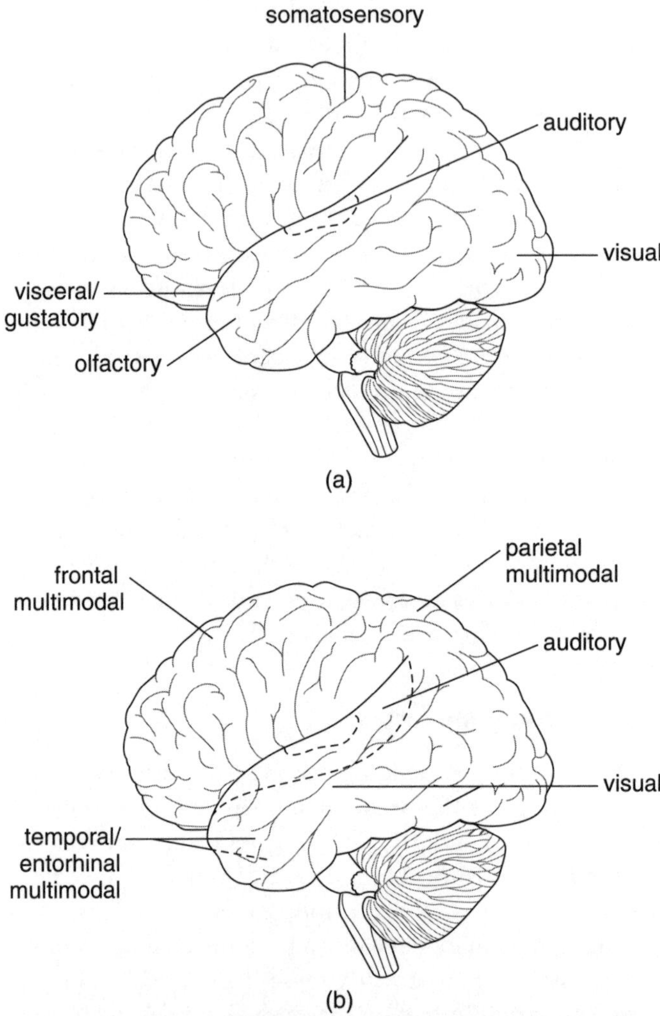

Figure 5-8 (*a*) Primary sensory areas and (*b*) association regions of the human neocortex. Processing of external and internal sensory information proceeds from the primary to the association neocortical modules. The prefrontal neocortex receives input from all association cortices and may be an important region of convergence of information. *(After J.H. Martin, Neuroanatomy, McGraw-Hill, 1989; reproduced by permission of The McGraw-Hill Companies)*

heroic scientific research by Kuffler and by Hubel and Wiesel that initially elucidated the interrelated structure and function of the visual system.[6]

In the primary visual cortex, we find evidence of significant transformation of the information contained in the thalamocortical afferent projections. Neurons in these cortical modules do not have concentric receptive fields like those of the retinal ganglion cells or LGN neurons. The visual field stimuli that elicit the most activity in visual cortical neurons include rectangular bars of light and dark and the transition between light and dark (edges). These cells, termed *simple* cells, also preferentially respond to the spatial orientation of a line stimulus.

If one measures cell activity horizontally across a line of cortical modules, certain neurons in each module respond maximally when a straight-line visual stimulus is presented at a certain angle of rotation. This pattern of nerve cell activity is referred to as the receptive-field axis of orientation. Thus, as a recording electrode is moved from adjacent module to module, nerve cells are found that respond best as the stimulus in the visual field is slightly rotated around its central axis. This demonstrates another amazing correlation between the structure of the external physical environment (the angle of the line in space) and the way the brain maps it. A series of these so-called orientation columns shows a stepwise maximal response to the rotation of a visual line stimulus throughout a cycle of 180 degrees. The structural and functional components that drive this computational process may include a synaptic field arrangement whereby a single cortical module is innervated by a group of LGN neurons whose receptive fields collectively "line up" at a particular axis of orientation. Thus, a convergence of information to produce a new representational order observed in cell response patterns is seen in the neocortical modules. Most simple cells are found in layer IV of each column and appear to be nonpyramidal or stellate neurons.

Complex cells also respond to bars or edges of a particular rotational axis. In addition, these neurons sustain a high nerve impulse rate when a particular stimulus is moved in the visual field, but the movement must proceed in a specific direction. If the same stimulus is moved in the direction opposite to the direction of maximal response, the complex cell's rate of discharge will be reduced. Conceptually, it can be seen how the synaptic convergence of a group of simple cells within a cortical column could result in the properties of the complex cell. Complex cells and even more stimulus-specific *hypercomplex* cells are found in layer III or V, and thus above or below the layers of simple cells. In a selected cortical column, cells in each of the layers respond to the same axis orientation of the stimulus. And this preferential angle shifts slightly as the recording electrode measures the nerve cell impulse rate from module to adjacent module, across strips of visual neocortex.

Ocular dominance columns reflect another structure-function property of the primary visual cortex and are intimately related to the orientation columns. We recall that the LGN receives retina ganglion cell axons from both the left and the right eye, but it is crucial to understand that the combination of the nasal retina of one eye and the temporal retina of the other eye produces a retinotopic map of only one-half of the visual field. Neurons in the LGN respond only to stimulation of one portion of the retina; no cell in the LGN will respond to the stimulation of any other retinal area. Thus, the LGN cells are considered strictly *monocular* in their stimulus-response properties. It is in the striate cortex that cells begin to respond to stimuli presented on either the right or the left retina; they are termed *binocular* cells. In a horizontal series of contiguous cortical columns, all cells in layer IV have the typical monocular response. But, as with the complex cell arrangement, in layers III and V, neurons respond to one retinal portion with a high discharge rate, but will also generate nerve impulses in response to stimulation of the contralateral retinal portion. These cells are said to display binocular properties, but with ocular dominance—that is, they still have a preferred side.

Across strips of visual neocortex, an adjacent series of ocular dominance columns with left eye preference is immediately followed by a matching series of columns with right eye dominance. This alternating sequence is repeated in row after row across the entire primary visual cortex. Again, the brain is genetically structured to physically map the external stimulus world in a location-specific manner at the micrometer (cortical module or column) scale of measure and with a constrained degree of resolution. These findings, which resulted from decades of highly difficult work, mark an unprecedented achievement in scientific research. Along with the results of many other experimental manipulations of the visual system, they unequivocally demonstrate the interrelationship between the structure of a complex volume of neural tissue and its computational (functional) activity, as neocortical modules that span the brain's convoluted surface.

The LGN cells that have color sensitivity likewise send axons into layers of the primary visual cortex. In brain tissue preparations of this region that show the microscopic location of an enzyme called cytochrome oxidase, a series of ovoid *blobs* is visualized in layers II and III. Electrophysiological studies have shown that cells in these blob areas have interesting center-surround receptive fields that respond to one wavelength in the center and a second color in the surround, and also to black-white combinations. The blob organization may represent another parallel system through this cortical region, as it does not appear that color is integrated into the other visual field information. The merging of color with shape and motion does not appear to take place until visual information is processed through regions of association neocortex.

We will make note here that the receptive field of the complex and hypercomplex cells is larger than that found in retinal ganglion cells or LGN cells, which may reflect an important fundamental biophysical property. Each wave of afferent activity entering the neocortex contains all the possible energy, order, and thus information about the transduced sensory environment. Any additional order or information that is derived from the original afferent flux comes at a cost in energy, thus order, thus information. As multiple fibers carrying nerve impulses from many LGN cells converge on a single cortical column (or a small number of columns), other neurons of the column become more active to integrate this informational input through the electrochemical activity within the local structure. To derive this new information about the complexity of the visual world, information related to the acuity or resolution of the stimulus environment must be subtracted from the total order in the input source. This cost, partly expressed in the larger receptive fields of the complex and hypercomplex cells, will be found throughout each neocortical region and, as we will see, is an important constraint in the model of consciousness.

The 2D surface area of the primary visual cortex contains the 2D retinotopic map (one-half of the visual field per hemisphere). New representational order is created within the third (volume) dimension of the functional cortical column; in other words, it is in these neocortical modules that the new properties of shape and motion are added to the objects in the visual field. The efferent output of these cortical columns, the *final computational product*, encodes this new information in activated axonal arrays, and a transformed representation of the visual world is thus sent to additional regions of cortical modules for further processing.

The Auditory Cortex

The MGN afferent fibers (the auditory radiation) synapse in two regions that make up the primary auditory cortex: the transverse gyrus and the caudal portion of the superior temporal gyrus (called Heschl's gyrus). The tonotopic organization of afferent synaptic zones is reflected in the electrophysiological response of the cortical neurons. In a structure-function relationship analogous to that of the visual cortex, all recorded neurons within a vertical column of cells in the auditory cortex respond to the same frequency range and represent a receptive field for auditory stimuli. A second map of the frequency spectrum is generated by fibers of the auditory radiation in cortical regions surrounding the principal region of termination. The tonotopic maps also appear to represent the binaural sensory environment, perhaps as a result of the crossing fibers in the brainstem or of axonal projections from the contralateral neocortex. A definite hemispheric dominance (laterality), in which the left-side gyrus is larger than the right, is present in most human neocortices. In a series of groundbreaking studies, Penfield and colleagues stimulated the cortical regions of lightly anesthetized patients undergoing neurosurgical procedures and recorded a fascinating collection of verbal reports of internal auditory experience.[7] Stimulation of the superior temporal gyrus caused the patients to report hearing brief, sharp sounds such as a bell or clicks, usually in the contralateral ear. The sounds did not include words or conversation. The transformations of the auditory information in the primary neocortex therefore do not appear to be significantly complex. The efferent projections from the primary auditory cortex synapse on more rostral regions of the temporal lobe, parietal neocortex, and insular cortex.

The Somatic, Visceral, Vestibular, and Gustatory Sensory Cortex

The postcentral gyrus of the parietal lobe receives the sensory information from the VPL, VPM, and VPI of the thalamus and is generally referred to as the primary somatosensory and viscerosensory cortex. The entire internal world of sensory information, as well as the vestibular and gustatory sensory projections, all enter the cerebral cortex in these regions. A topographic map of the entire body, the face, and all internal viscera is found in the structure and function of this cortical region. The well-known sensory *homunculus*, the distorted depiction of the human form drawn atop this region of neocortex, represents the relative amount of cortical tissue that appears to be involved in processing motor (muscle and joint receptor activity) and sensory (mechanical, chemical, and thermal receptor activity) information from each part of the body. Thus, the fingers and the tongue (which are drawn disproportionately large on the homunculus) have more neurons subserving their motor and sensory representation than do the wrist and the knee (which are depicted as relatively small). This type of pictorial mapping reflects the relative size of the receptive fields for each body location, on the millimeter scale of measure. The larger the relative size of the homunculus body part, the smaller or more discriminative the receptive fields.

The visceral structures, vestibular information, and the gustatory projections are mapped in the most ventral portion of the postcentral gyrus, the parietal *operculum* and the adjacent *insula* cortex. The somatotopic maps of the primary sensory cortex represent only the contralateral side of the body, except for those for the face and tongue, which are bilaterally represented (recall that the trigeminal nerve has bilateral afferents to the VPM), and the nonlateralized midline structures of the genitals and rectum. It is interesting that the tongue and throat regions of the body are mapped in the ventral region of the cortical strip, near the internal viscera and taste representations.

The cortical modules in vertical organization appear to process different sensory receptor information, maintaining a separation of basic stimulus sources over a given receptive field (e.g., stimulation of skin by pressure, movement of a hair fiber, temperature change, stretching of bowel tissue, etc.). Neurons in each lamina of a discrete cortical column respond to only one type of sensory receptor. The size of the neocortical receptive field is larger than the size of the receptive field at lower levels of the neuraxis, again as a result of the convergence of axonal arrays onto fewer neurons in the cortical column. One map of the body and viscera is based on the distribution of the light-touch receptors, whereas an adjacent, parallel map represents deeper pressure, and another corresponds to the location of joint and muscle receptor information. Thus, it does not appear that significant convergence of sensory receptor types occurs in this initial afferent projection. Neuron responses in this region are mostly limited to one type of sensory stimuli, and a separation of information from cutaneous or surface receptors from that from deeper body tissues is preserved. No map of the specific thermoreceptor information has been constructed. The gustatory projections also appear to be processed separately from the other sensory receptor information in this brain region. Little is known about the mapping of the vestibular information onto the cerebral cortex or its transformation through the computational networks. However, clinical and research observations indicate that significant sensory information about rotational and inertial changes reaches the neocortex, by the reports of the *vertigo* sensation.

The primary somatosensory and viscerosensory cortex sends a significant efferent output to the adjacent parietal cortex. From here on, each subsequent cortical-to-cortical progression of transformed somatosensory information is based on the original projection into the primary sensory cortex.

The Olfactory Cortex

Unlike those from all other sensory systems, the axons from the human olfactory bulb project only to other telencephalic regions. No other part of the human brain receives direct information about odorous stimuli. All projections from the olfactory bulbs are to primitive regions of the cortex, collectively called the piriform cortex, and the amygdaloid nuclei. The regions of piriform cortex, a three-layered *allo*cortex, lie near the anterior tip of the ventromedial temporal lobe in an area called the *uncus*. The synaptic zones form topographic arrangements, but the exact nature of the informational processing is unknown. The principal outflow of olfactory representation is carried to the nearby entorhinal association cortex, which returns reciprocal fibers. The anterior commissure contains axons that interconnect the two primary olfactory areas.

Toward the Association Neocortex

The primary sensory neocortex demonstrates a continuation of parallel processing between sensory modalities, and even within each modality (e.g., the separation of color and shape in visual information streams). This divergent pattern of stepwise progression from cortical column to cortical column and from region to region will continue in the neocortex to a great degree. However, convergence of information between and within modalities begins to occur in a select few neocortical locales. We will quickly see how complicated it will become to follow a path of multimodal sensory processing and still maintain a simplified language of clear, descriptive terms. To develop an understanding of this level of sensory information associations, we will present some of the higher-order, integrated, complex behaviors that we attribute to computational functions within and between association neocortices. Our examples will necessarily be basic and brief and will omit a great amount of information from the literature (which contains its fair share of contradictions and disagreements) regarding the function and dysfunction of these neocortical regions. For, when one attempts to describe complex animal or human behaviors and their relationship to the structure and function of the nervous system, the seemingly simple and logical trek from anatomy to physiology, to systems operation, to behavioral manifestations becomes a complex and tortuous odyssey. And to date, most of the signposts along the way remain written in an inconsistent anthropomorphic lexicology.

The Association Neocortex

As we move through these specialized neocortical regions and follow the flow of sensory representations, we will encounter biocomputational associations between two or more primary sensory modalities. These regions of true multisensory or multimodal association neocortex are found primarily in the frontal lobe, but also in the parietal and temporal lobes. It is in these areas that the full measure of our concept of binding in time, as the basic within-system function of neural activity, may be realized. It is in these modular fields that we will see the convergence of sensory representations from distant regions of the internal and external receptor organs, from different classes of sensory energy sources, and from different moments of sensory transduction activity. It is in these coalescing afferent synaptic zones that the disparity computation for phase differences in space and time will be performed to a degree not possible at any other point along the neuraxis.

The mature human cerebral cortex and the regions of the occipital, parietal, temporal, and frontal lobes that may be considered predominantly association areas are illustrated in Figure 5-8. It must be noted that the descriptive name "association" cortex reflects a relative condition. The associations, such as they may be, remain primarily within one sensory receptor class; when more than one sensory modality is associated, one is highly dominant in terms of relative informational content. These regions are, however, associative in the sense that they strongly interconnect with the contralateral hemisphere though the commissural projections, and with other contiguous and distant areas of neocortex through a truly staggering number of reciprocal axonal projections. Moreover, the significant two-way exchange of sensory representations between the neocortex and the thalamic nuclei in reentrant pathways creates another type of critical associative function.

Sensory Representation in Association Neocortex

Each primary sensory region of neocortex sends an efferent output to a nearby region of association cortex. In each cerebral hemisphere, the unimodal sensory information is thus kept alive to undergo additional transformations in fields of modular synaptic zone activity. The binding of the contralateral sensory world becomes more prominent in the association regions, as the fibers of the corpus callosum and anterior commissure bring representations of similar sensory energies and similar peripheral receptor locations to converge with the homologue representations formed on the other side of the body. Additionally, each association region sends and receives sensory information to and from thalamic nuclei, and also projects to many other forebrain, midbrain, and hindbrain nuclei. We will focus primarily on the corticocortical association pathways on one side of the cerebral hemisphere, and only briefly refer to other afferent and efferent projections. Jones and Powell (1970) conducted the seminal neuroanatomical studies of primate association cortex that form the basis of our current understanding.[8]

Visual Representation

Visual information is processed in many parallel paths that possess partial aspects of the total photon-driven sensory world and that travel through the modular fields of visual association cortex and into the true multimodal neocortical areas of the temporal, parietal, and prefrontal lobes. Movements of objects in the visual field appear to be a principal source of afferent information in the border regions where the occipital, parietal, and temporal lobes meet, whereas specific shapes of objects are more prominently represented in the visual areas of the inferior temporal lobe. Color as an individual, quantitative information source is processed in the blob regions, and objects integrated with their color properties appear to begin to merge at the confluence of the temporal and parietal lobes.

As we move along the inferior temporal cortex toward the anterior pole, neurons will selectively respond to more complex features of objects. These sequential representational transformations bring a convergence to basic visual information and encode higher-order properties and dimensions in the axon fiber arrays that interconnect the contiguous regions, contralateral homologues, and other neocortical areas. In more rostral regions of the temporal cortex, cells and modules are selective for combinations of shapes, textures, and even color. A large percentage of cells will respond only to such objects as hands or faces.

This massive integration of basic visual sensory information into local fields of specific and complex object selectivity comes about in regions that are highly interconnected with both visual hemispheres by the commissural pathways and with other visual cortex and thalamic nuclei by reciprocal or reentrant pathways. As we have discussed, there is a metabolic and informational cost to these representational transformations: Metabolic energy is expended to sustain the computational function of tissue volumes of the cortical modules, and a degradation in visual field resolution is the cost of higher-order organization of information. In fact, for regions of neocortex that integrate very complex sets of visual stimuli, the basic retinotopic information is lost. The receptive fields of these cells and modules span virtually the entire retina and can include regions of the visual field on both sides of the midline. In this and many other examples across all sensory modalities, we see the evidence of a general model: representation transformation and convergence of basic aspects of the stimulus worlds at the cost of acuity or resolution, relative to the maximal potential information encoded in each afferent nerve impulse wavefront.

We have now reached a stage in sensory representation where our descriptive language must include terms like *object, hand,* and *face,* and it must be remembered that *we, the observers,* are imposing the organization and nomenclature on an immense number of points of photon energy across many moments of sensory transduction and neural transmission, and through several regions of computational activities. In the neocortical modules, every object and its various qualities and motions is represented by a pattern of afferent arrays that form structured synaptic zones and drive a pattern of cellular responses for a moment of computational activity within one or more vertical columns. It is only from our unique point of view in consciousness and memory that we *see* and *name* a hand, a face, a monkey, or a grandmother.

Up to this point in our examination of how the nervous system binds in time sensory information, all representations of the sensory worlds can be geometrically projected onto a 2D surface. The location of an object in visual space, a single sound in auditory space, or a location on the body surface can be mapped on a flat surface of coordinate points. We have not discussed the explicit derivation of the third spatial dimension, volume or depth, or the one temporal dimension that is theoretically embedded within any two sets of sequential spatial coordinate information.

The final two dimensions, depth and time, were implied when we referred to binaural sound location; to complex objects with volume, such as hands and faces; or to stimulus properties such as motion. The biomathematical vector analyses that can derive two, three, or four dimensions will be discussed under the general term of phase disparity computations. We initially described how this might occur in the superior olivary nuclei of the brainstem for binaural information [$3D = f(2D_{left}, 2D_{right})$] and it is also an important operation in the inferior and superior colliculi as they direct head movements (motor vectors) toward auditory or visual stimuli, and in the cerebellum in its highly complex computation of fine motor movements across space and time. At these levels of the neuraxis, the sensory representations upon which the phase disparity computations are performed are of a basic, but highly resolved, quality. This may allow for fast effector actions to promote survival and homeostasis.

In the visual system, at the level of association neocortex, we may now observe the biomathematical creation of the novel 3D product of depth, experienced in the phenomenon of *stereopsis*.[9]

In evolutionary time, animals developed bilateral symmetry, forming a midline axis that gave an orientation of top, bottom, front, and back. From the perspective of genetic material, this development created a "two (hemispheres) for the price of one (basic genetic code)" situation. The sensory organs, including the photoreceptors of eyes, that developed on each side did not merge their sensory information until axons that crossed the midline, commissural fibers, interconnected them. Moreover, when in mammalian evolution the two eyes achieved a relative position on the body surface such that both retinas transduced light coming from a common midline region of the external world, the moment-to-moment computation of the third dimension, depth, become biophysically possible.

We noted that Hubel and Wiesel found some neurons in the primary visual cortex that had a binocular sensitivity, but they detected even more in adjacent association areas. These cells responded only when a stimulus was present in a region of the visual field that was transduced by receptors in both retinas. As Hubel, Wiesel, and other pioneers in this field of research have remarked, it is truly amazing how much specificity of connectivity exists in the commissural fibers that link the cortical columns for the receptive fields of one retina to the same ones on the other side of the brain![10] The neurons and modules that receive afferent input from both sides of the overlapping portions of the visual field form receptive fields that span this vertical midline (the vertical meridian). It is in these integrative modules that the position of a stimulus relative to other stimuli along a spatial dimension of near or far can be calculated. The relative depth location of an edge or a line, or the detailed volume properties of a convoluted shape such as a face, can be derived in caudal and rostral visual associative cortices, respectively.

Disparity refers to the points on two maps representing a similar space that do not have exact correspondence. It is the relative difference between two overlapping point distributions in either 2D or 3D space. The exact set of equations that would provide a mathematical understanding of how the next higher dimension is derived from two similar, but disparate, data sets is unknown. Much brilliant work on the mathematics and neurobiology of such a computation has been conducted, and this is an active area of research (refer to Marr, Poggio, Zeki, Julesz, Pellionez, and others).[11]

In the human nervous system, visual depth or stereopsis becomes part of the sensory representation when the overlapping retinal images are within 2 degrees of horizontal visual space apart, or about 0.6 mm distance across the retina. The vertical alignment must also be very close across the two retinal images (the distance should be measured in seconds of arc in the vertical direction). An individual may sense depth or volume when stimuli are within these parameters. If the visual overlap of the two fields is experimentally reduced beyond a *critical threshold*, the representation of depth is lost; adequate information is thus not available to the computational modules in the neocortex. In nonhuman neuron recordings, *disparity-tuned* cells change impulse rates when a properly placed stimulus is moved toward or away from the retinas. These cells are classified as *near* cells or *far* cells.

In stereopsis, at a critical threshold, when two similar but somewhat disparate afferent wavefronts of visual sensory representation simultaneously merge in neocortical modules, the computational function derives the next dimension and encodes this information in its efferent output projections. *A biocomputation fusion of 2D information creates a novel product of 3D order.* Stereopsis is a perfect, explicit example of a nervous system structure-function relationship that includes anatomical localization, information convergence, and the biomathematical derivation of a new dimensional product by disparity computation.

It has been known for a very long time that photographic images can trick the brain into performing this binocular fusion. In 1938, Sir Charles Wheatstone's *stereoscope* used angled mirrors to project two horizontally disparate photographs of the same visual scene onto the retinas of the viewer.[12] Seemingly by magic, a sensation of depth appeared to jump out from the two flat pictures. Widely popular for many years, and now undergoing a current revolution using integrated circuit technology, this use of disparity computation to derive higher dimensions is finding many practical applications.

A related and fundamental insight into nervous system function came out of quantitative psychophysical, mathematical, and neurobiological research into stereopsis. In 1971, after many years of work on this subject, Bela Julesz produced the *random dot stereogram.*[13] Julesz first created a computer-generated square field of random dots on a page of paper. By taking a small square out of the middle portion and moving it slightly (only a few degrees) to the left on one page and to the right on another, then filling in the background with more random dots, a complete functioning stereogram was created. The simple genius of this work is shown in Figure 5-9*a*. When the two images are fused in the visual field, a viewer sees a tiny square floating above the flat surface background (or below it, depending upon the direction of the relative shifts). The brain conjures up a 3D image from a random pair of 2D stimuli. Though there has been much research into the parameters of this effect and its mathematical and neurobiological foundations, we still do not know how it happens at the mathematical level. However, for this present work, we note that the random dot stereogram may provide an insight into nature's eloquent methods of neural-based computational algorithms.

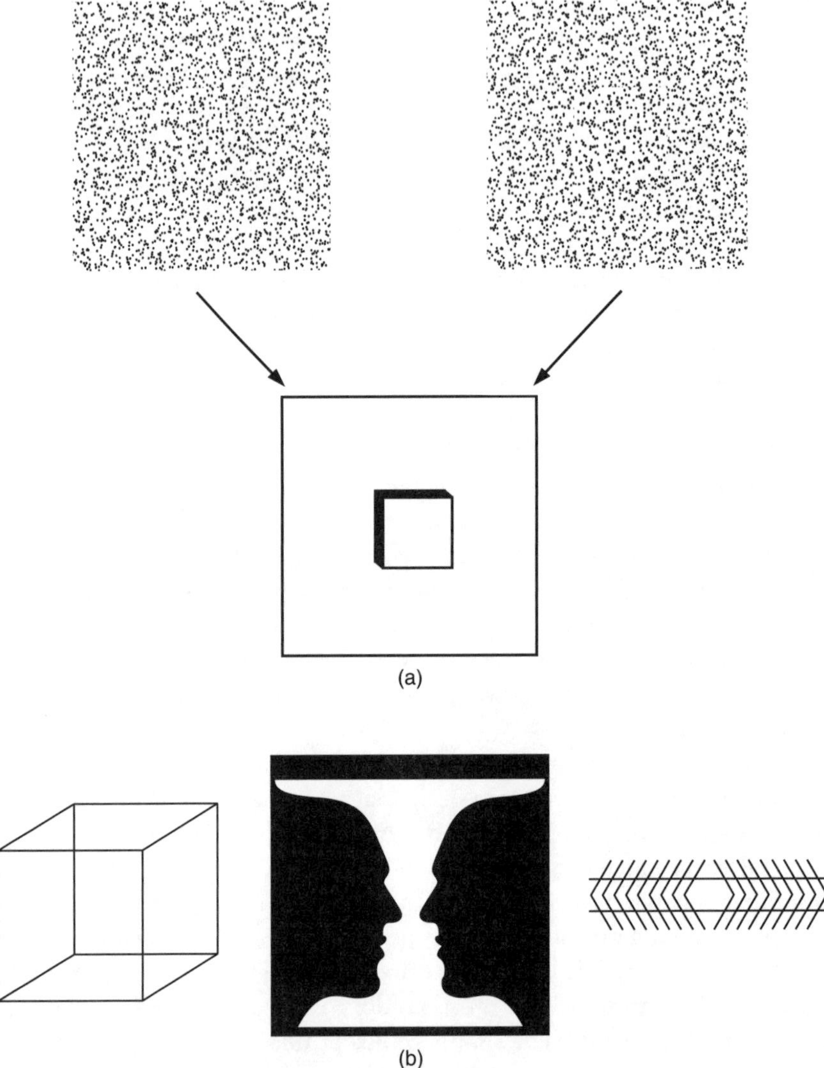

Figure 5-9 (*a*) The random dot stereogram. When the two squares are visually fused, a new figure appears to emerge that possesses the third dimension of depth. Prior to visual fusion, the new figure cannot be determined. (*b*) Simple figures that illustrate the computational operations the brain performs on sensory information to derive new dimensions. The "solutions" that the brain derives may undergo change (the cube may be seen to change its front edge, and one may see a face or a vase) or be incorrect (the two lines are not curved).

In the random dot stereogram, information about a third dimension cannot be found or used until the brain performs a computational fusion of the two 2D stimuli. The information is there, but neither the nervous system nor any outside observer can see it until the disparity computation is performed in the neocortex. It thus appears that a disparity computation may be a default function of visual integrative neocortical modules. Perhaps any two 2D input will be fused in disparity computation functions of the visual associative neocortex, and a higher-dimensional output will be generated. In a simple fashion, for this region of neocortex, the functional equation may read $3D = f\,(2D_{left}, 2D_{right})$. A biomathematical integration or function (f) is performed on two similar, but not identical, spatial arrays ($2D_{left}$, $2D_{right}$), and a three-dimensional spatial output (3D) is the solution—exactly the same operational method that we suggested occurred in the brainstem and midbrain regions for auditory stimuli.

If we can generalize this functional aspect of certain brain networks, then it should not matter what the stimulus input consists of, as long as certain parameters of spatial arrangement are met. That is, if you replaced the retinal photoreceptors with thermoreceptors, you would derive a 3D product of the external temperature field. Furthermore, the psychophysical literature contains many examples of possible ways in which certain brain regions attempt to perform a disparity computation on all stimulus input that enter through the appropriate afferent synaptic zones. Any three lines that form a corner create a sensation of depth, even though not all the lines of a cube are present and the lines are drawn on a 2D surface. There are many visual drawings that evoke a flickering sense of volume (like a cube), a shifting perception of foreground and background objects (the face-vase drawing), or an erroneous bending of straight lines as the brain derives depth across many intersecting lines (Figure 5-9*b*). Visual illusions of this type may serve to illustrate and elucidate not only a fundamental operation of the neocortex, but also a powerful constraint on the ability of the nervous system to construct a consistent reality.

The visual association cortex and the multimodal cortical regions may derive the shading, texture, tones, colors, and motions of objects in the visual field through modular computational activity. We can imagine the letter A residing in the visual association cortex, or the written word FIRE, or the 3D shape, color, and texture of a pencil, and faces, too. However, there is no *sound* of the word FIRE, no *name* for the letter A, no *name* for the pencil, and no *emotions* about a face here. And what about a red apple that has been cut open to expose its core, containing small brown seeds?

This complex visual image has just been evoked by a string of written letters! The additional complexities of our experience in consciousness, which involve names, feelings, and sensory representations from one stimulus source evoked by an entirely different pattern or even class of sensory stimulation (e.g., a visual object evoked by visual letters or by auditory words), involves the integration of several sensory modalities and the integration of the past and the present. All this may occur in the functional interface of several of the multimodal systems of the neocortex, and it may be as much a default computation as is binocular disparity.

Auditory Representation

The progression of sound processing in the auditory association neocortex is difficult to research, as only humans utilize words and music. Much of our knowledge comes from clinical evaluation of patients with damage to various areas related to auditory function. Penfield and Perot's classic brain stimulation studies of alert neurosurgical patients produced many reports of what these patients say they heard while having various portions of the auditory cortex electrically stimulated.[14] More recently, Ojemann and colleagues have extended this demanding experimental approach and have advanced our understanding of cortical sensory processing.[15] Neuroimaging studies using PET (positron emission tomography) and fMRI (functional magnetic resonance imaging) techniques have measured relative changes in certain parameters of brain metabolic activity in response to auditory stimulation and thus revealed maps of cortical areas that appear to be involved in processing this type of sensory information.[16]

The binaural sensory information that reaches the primary auditory cortex in each cerebral hemisphere creates tonotopic maps of the acoustic world. The module-to-module pathways that serve to reorganize and recombine auditory information, highly interconnected with thalamic reentrant circuitry, lead into the multimodal regions of the temporal, parietal, and prefrontal neocortex. As we move along the superior temporal gyrus from the primary sensory region toward the anterior pole of the temporal lobe, more complex organizations of basic acoustic components are formed. Sounds described as clicks, buzzes, and bells were frequently reported by patients whose anterior superior temporal gyrus was stimulated under surgical conditions. These complex aggregates of basic sound frequency and intensity stimuli may correlate with the convergence computations that produce the complex and hypercomplex neurons in the visual system.

From the perspective of the nervous system, the human concepts of words, sentences, and melodies are in fact massively organized and aligned discrete moments of sound processing: a field of frequencies and amplitudes that may be integrated to derive the more complex properties of pitch, tone, sequence, and location. From sounds to syllables and words or musical notes and triplets, to sentences or melodies, to stories or songs, it is the human observers that provide the aggregate conceptual organization to the underlying patterns of neural activity.

The stepwise auditory disparity computations of the neocortical modules along the caudal-to-rostral regions of association cortex in the temporal lobe produce more complex arrangements of sound qualities and their temporal relationships. Axon tracts from these modules enter the true multimodal regions of the anterior temporal pole and parahippocampal/perirhinal cortex. A second pathway leads from the primary sensory cortex to a multimodal region formed at the confluence of the superior temporal gyrus and the inferior parietal cortex. A rich multimodal convergence in this region integrates somatosensory and viscerosensory information with auditory and visual representations. The third pathway of auditory representations leads to the prefrontal cortex. In one location along the inferolateral convexity (Broca's region), important sequencing parameters of the final motor output of speech are created. All of these regions are heavily interconnected with the forebrain memory system, which provides the ability to maintain a temporal linkage between moments of real-time auditory experience and more distant memories of the categorized sound sequences that we call words and melodies.

Parietal Multimodal Neocortex

At the confluence of the inferior parietal, posterior temporal, and rostral occipital cortices, in the area of the superior temporal sulcus, lies the parietal multimodal neocortex. This region receives visual, auditory, somatosensory, viscerosensory, and perhaps vestibular afferents from each respective association cortex. The synaptic zones in this region form interlaced mosaics of unimodal representations, but there are also regions in which synaptic terminations from more than one sensory modality converge upon the same modules and neurons. The transformational flow of information through these integration modules appears to create novel representations of both the internal and external sensory worlds. Specifically, the parietal neocortex derives information related to our sense of our bodies and our place in the local 3D environment. It also functions to bring together all the sensory qualities of objects that enable us to identify them with names by their shape. Certain mathematical abilities also appear to be dependent upon the normal operation of this brain region. This parietal multimodal neocortex is highly interconnected with the contralateral hemisphere, the multimodal memory system of the temporal lobe, and the thalamus.

The computational products of the parietal neocortex outlined previously reflect yet another level of representational intricacy and order that is achieved by the nervous system and require us to further employ the language of large-scale behavioral description (e.g., our sense of our bodies or mathematical abilities). Just as the nervous system loses degrees of resolution as the cost of integrative representation, so does our language lose degrees of specificity in the description of complex constructs that involve multiple sensory systems converging across multiple processing cycles. The particular system upon which entropy exacts its toll is irrelevant.

Thus, in the parietal multimodal neocortex, we find that basic sensory representations of pressure, temperature, vibration, and joint movements are integrated into patterns of activity that reflect the physical properties of external objects that come into contact with the body. In other words, the homuncular representation now has overlapping properties of location, volume, movement, and multimodal sensory information, derived from real-time neural activity and coordinated memory system input.

A cold metal key held in the hand may evoke a local pattern of modular activity that contains the full dimensional and sensory properties of the key; moreover, the visual and auditory patterns from the memory system that correspond to the key's image and name may also be simultaneously activated. Without the object's being seen, its collective qualities, transduced moment to moment as it is moved and perhaps rotated in the hand, may create a representation in multimodal neocortex that endows its human handler with information about its three-dimensional form, its temperature, its metallic composition, and, if this was learned from past usage, its image, how to use it, what lock it works in, what sound it makes as it is pushed into the lock, what door it opens, and so on. We say that there is a *global* representation or knowledge about this object in the hand.

Knowing (*gnosis*) about the body, its position in space, and what comes in contact with it appears to be a critical function of this brain region. *Stereognosis* is the term used to describe the ability to name and recall information about an object that is in contact with the body. This ability may be demonstrated not only for objects placed in the hand, but also for objects held against a cheek or placed in the mouth. Also, if a letter or number is traced with a pin on one's arm, leg, or back, the letter or number can be identified by integration of the somatosensory, visual, and auditory (from memory) information. Astereognosis is the diagnostic term for the clinical deficit of this ability following damage to parietal multimodal neocortex. Losses of knowledge, or *agnosias*, of unimodal and multimodal complex representations may be found after discrete damage to various locations within this neocortical region.

The ability to recall the names of objects or their properties may also be impaired (*anomia*) by lesions in specific modules in this area. The anomias that are clinically documented include interesting patterns of deficits, from tactile anomia, where the patient cannot name an object from its feel, to color anomia, where he or she cannot name its color. Other clinical syndromes found include deficits of language (dysphagia/aphasia), movement (dyspraxia/apraxia), math skills (dyscalculia/acalculia), reading (dyslexia/alexia), and writing (dysgraphia/agraphia). Gerstmann's syndrome represents a unique cluster of clinical observations in certain patients with inferior parietal lobe lesions. The deficits include confusion of left and right, finger agnosia, dysgraphia, and dyscalculia. Deficits of this class reveal the dominance of one hemisphere of the brain over the other; lesions on the left side primarily affect language, and right hemisphere damage may more often result in deficits that involve the integration of body location and spatial relationships. Difficulties in drawing complex figures (constructional apraxias) and lack of math abilities may thus be found. The fascinating *neglect* syndrome may also be observed, in which a patient may not treat one of her or his arms or legs as her or his own, or may neglect to wash or dress one side of the body.

Detailed experimental analysis has shown that neurons located in the parietal multimodal region increase their response rates when learned visual stimuli are placed in specific regions of the external spatial environment relative to body position. Other cells may respond only to specific stimuli moving toward or away from the body location. Some neurons appear to be more sensitive to the spatial location of sounds and their motion in the environment. The receptive fields of these multimodal cells are typically large, again reflecting the information cost in acuity to gain order. PET studies have demonstrated an increase in metabolic function for this region when a test subject is requested to mentally rotate objects, suggesting that an integration of shape, form, motion, color, size, orientation, spatial location, sight, sound, touch, and memory may occur to various extents in this multimodal region of neocortex.

Temporal Multimodal Neocortex

The forebrain memory system is functionally embedded in a group of heavily interconnected multimodal regions of temporal neocortex, the hippocampus, and their reciprocal projections with other cortical and subcortical structures. The anatomical and physiological convergence in these areas is unlike any other seen to this point, and it results in profound behavioral abilities that fall under the general concept of memory. The temporal multimodal neocortex includes the temporopolar region of the anterior tip of the temporal lobe, the parahippocampal gyrus and perirhinal cortex on the medial surface of the temporal lobe, and the entorhinal cortex that lies more anterior to the parahippocampal region. The additional telencephalic structures of the hippocampus, amygdala, and subiculum are vital to any discussion of the functionality of the temporal multimodal areas.

The concept of memory has captured attention since the dawn of human discourse, and libraries have been filled with fiction and nonfiction writings about its many qualities. It will certainly continue to be an exciting field of research and an enigmatic construct long into the future. For our purposes in this section, we will operationalize memory to reflect a representation of sensory information. Thus, memory is defined here as a product, from a simple unimodal computational outcome to the most complex multimodal construct. A memory is a biocomputational solution that has been converted (i.e., transduced and structurally consolidated) into a more permanent molecular property of a local region of neural tissue. Furthermore, we operationalize a memory to have an additional quantitative constraint in that it is the product of one moment of computational activity within a defined network or module of neural tissue. This sets a theoretical limit on the amount of information that may be contained within a single memory product, both in its initial computational formulation and in its more stable consolidated state. Memories may be combined or modified to reflect an update or modification, but these novel products are still constrained by informational limitations. Memories, as products of past experience that are evoked by sensory events to participate in current computational operations, thus become manifest in a pattern of afferent synaptic zone activity.

The temporopolar cortex receives a very complete convergence of sensory projections. Not only does the parietal multimodal cortex send axons to this region, but the visual, auditory, and olfactory association neocortices also do so. Additionally, the insula neocortex sends information about gustatory and visceral sensory experience to this region. Here, then, is a region that contains information about virtually the entire sensory universe. There is an important reciprocal connection between the temporopolar cortex and the amygdala, imparting complex visceral-autonomic information that is critical to the proper function of the memory system. A large reciprocal innervation with the prefrontal cortex is formed through an imposingly massive fiber bundle. Finally, this region is interconnected with the other regions of the temporal multimodal neocortex and sends subcortical efferent fibers to thalamic and hypothalamic nuclei.

The parahippocampal/perirhinal areas also receive sensory information from virtually all association cortices and have reciprocal pathways to the cingulate neocortex, as well as to the amygdala and entorhinal cortex. The entorhinal cortex, hippocampus, and subiculum will be discussed as an interlinked pathway of multimodal sensory information that serves as the foundation of the forebrain memory system. Van Hoesen, Pandya, and colleagues performed detailed anatomical studies of these regions in the primate.[17]

The exact nature of the sensory representations, the information that enters the modules of the entorhinal cortex, what transformations are performed, and what the efferent products contain are unknown. There are definite anatomical patterns to the afferent projections that create the synaptic zones in this region of neocortex. Thus, there are maps that may reflect a homunculus of sorts, where each point on the internal and external body rendering is dense with overlapping sensory information about several classes of stimulus energy: their relative strengths, locations, and directions of motion; the volume space nearby and its sensory properties; and information regarding the internal state of homeostatic processes related to hunger, thirst, and temperature. Moreover, the representational maps entering this region, or perhaps the computational outcome or efferent product, may contain the interrelationship between the external locations of places and things that influence the internal homeostatic condition, such as food, water, and heat sources. The possible computational nature of this region becomes more evident when we look at the primary efferent projection from the entorhinal cortex to the hippocampal formation (the so-called perforant path) and its functional operation. The hippocampal formation receives sensory information only from the entorhinal cortex; thus, it is virtually isolated from any information about the stimulus environment, except for this single source.

The simplified pathway of sensory information through the hippocampus leads from the dentate gyrus granule cells to the large dendrites of pyramidal neurons in the CA3 field (*cornu ammonis* or ram's horn, reflecting the curled anatomical profile). From here, in unilateral progression (with feedback fibers), the CA3 neurons project to the next field of pyramidal cells (CA2) and then from CA2 to CA1, and from these neurons a projection emerges that is sent out to several regions of cortex (the subiculum, entorhinal cortex, and prefrontal neocortex). The subiculum interconnects with the cingulate gyrus, entorhinal cortex, parahippocampal/perirhinal regions, and prefrontal area. The subcortical efferent output of the hippocampal formation is carried by the myelinated *fornix* fibers that travel to the forebrain septal nuclei and to the mammillary bodies of the hypothalamus. The nearly closed looplike connection between the entorhinal cortex, the hippocampus, and the subiculum, along with its afferent-efferent connections to the amygdala, septal nuclei, thalamus, and hypothalamus, has drawn the attention of anatomists for many decades, and led James Papez (1937) to hypothesize that this region served as the substrate for emotions.[18]

A number of published clinical cases have helped us to understand memory in human brain function and have indicated that the hippocampal formation is an important anatomical region. In 1947, Grunthal (as reported by Gloor) described a postmortem examination of a patient with severe memory problems in which bilateral hippocampal damage was discovered.[19] A second case report, by Glees and Griffith (1952), discussed a patient who had difficulty with memory for recent learning and also had hippocampal damage.[20] However, the seminal paper that brought the hippocampal formation and its role in memory to worldwide attention was that of Scoville and Milner (1957).[21]

The now famous patient discussed in this paper, referred to by the initials H.M., was a young man with intractable epilepsy. Scoville, a neurosurgeon, removed portions of his anterior temporal lobe on both sides of the brain. This dramatically reduced his seizure activity, allowing him to live a more normal life. Equally dramatic, however, was his newly formed inability to retain any facts about the recent past or to learn just about anything new. His overall awareness of the environment and who he was remained intact, but he could not hold onto moments of experience as they faded into the past. H.M. could recall and recognize people, places, and events of his life before the surgery, but without his two hippocampi and portions of the anterior temporal lobes, he had no recent memory. He was locked into an eternal present.

Brenda Milner and her colleagues produced an unparalleled and landmark body of research into H.M.'s unique condition, demonstrating that H.M. could learn new motor-based, repetitive tasks, but was virtually unable to learn any new concepts, dates, or facts.[22] Since H.M., many other patients who have suffered bilateral hippocampal or parahippocampal and entorhinal damage have been found to have basically similar memory difficulties. Larry Squire and his colleagues devised an ingenious set of experimental approaches to study and thoroughly document the various types of learning that may be preserved in these patients.[23] But the saved abilities pale relative to the robust, effortless memory of the immediate past that we take for granted.

In concert with our model, it may be proposed that the forebrain memory system serves to provide a structural representation of the past, so that disparity computations between similar representations of the present and past may be performed to derive solutions concerning the next moment of behavior. A cold metal key in the hand may evoke a similar pattern of neural activity from the memory system. Across many millisecond cycles, the real-time disparity computations in the parietal multimodal integration modules may produce efferent products that, in turn, elicit additional memory information regarding the name of the key, its function, and perhaps images of the food and warmth that resulted from its past use—with all this multimodal experience resulting from an ongoing computational comparison between real-time sensory stimuli and a large store of moments of past learning. Without a functioning forebrain memory system, all or part of this process is disrupted, and one may be lost in past time, unable to update the ongoing reality of a changing external sensory world or of the changing internal sensory world known as the self.

A neurophysiological study of rodents by O'Keefe and Dostrovsky (1971) found that certain neurons in the hippocampus respond to the 3D spatial location of the animal in real time.[24] It did not matter what the animal's body position was or what specific objects were nearby; the only thing that mattered was the coordinate place, defined absolutely by the external environment. These *place* cells have been enthusiastically investigated since that time, and indeed they appear to have a receptive field that represents a place in the local space that is not dependent upon physical orientation or the surrounding context. Collectively, they appear to map local 3D space in real time. A compelling model of hippocampal function based in part on these findings was produced (O'Keefe and Nadel, 1978), and it remains a vital and valuable formulation.[25] The discovery of place cells provided us with a physical location where we could envision a real-time map of the sensory environment. Indeed, it is a highly ordered multimodal map, as only this level of complex information may reach the hippocampal fields via the perforant path fibers!

Now, if within this real-time map of multimodal space, the hippocampal and memory systems integrate past experiences that occurred in the same places, a disparity computation could produce an informational update about the current situation. In other words, if the local environment stimulated memories that contained information about a specific coordinate location where food was once found, then the computational comparison of the past and present stimulus environment may product an efferent product that initiates movement toward the remembered location of food. Thus, as a simplified general model, we can see how the comparison of a present 3D context with related past experience would provide a powerful method by which to determine what to do next.

The formal scientific study of animal and human behavior, which has now been going on for well over a hundred years, is to a large part predicated upon trying to understand what forces cause an animal or person to determine what to do next: How do we decide, choose, or will the future? In two experimental settings nearly 40 years apart, the simple observation of healthy laboratory rats moving through space and time has provided us with deep insight into the function of the hippocampus and the forebrain memory system and the powerful ability it has to determine behavior in complex settings.

In the 1930s, behavioral scientists were examining virtually every type of animal activity in experimental settings in a search for the limits of intelligence (and consciousness). They devised and constructed many types of testing mazes in an effort to quantify the capacity for learning and memory and the ability to correctly determine what to do next. One of the most brilliant scientists of this era, E. C. Tolman (1932, 1948), made the casual observation that some of his rodent subjects, after learning a particular maze route, would tend to climb on top of the maze, proceed straight to the place where the food reward was located, and then climb back down and eat the reward.[26] It appeared to Tolman that his little friends had somehow acquired a cognitive map of the maze as a whole. They knew the absolute 3D spatial location of the food reward without being able to see it, so they didn't have to negotiate the maze again.

We now fast-forward to the 1970s, when David Olton (1977, 1978) first documented a remarkable observation related to Tolman's insight.[27] If a laboratory rat was placed on a open platform maze (constructed in such a way that a number of paths radiated out from a central region, like spokes from a hub), it could forage for a hidden food reward at the end of each arm without making any repeat trips down paths it had already visited. The incredible, almost unbelievable part of these food-gathering behaviors (similar to what ethologists had documented in birds and certain mammals in their natural settings) was that a rat could successfully perform this task on

8-, 16-, or even 32-arm mazes when delays of considerable length were interposed between the foraging trips. There were very few repeat visits, and, almost miraculously, no particular pattern of foraging was consistently employed. That is, the rat or mouse did not just start at one arm and use a *go-left* or *go-right* strategy.[28] To this day, we hear scientists express wonder about how these rats perform memory tasks that they themselves would have difficulty doing as well!

Place cells, memory for spatial locations, and foraging behavior are all perhaps related to the hippocampal formation and the memory system. In fact, it is well established that bilateral damage to the hippocampus or related structures impairs the ability of animals and humans to perform such memory tasks. But how does a laboratory rat, or a bird in nature, remember for such a long time where it has been and where the remaining food may be? What exactly must be remembered during such delays? How does the animal maximize its time and energy to obtain food in as few trips (choices) as possible?

The answers to these questions lie in an understanding of the type of sensory representations that are being transformed in the forebrain memory system and the function of the hippocampus in generating a real-time coordinate system of the local 3D spatial environment. We can imagine the computational operations of the hippocampal regions keeping a map of the current spatial context that is updated through the information contained in moment-to-moment afferent inputs. This is a map of the real-time space around the animal; it is not a memory construct. However, particular sensory stimuli in the current environment may elicit information from the memory system. The visual context, sounds, tactile cues, and internal states of hunger or thirst may all combine to evoke patterns of previously learned places within the overall spatial environment. In our example of the radial-arm maze, the learned places are the ends of each arm, where food may be hidden from direct view or smell. As the animal treks down one of the arms and consumes the food, the multimodal sensory component that is integrated with that particular place on the spatial map may lose some of its homeostatic attraction, or statistical weighting, because the food is now gone.

When the animal is allowed to make another choice, perhaps after a delay, and two potential pathways are in sensory view, the updating function of the spatial map and the integrated multimodal component conveying information about attraction or hunger may enter into disparity computation. In a few computational moments of millisecond duration, the real-time spatial map of two possible pathways—the long-term memory of the learned behavior of "pathway equals food" and the short-term memory of one "path just visited"—may converge into a disparity analysis that will lead the animal to move down the "path less traveled" during this particular foraging time frame. When viewed in this sequence, the incredible memory task becomes one of a two-point choice, repeated at each moment of reentry into an arm, for the total number of choices in a session. An 8-, 16-, or 32-location problem reduces to a *yes-no* choice at a series of 3D spatial intersections. If two adjacent paths are both empty of food, that double negative, *no-no*, can be learned and can induce a slight shift until a *yes-no or yes-yes* choice comes into sensory view and computational activity. Thus, the entire meal may be obtained without having to remember every place at every moment.

Several summary points are important. First, there are limits to these behaviors. If the 3D spatial context is not stable, more errors will occur. If you place a distinct visual shape at the end of each arm and randomize the larger spatial context, no animal will be able to perform even a four-choice task. Animals cannot read or remember a list of 2D symbols. It is only the stable 3D spatial setting, the stimulus context as transduced by the animal's sensory receptors, that provides information from which they can construct places and their relative importance.

Second, there is a temporal decay function for this unique short-term memory task. If the delay extends to hours, the differential weightings of the paths are lost: The map is cleared. This class of short-term spatial memory has been called spatial working memory, or just *working memory*. Much has been written about the topic of working memory, and it can be a confusing subject. For the purpose of this discussion, it should be remembered that it is only when an animal is within a specific spatial environment and remains within that 3D multimodal space that these working memory abilities, as remarkable as they are, exist. The real-time 3D spatial setting, generated as a place map in the hippocampal system, permits the disparity computations that determine what to do next. The 3D spatial map provides the neuronal framework upon which time-limited weightings of *go, no-go* choices may be supported.

The working memory is wholly dependent upon the construct of a spatial map, and thus upon the hippocampal system. And nearly all long-term learning is dependent upon the hippocampal formation functioning in an integrated forebrain memory system. Thus, while behavior in the relatively short term may function with the assistance of the working memory system, any complex neural pattern representing new integrations of sensory information must be converted into a long-term structural system, a memory, if it is to be available for use in the distant future. The subject of memory *consolidation*—the temporal parameters, the physical processes [such as long-term potentiation (LTP) and structural changes to membranes and receptors], and the theoretical limitations—has always been, and will for a long time continue to be, a most important area of research. We are just touching upon a few important items in this chapter; we will discuss this in more detail in later chapters.

We noted previously that it appears that most behaviors related to the external and internal sensory worlds can be conducted to a great degree without the neocortex. The behavioral impairments linked to damage to a region of association cortex or multimodal cortex primarily involve a learned aspect, a memory component. Now we see the critical role of this system in forming a permanent trace of multimodal experience. Without the forebrain memory system, we cannot hold onto the present as it becomes the past and use those moments to update and understand the current present, the now. H.M.'s memory impairment was a result of the loss of a critical link in this forebrain system. Learning, through memory, is an ongoing, reiterative process that results from disparity computations between a real-time complex sensory representation and similar representations from past moments. The disparity—the difference between afferent representations—may indicate the location in 3D space where food was found, the situation in which a past injury occurred, or the name associated with a face. The efferent output products of the forebrain memory system may influence motor systems to initiate movement toward food, to initiate movement away from injury, or to speak a word. They may alter the internal visceral-autonomic conditions as well. Neural computations are of course performed on a millisecond-to-millisecond basis as new representations converge in synaptic zones at each modular locale. Behavior, as we have stressed, may appear to be fluid over seconds or minutes of time, but the neural activity underlying its expression, including that related to the memory system, proceeds in a millisecond time frame.

Frontal Motor Neocortex

Three regions of the frontal lobe make up the motor neocortex: the primary motor area, the premotor area, and the frontal eye fields. The primary motor area is located on the anterior portion of the central sulcus and the precentral gyrus. It continues onto the medial side of each hemisphere and down each lateral convexity to the most inferior extent. As implied by the name, this area is involved in effector output through muscle actions.

However, as we have noted, there are many points along the neuraxis where descending fibers from many brain nuclei and neocortical regions reach muscular control areas. Thus, this frontal neocortical region may function only in more subtle adjustments or modifications to the ongoing motor outflow of highly complex behaviors.

The frontal eye fields consist of the frontal neocortex immediately anterior to the premotor area. In addition to afferent fibers from the premotor area and all of the sensory association cortex, there is a large reciprocal connection with the dorsomedial nucleus of the thalamus. This region appears to be involved in eye movements elicited by verbal commands such as, "Move your eyes to the left."

We have traced the flow of sensory information through the brain, and now we are approaching the rostral-most extent of the neocortex, the frontal lobes. It is in the structure and function of this region that we will observe the emergence of consciousness as a novel frame of reference.

The Prefrontal Multimodal Neocortex

The unique functional role of this brain region, in concert with the entire nervous system, is to create the frame of reference of consciousness. The basic structure and the functional innervation patterns of the prefrontal area appear to be like those described in other regions of the neocortex. Thus, while this area of the brain is the most recent in evolutionary time, it appears to retain the general operational parameters of integration, convergence, and disparity computation. Many scientists have devoted themselves to the study of this brain region, from its anatomy, to physiology, to biocomputational theory and behavior. Mountcastle, Eccles, Nauta, Jacobson, Mishkin, Pribram, Jones, Powell, Passingham, Goldman-Rakic, and Fuster, and their colleagues must be mentioned prominently for their past and present work in understanding the functional neurobiology of this region.[1]

The major connections of the prefrontal multimodal neocortex include afferent projections from all association cortices and from all multimodal regions of the temporal, parietal, insular, and cingulate cortex, and outputs of the hippocampal system. Thus, underlying the six layers of the neocortex is a series of massive axon bundles which carry information between the cortical regions and between the cerebral hemispheres of the prefrontal cortex. These so-called white matter tracts include the corpus callosum, the cingulum, the superior longitudinal fasciculus, and the uncinate fasciculus.

The prefrontal region is also interconnected with the dorsomedial nucleus of the thalamus. This topographic, reciprocal connection appears to be the only neocortical projection from this thalamic nucleus. The anatomical boundaries of the afferent fibers from the dorsomedial nucleus provide one method by which to define the limits of the prefrontal region (Fuster, 1997).[2] Within the prefrontal region, two divisions have been identified: the orbitomedial and the dorsolateral. In the thalamus, the lateral dorsomedial nucleus contains (parvocellular) layers of small neurons that project to the dorsolateral prefrontal cortex; while the medial thalamic nucleus contains large (magnocellular) cells that send their axons to the orbital and medial prefrontal area. In general, the gustatory, olfactory, and visceral-autonomic sensory representations converge in the orbitomedial division (including the cingulate region), and the visual, auditory, parietal, and temporal lobe information converges in the dorsolateral area. The efferent output of the two prefrontal regions also reflects a functional distinction. In addition to the differential connectivity with the dorsomedial thalamus, the orbitomedial region has a significant efferent projection to the amygdala and other subcortical nuclei, whereas the dorsolateral region has significant projections to the temporal neocortical regions involved in multimodal representation and memory function.

The patterns of sensory representation created by afferent synaptic zones in the prefrontal regions reflect both parallel processing of individual projections and a true convergence of several sensory modalities, especially in the dorsolateral division. Thus, there are regions in the prefrontal area where several of these individual sensory maps overlap in common integrative modules. A hypothetical depiction of converging sensory representations as interlaced regions of information processing is given in Figure 6-1. These prefrontal integration modules may create fields of ultimate multimodal convergence in both cerebral hemispheres. Goldman-Rakic (1982) found an interesting columnar organization of afferent projections from the parietal lobe in the monkey.[3] A topographic map of the parietal lobe in which afferent fibers from one side of the cortex alternated with the homologous projections from the contralateral prefrontal region (by fibers of the corpus

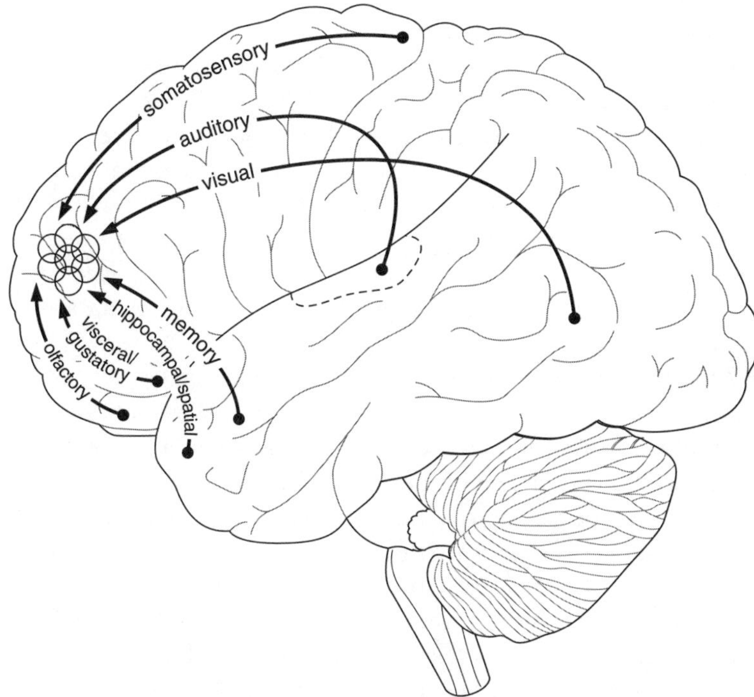

Figure 6-1 Modular regions of the prefrontal neocortex may receive a convergence of many multisensory pathways. Such regions may repeat across the prefrontal brain.

callosum) was found in repeating columns several hundred micrometers in diameter. Other studies have indeed demonstrated that several different sensory modalities converge onto neurons within small columnar regions of prefrontal cortex.

Many theories regarding prefrontal cortex function are derived from the impressive amount of knowledge on the electrophysiological response of prefrontal neurons that has been compiled from primate research (Fuster, Goldman-Rakic, Mishkin, Pribram, and others).[4] One of the most interesting and replicated findings is that cells of a type found primarily in the dorsolateral regions appear to alter their nerve impulse responses during complex, multimodal behavioral situations when a delay is imposed between two parts of a highly practiced behavior sequence. The key factor driving the change in nerve impulse activity appeared to be the delay itself, the time between behavioral actions. This type of neuron has been named the *memory cell* (Fuster and Alexander, 1971).[5]

Significant research has been directed toward understanding the memory cells of the primate prefrontal cortex: the type of sensory modalities that stimulate their activity, the type of delay to which they respond, what limitations are involved, and what their behavioral significance may be. The classic experimental paradigms of delayed matching to sample and delayed nonmatching to sample have been employed over a wide variety of settings, stimuli, and interposed delay conditions. In a delayed-matching-to-sample (or DMTS) test, the subject must hold a place or complex stimulus in short-term memory so that after an imposed delay, he or she will be able to choose either the same place or the same stimulus. In a delayed-nonmatching-to-sample (or DNMTS) test, the subject chooses an alternative place or stimulus to obtain a reward. These procedures are typically done with a monkey. The monkey extends an arm to retrieve a piece of food from one of two wells. After this act, the wells are removed from view and a piece of food is placed in either the same well or the other well, Both wells are then covered and presented again to the subject, in the same spatial setting, and the subject is allowed to choose one of the wells. Many hundreds or thousands of training trials may be run, in which the first phase involves teaching the subject to select either the same well (matching to sample) or the other well (nonmatching to sample); the sample refers to the initial selection. After the task is mastered, delays of increasing length are successively introduced between the first and second choice behaviors, with the monkey's success rate declining as the time between the choices gets longer.

Years of high-quality primate research have demonstrated that successful learning of these tasks is correlated with the presence of neurons that respond to the delay.[6] If the neural functions of the prefrontal areas containing the delay-responding cells are disrupted, the subject will fail to successfully perform the nonmatching- or matching-to-sample task. We must note that other regions of the nervous system, such as the temporal lobe memory system, must also be functioning normally for the initial learning of the procedure and its successful execution to take place.

It is possible that portions of the prefrontal neocortex map real-time three-dimensional (3D) multimodal space and flexibly weigh biologically important, learned places within it. From an evolutionary perspective, it is intriguing that this functional description of the prefrontal neocortex is analogous to the hippocampal spatial map and working memory system in which short-term memory combined with continual sensory input from the environment produces a 3D map, as we saw with the rats in the maze. The differences are that the prefrontal neocortex is arranged in modular fashion and that this region receives afferent sensory information from many other areas of the brain, including the hippocampus itself. Perhaps the level of complexity of sensory representation derived in the multimodal disparity computations of the prefrontal cortical modules is of a higher order than that of hippocampal information. Perhaps, then, in the prefrontal modules, more combinations of, or more subtle variations in, multimodal properties of the 3D sensory worlds may be interrelated, compared, and linked to produce efferent behavioral sequences that span a large temporal frame. And that time frame of active retention, the working memory component, may serve to physically bridge segments of a complex behavioral sequence, even when the segments are partitioned by imposed delays.

We must not forget that the primate behavior displayed in these delay tasks, like all learned behavior, is created, stored, and evoked from memory as a sequence of thousands to millions of millisecond computational products. The stream of moment-to-moment memory information is elicited by the real-time processing of the internal and external sensory environments related to the testing session. In the prefrontal integration modules of the nonhuman primate, past behavioral sequences are revived in the present situation, compared with the specific stimulus conditions of the current task, maintained across interruptions in the sequential flow, and finally brought to completion by changes in the external stimulus conditions.

We must then ask an important question: How much order, complexity, or dimensionality must be present for a particular stimulus type to be maintained across the temporal delay by the internally generated 3D spatial map? In the hippocampal system, a complex 3D place may be represented in the nervous system and held over time to play a role in choice behavior. In the nonhuman primate, it may take a highly learned complex stimulus—one that is strongly embedded in memory structure—with its own 3D place component to elicit a correct behavioral sequence across delay periods. If this is so, it begs this simple question: Can a nonhuman primate perform a similar delay memory task with only a 2D stimulus set when all learning takes place within an inconsistent 3D external setting? Recall that rats needed a stable 3D external testing environment to successfully perform delayed learning tasks. Is this different across species? Can a human do these tasks with less stimulus information, less stimulus dimension, and across longer delay periods? Why? Does consciousness have something to do with these considerations? We will answer these questions in this chapter, and further examine them in a later one.

Work with human patients who have suffered damage to the prefrontal neocortex reveals behaviors similar to those studied experimentally with animals. Fuster (1980) noted that the overall function of this region was "the formation of temporal structures of behavior with a unifying purpose or goal."[7] It was also noted that the cognitive functions of short-term working memory, attention, and inhibitory control appear to be created in the prefrontal areas. In animal research, it has been reported that prefrontal damage results in learning impairments, especially when temporal delays are present. Such subjects may be hyperactive, distractible, impaired in shifting between learned tasks, slow to adjust to changes in the environment, disinhibited, and socially and emotionally dysfunctional (reported in primates). Similarly, human patients may be hyperactive or hypoactive, have decreased awareness, be distractible, or be impaired in future planning and working memory. Other human case reports note speech problems involving fluency and a reduction in spontaneous speech. Apathy, depression, euphoria, hypersexuality, and a loss of the moral or social rules of behavior have all been found in patients with damage to a variety of regions of the prefrontal neocortex. Orbitomedial lesions appear to be able to cause dramatic changes in basic personality, reflected in apathy, mutism, disinhibition, paranoia, and a reduction in the awareness of self. Dorsolateral prefrontal damage may result in many of the same syndromes reported with orbitomedial lesions, but may also include planning difficulties, short-term memory problems, and a *dysexecutive* disorder.

Since formal observation of nonhuman animals and humans with damage to the prefrontal areas began, it has been suggested that higher-order behavior functions include decisions, abstract intelligence, attention, awareness, cognition, choice, will, self, and consciousness. Perhaps we have always been correct in these observations. Perhaps we have been partially correct, but not entirely so. Of course, as we have stressed, the operational definitions of these large-scale behavioral terms are critical in determining what behavior is being observed, what neural operations support its expression, and where they occur in the brain. It is now time that we formalize our model of prefrontal integration module function and the generation of consciousness.

The Prefrontal Integration Module

The neurobiological model of consciousness rests upon a foundation of structure-function relationships. The cornerstone of this foundation is the prefrontal integration module (PIM). The construction of this term reflects the neocortical region of interest (prefrontal), indicates the general biophysical computational function (integration), and honors the generally accepted interlaced columnar design of the neocortex (module). Since we cannot fully define the exact dimensions, cellular components, synaptic patterns, informational content, or specific biomathematical operations performed in the PIM, it must ultimately be viewed as a heuristic construct. The PIM, as envisioned, is a repeating structure within each hemisphere of the prefrontal area in which afferent fibers conveying several informational products topographically converge; it is a living, structured, multimodal information space. Indeed, it is a location where the other true multimodal representations, constructed in parietal, temporal, and frontal cortices and in the hippocampal system, may be further transformed into even higher-order representations. The efferent output of each PIM thus contains a representation of this ordered information for dissemination to other regions of the neocortex and to the entire neuraxis.

Based on the neuroanatomical, physiological, and behavioral evidence, we visualize the basic component inventory of potential afferent axon sources reaching PIMs as including (Figure 6-2)

1. Unimodal sensory projections from each association cortex
2. Multimodal sensory projections from the parietal, temporal, and prefrontal cortex
3. Hippocampal fibers from the CA1 neurons
4. Memory system projections from the subiculum, entorhinal, and parahippocampal regions
5. Dorsomedial and other thalamic fibers
6. Brainstem reticular nuclei and basal forebrain projections

The topographic functional information that may converge in these modules during a moment of stimulus processing could include

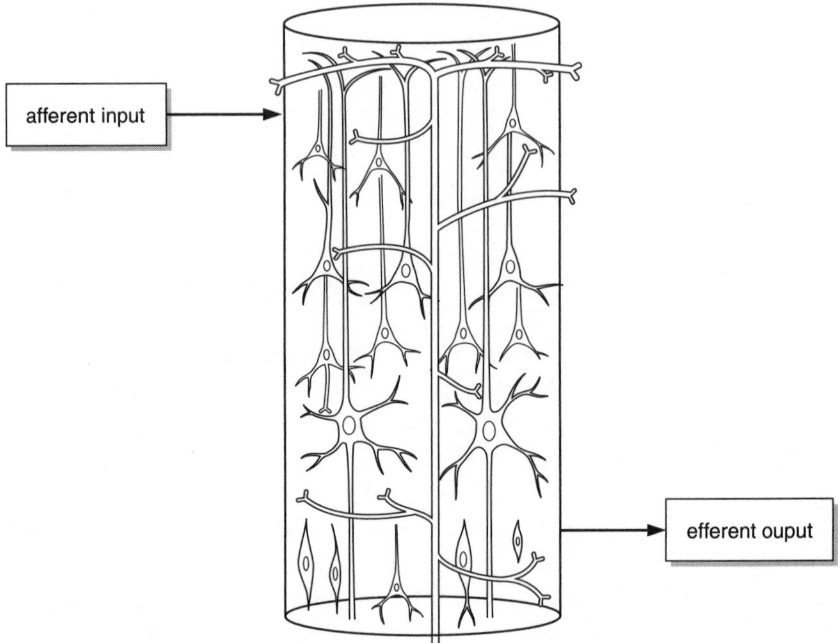

Figure 6-2 The prefrontal integration module (PIM), a hypothetical construct in the prefrontal neocortex in which the majority of all sensory modalities are represented by afferent wave convergence. PIMs represent the locations in the brain where the external and internal sensory worlds reach their highest degree of multisensory integration per moment of biocomputational activity.

1. Representation of the unimodal external and internal 3D sensory worlds
2. Representation of the multimodal external and internal 3D sensory worlds
3. Representation of the real-time 3D spatial environment
4. Representation of recent and distant past sensory moments (memories)
5. The timing and coordinating influence of the dorsomedial thalamus
6. The activity and coordinating influence of the monoaminergic nuclei

The efferent projections that arise from various PIMs could include

1. Corticocortical fibers to adjacent PIMs
2. Commissural axons to the homologue PIM in the contralateral hemisphere

3. Projections to neocortical regions
4. Projections to the entorhinal-hippocampal spatial map system
5. Projections to the memory system cortical areas
6. Projections to subcortical nuclei in the thalamus, basal ganglia, amygdala, and all descending targets

We conceptualize a PIM as a functionally defined volume of prefrontal cortex that can simultaneously receive a majority, if not all, of the afferent influences listed above. There may indeed be a differential weighting of the various representational influences across a field of PIMs and across moments in stimulus processing. It is in these cylinders of neocortical tissues that we see the most complete representation of the sensory worlds, the ultimate *point representation* that can be achieved by nervous system computation, the most comprehensive *binding in time* of 2D and 3D stimulus information possible.

A simple equation provides us with a bookkeeping tool for all the various representations that converge in the PIMs, undergo transformation, and become encoded in output axonal arrays. The maximum sensory representation (R) of the real-time external and internal stimulus environments that may be present in a single wavefront of afferent (a) synaptic zone activity is designated as R_a (representation from afferents). This potentially includes each afferent representation from unimodal and multimodal neocortical regions, the hippocampus spatial map generator, and the moment-to-moment thalamocortical and monoaminergic influences. The time designation that corresponds to each millisecond-scale R_a flux will be t, and $_n$ (an integer) will denote the sequence of processing moments. $R_a t_n$ is the maximum point representation of the current sensory environment at a given moment as it enters a given PIM.

We must include two related terms that account for the additional afferent projections that may enter a PIM at each operational cycle. First, the corticocortical projection from one PIM to an adjacent PIM contains representations that are similar in informational content to the R_a entering the neighboring PIM, because the basic afferent sources are so anatomically close. The designation R'_a indicates input from another PIM that is processing a similar but not identical afferent representation. Since we must follow the flow of information across many modules and over many transduction moments, it is necessary to adopt a convention in which we designate a reference PIM as the one receiving $R_a t_n$. The time reference t_n indicates the present moment (the *now*) of sensory integration through the neocortical module. Integration cycles prior to and following t_n are designated by a single integer change per sensory integration moment. In this manner,

t_{n-1} refers to the sensory integration cycle immediately prior to the reference, and t_{n+1} refers to the next cycle following the reference. Thus, afferent information that reaches the reference PIM through axons that originate in an adjacent PIM that is only one synaptic system away is termed $R'_a t_{n-1}$. This is a similar afferent representation of the sensory environment, but it is one neocortical processing cycle out of phase and thus is in the past relative to the designated reference PIM.

The final term for the afferent influences on the reference PIM refers to the representation of the recent and/or distant past, the memory input. Since stimuli of the current external or internal environments evoke past memory information, we consider the representational components to also be similar to some degree to sensory information entering the prefrontal modules from other neocortical regions. Therefore, the designation for the memory afferent influence is $R''_a t_{n-x}$, where $n - x$ represents the now minus the time (x) before the current afferent processing moment when the memory was laid down. The value of x is therefore greater than 1 and could represent many hours, days, or even years of processing cycles in neural activity.

For a single millisecond-scale flux of afferent activation of all synaptic zones in the tissue volume that makes up the reference PIM, the computational operation may be represented by the simple expression $f(R_a t_n, R'_a t_{n-1}, R''_a t_{n-x})$, with the function f indicating the largely unknown biological transformations performed on this immense data set contained in the flux of neural activity. We may now begin to appreciate the incredible density of information that is captured in this representational tapestry for only a single moment—a fraction of a second—of physical existence.

The maximum possible output product of each PIM computational moment is designated as the efferent representation R_e per operational cycle: $R_e t_n \approx f(R_a t_n, R'_a t_{n-1}, R''_a t_{n-x})$ and is encoded in the structure and nerve impulse activity of the axonal fibers. Some fraction of the representational information contained in $R_e t_n$ reaches nearby PIMs, the contralateral homologue PIMs, the association cortical regions, and the hippocampal and memory systems. There is undoubtedly a variable distribution of information across each of the potential efferent targets, but we do not yet know what the partitioning entails.

We propose that the region defined by a PIM operates in essentially the same way as any other neocortical column or module. The physical components may involve many interlaced vertical columns, or perhaps an even more distributed volume design, but the synaptic-driven processes remain the same across all cortical regions. Therefore, as each wavefront of afferent neural activity enters the synaptic zones of a module and initiates the integration operation, a disparity computation is performed for the 3D spatial and 1D temporal phase differences contained within the representational order. The computational solutions, expressed in the collective efferent output array $R_e t_n$, contain a novel representation derived from aspects of the present sensory worlds ($R_a t_n$), the previous moment's integrated representation ($R'_a t_{n-1}$), and the more distant past's computational products from memory ($R''_a t_{n-x}$). In other words, it very much appears that these integration modules are capable of comparing the past with the present and computing information about what to do next. This certainly reflects much of what we have presented for the known anatomy, physiology, and behavior of this brain region.

The sensory information within the total afferent synaptic array reaches a complex state in the PIM across the millisecond process of neurotransmission. We therefore propose that *the maximal degree of sensory experience that the brain may achieve (for that biophysical computational moment) is represented in the PIM*. The computation performed in the synaptic field of a PIM (a region of electrochemical, and thus electromagnetic, graded current flows) is proposed to be an integral function created by the biophysical structure of the sustaining cellular and extracellular system of the organic brain. This model suggests that the biophysical methods by which the brain derives information from sensory processing may be radically different from the many theories that relate the brain's operations to those of electric circuits, computers, or point-to-point so-called neural networks.

The complex, but constrained, biochemical energy field within the boundaries of the PIM possesses a force (as does any electromagnetic field), and this ordered volume of charged organic tissue initiates a nerve impulse code as the physical solutions of the disparity computations, that is, the efferent output products ($R_e t_n$). These efferent wavefronts (also volume-encoded fields of organic materials) may carry novel information related to the probable next moment of higher-order sensory-behavioral experience. *Thus, the functional consequence of PIM activity may be seen as reinforcement or inhibition of ongoing behavioral and homeostatic activities, in addition to a contribution to the memory system.*

The PIM may be seen as a complex statistical weighting system for the totality of the momentary experience of the neocortex, and thereby for the animal. It may be seen as providing a temporal link between moments of external behavior or internal states. We note that some regions of PIM activity will receive more afferent influence from a particular subset of sensory information than others; that is, some PIMs will be more visual-dominated or more autonomic-dominated than others, and so on. Furthermore, many PIMs are simultaneously, in parallel, processing many different sensory combinations with a range of internal weightings for each afferent component. And it is vital to comment here (and we will return to this point often) that the effect of this *gestalt* computation of past and present representations is usually collapsed to a minimal behavioral impact by the overwhelming demands of the stimulus environment and the metabolic imperatives of the internal systems. What we mean by this is that all the myriad computational output at each neural processing moment that is produced by nonprefrontal cortical regions, subcortical nuclei, and peripheral ganglia in response to the transduced sensory worlds actually determines the behavior of all biological systems. The ongoing interaction of incoming sensory influence and outgoing effector-initiated actions has a pace and progression that is set in motion by the genetic code, the developmental modifications, and the real-time composition of the stimulus environments. No additional information or computational analysis is necessary for the nervous system or any other system to continue its moment-to-moment function. Nevertheless, when the conditions of the internal and external sensory worlds permit or demand it (e.g., when a behavioral sequence must be maintained across time during delays, or when an action involves a higher-order multimodal informational comparison of context and memory that cannot be performed anywhere else in the nervous system), the PIMs' computational output may create an efferent code that has a significant biasing role in the ongoing behavioral flow of life.

We may therefore view the efferent outflow of a PIM as either reinforcing various behaviors or internal functions, modifying them, or, at most, inhibiting the continuation of a previously ongoing behavior or internal process as a result of a significant change in one or more representational components of the afferent sources. In other words, a PIM compares aspects of past and present behavior or past and present internal conditions, and its efferent output solutions (as physical products encoded in axonal array activity) may influence the next moment of behavior or homeostasis in a manner that either promotes the current state, moves it toward another state, or retards its progression.

The basic output effect of a PIM, irrespective of its specific informational content, may at its most simple articulation be conceptualized as a graph of a sigmoid function curve (Figure 6-3). The vertical axis represents the gestalt disparity computation within a given PIM as a simple correlation function: The afferent representations of the past ($R'_a t_{n-1}$ and $R''_a t_{n-x}$) are thus corre-

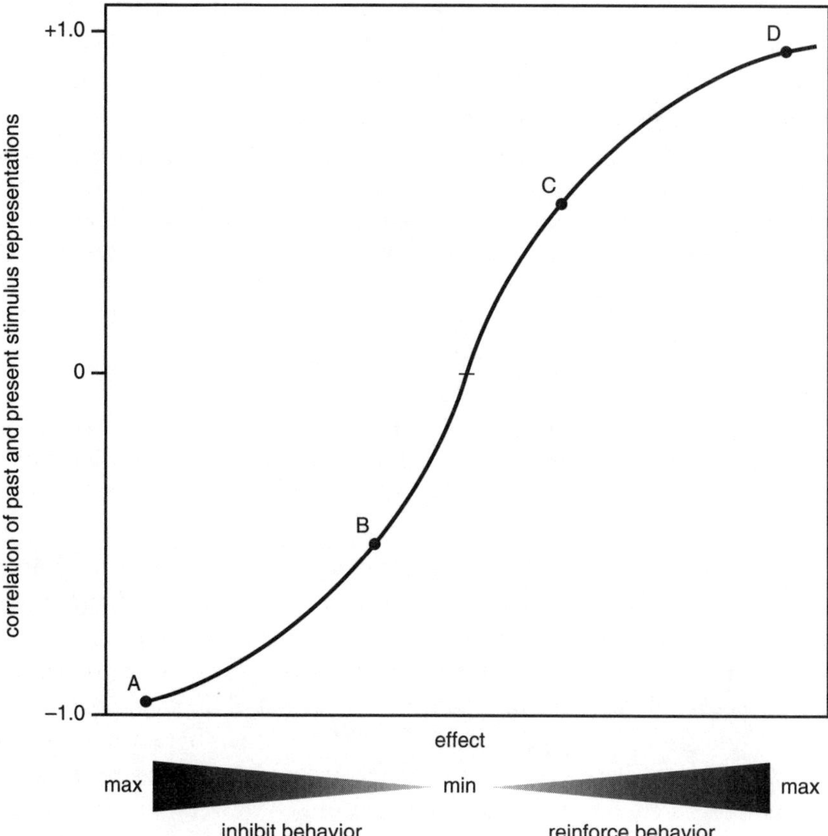

Figure 6-3 The modifying influence of the efferent output of a PIM on behavior. The computational outcome of comparing the immediate past sensory moment with the present moment, within a PIM, may result in a range of influences on the actions of the animal. PIM efferent output may thus inhibit (A and B) or reinforce (C and D) behavior.

lated with the present moment representation ($R_a t_n$). The converging past and present information may be highly similar and thus produce a positive correlation between representational moments, with +1.0 representing the theoretical limit of complete agreement. At the other extreme, if the afferent input of past and present contains very different or contradictory representations, a negative correlation is computed; −1.0 is the maximum limit of this disagreement. Each point on the S-curve reflects the relative similarity between informational components of the past and present point representations for the organism and the basic manner in which the computational solutions encoded in all efferent projections influence the behavioral progression. The mathematics of S-shaped functions indicate that the extreme limits of absolute similarity or disparity are not easily (if ever) reached, and thus the curve flattens out as it gets nearer this theoretical limit.

Again, we so very much belie the staggering informational and computational processes that can be occurring in these prefrontal modules. But it is necessary to bring a conceptual framework to this daunting enterprise if we are to differentiate and perhaps better understand how consciousness emerges from neural activity and what behavioral manifestations may reflect its existence. A simple narrative of the key points (*A* through *D*) along the S-curve will serve at this time to hint at the grand nature of the prefrontal computational products.

Refer to Figure 6-3 for the positions of the following scenarios on the S-curve. The output of PIM function may act to influence behavior in the following manner:

A. *Strongly inhibit.* A child moves her hand toward a slightly familiar object. When her hand gets beyond a certain critical sensory boundary near the object, a memory ($R''_a t_{n-x}$) of a previously very painful outcome of touching the object is elicited. The past, a condensed gestalt of many sensory moments arising out of the memory system, merges with the present in the PIM, and the efferent output can contain a code to cortical and subcortical targets that strongly supports a change in the next moment of behavior: that is, Stop!

   As the child's hand nears the object, a candle flame, the temperature change and the overall spatial relationships of body, hand, and candlelight are all being processed at many levels of nervous system activity. At a critical threshold of representation, the memory sequence is initiated, and its influence also begins to affect the nervous system. Even before the PIMs make the computational products, other cortical and subcortical systems may have already begun to shift the flow of behavior with respect to the heat energy increase, perhaps through direct memory-output effects to subcortical nuclei (through the amygdala, hypothalamic, basal ganglia, or other pathways). The PIM efferent influences may support these millisecond-earlier shifts in behavior and bring a more rapid or perhaps a more context-appropriate change in action. That is, the child may quickly, but gently, move her hand toward another, less harmful object in a smooth manner that would not bring the attention of her nearby parent.

B. *Slightly inhibit.* A man is enjoying a meal and has a large amount of food left on his plate. In his sensory worlds, several complex stimuli are changing. The internal environment is adding sugar and then insulin to his bloodstream, his stomach walls are beginning to distend, and his blood pressure is rising. At a critical point, a memory of heartburn and its context properties and visceral-autonomic qualities is elicited. Simultaneously, the man notices a clock on the wall that indicates that he has plenty of time before he must stop eating, and he surveys the appealing assortment of food that remains to be sampled. In moments of prefrontal module processing of these higher-order sensory representations, along with the lower levels of nervous system activity, the computational compromise from these competing afferent representations may result in a slower pace to his ingestion. Slow down, but don't stop is the overall gradual behavioral shift that occurs after many seconds of computational activity comparing the converging representations from virtually all sensory modalities and memory sources.

C. *Slightly reinforce.* A young male lion has been assaulted twice by the pride leader when he approached a particular location close to the only available pond. A day thereafter, the young lion finds himself downwind of a female lion that has entered a fertility cycle. The olfactory, visual, and auditory sensory representations add up to initiate a very strong behavioral sequence! However, in this particular instance, the female lion is crouching in the exact place where the young male was twice mauled. As he approaches the location and the female lion, the spatial place elicits his learned response to avoid it. The push-pull dissonance of this complex behavioral situation is represented in moments of PIM activity. In this case, the absence of an important 3D, 400-pound, large, loud, pungent stimulus results in an outflow of efferent activity that does not inhibit the reproductive behavioral sequence with a stop influence. The place-memory weighting does not even result in a retardation of the ongoing behavior; it just alters it slightly by initiating more scanning eye and head movements, or perhaps more crouching behavior as he approaches the specific spatial location. As each moment goes by and the pride leader remains out of sensory range, the current mating behavior sequence is reinforced. Proceed, but change the hard-wired behavior sequence a little is the efferent influence of PIM activity over many seconds of processing time.

D. *Strongly reinforce.* A concert pianist is performing one of her most loved and most practiced pieces. The long behavior sequence has begun, the conductor is smiling, the orchestra sounds as if it is reading her mind, and the faces in the front row look joyous. The pre-

> frontal modules are receiving this flood of multisensory information of higher-order representation in real time. The integration cycles comparing the current sensory environments (internal, motor, somatosensory, visual, auditory, and so on) with those just past and with the ongoing memory input of similar, successful performances create an efferent influence that does little to alter the progression: that is, Go! We note that any significant efferent influence that might result from higher-order prefrontal comparisons might actually impair this level of performance. As with many highly practiced (and thus strong) memory behaviors in music, athletics, and dance, sometimes it seems that the prefrontal influence can be more detrimental than helpful—at least during moments of so-called flow conditions.

The fields of PIMs thus produce a millisecond-to-millisecond influence on the existing state of overall nervous system operation. From one perspective, it may be said that the prefrontal influence is just a biasing or weighting factor: It doesn't seem very controlling, or much of an executive! Most behavior and changes in behavior occur before the PIM even gets a chance to decide what to do. Where, it may be asked, is the real guiding force for which behaviors are chosen and which are discarded?

On the other hand, we must keep firmly in mind that the nervous system is performing an incredible number of functions that bind in time various stimulus influences and produce effector responses that basically keep the animal alive for the next moment. To make all those functions dependent upon computational solutions produced in one region of neocortex would have obvious drawbacks. Thus, we propose that the prefrontal modules have the capacity to bind in time only a higher order of nervous system sensory representation—one beyond the basic transduced energies of light, sound, touch, or taste and beyond the brainstem, midbrain, and primary neocortical unimodal computational products of stimulus location, intensity, or vector. What occupies the PIMs is an informational structure carried in wavefronts of neural activity that conveys the current contextual parameters derived from virtually any 2D or 3D combination of internal and external sensory energies and their historical beneficial or decretory impact.

The PIMs produce solutions that may alter the next behavioral moment in a manner that further increases the probability of a beneficial outcome and that may also modify the memory of these interrelated contingencies for future recombination. Of all the homeostatic functions for living systems that evolution has produced beginning with the first cell, the activity of the PIMs is the most complex. The PIMs' only function is to create the highest order of 3D multimodal representation for each moment in the bound existence of the animal. Perhaps at some level this appears to play a seemingly minor role, but we must remain cognizant of the immense flexibility and complexity (as in the number of behavioral possibilities) that this activity bestows upon nervous system function. It is the vital function in certain higher-order behaviors that demand a contextual computation or a multimodal and multidimensional past-to-future movement vector calculation. It subserves all those nonhuman and human complicated activities that we invariably define with terms like *working memory*, *attention*, *cognition*, *understanding*, *social awareness*, and *moral judgment*. All of these are actions that involve rules, context, memory, and choices over time.

All of these actions are collectively the manifestations of thousands upon thousands of millisecond disparity computations performed in the prefrontal region of the neocortex. All the computation products, encoded in the efferent axonal outputs, have influence on the system through complex manifestations of millions to billions of synaptic zone activity moments that we, the observers, organize into definitional categories of large-scale, high-concept behaviors. Working memory, attention, cognition, understanding, social awareness, and moral judgment are all human constructs based on many internal and external multimodal behaviors that occur in patterns over extremely long time frames. In the nervous system, each of these behaviors reflects a fantastic number of serial and parallel computational moments, moments without necessary connection.

When does the nervous system *know* it is attending? When does the nervous system *care* that it has made a moral judgment? When does the nervous system become *aware* of delay periods, its next choice, and the consequences of its actions? We can ask whether the disparity computations of the PIMs ever become connected in any real, meaningful way, or whether the nervous system generates all behavior in discrete moments of time. Is all behavior just flickering waves of fading neural activity flowing through interconnected modules? For all their convergent and higher-order computational activity, where in the fields of PIM activity do we need to invoke a new reference system of consciousness?

An important concept in our model is that of a dominant focal region of activity that moves across the prefrontal fields over time. We will consider a single PIM (regardless of its ultimate size) as the unit of dominant focal activity. The dominant or focal PIM is operationally defined by a balance of influences that creates a region of maximum activity for each successive wave of afferent sensory information. These factors include the following:

1. *Competition.* The sources of sensory energy in the external and internal worlds are transduced by the neural receptors based on their relative intensity and duration. The within function of the nervous system binds in time these vastly different sources of stimulus energy, and thus a type of competition exists in the relative attention that a particular sensory source commands in the higher-order processing regions. The competition is also between locations of the body, and thus a multisensory combination of visual-auditory or visceral-autonomic sensory stimuli from a particular location in the external or internal world may create a focus of neural activity in the prefrontal regions.
2. *Bias.* The ongoing behavior of the nervous system has a momentum, an inertia that influences the probability concerning the location of the dominant activity for the next moment of synaptic zone activity. Once a certain path of behavior begins, it is likely that this path will remain the focus of neural activity for a certain amount of time. If a powerful sensory input is at odds with the current behavioral state, then a shift in PIM activity may occur that contributes to changing the behavior.
3. *Focus.* A timing and coordinating function of thalamic nuclei influences PIM activity in a manner that may stabilize and shift the focus across a region of processing modules. The lateral inhibition model may apply to this type of focusing activity, whereby modules around a dominant focal PIM are inhibited in their relative activity to provide additional bias to the active PIM. Modulating influences from the monoaminergic fibers may assist in this focusing activity.
4. *Output effect.* All of the previous factors may function to produce a dominant focal PIM for each moment in prefrontal sensory processing. The efferent output products emerging from that PIM in the PIM's axon array must also have some type of preferential effect, or nothing is gained from a behavioral perspective. The efferent connections of the prefrontal regions do not go directly to the primary motor neocortex or other motor systems, but are modulated by the premotor neocortex and the thalamic nuclei. Therefore, in a system-to-system coordination, the efferent output of the dominant PIM may have a relatively greater effector action, as processed through the thalamus, basal ganglia, and premotor cortex, than efferents from other modules. The same relative weighing function for the dominant PIM efferent information may apply to the projection into the forebrain memory system as well.

The remainder of the prefrontal neocortex (or any other region of the nervous system) does not sleep or stop working during the operating cycle of the dominant PIM. We must not forget that most behavior and homeostatic activities are ongoing and are only promoted or inhibited by the output of this neocortical region. Theoretically, every PIM, from the most dominant to the most inhibited, at each integration cycle, could have its own unique output influence projected onto the S-curve function of Figure 6-3. In parallel, each PIM has its own moment-to-moment effector impact on the nervous system. Because it takes time to transduce, transmit, and integrate sensory information, because it takes time to change an ongoing skeletal motor or digestive behavior, and because sensory environments tend to remain stable over many moments of neural activity time, the regions of prefrontal activity away from the dominant focus are most likely engaged in very similar (positively correlated) informational processing activity. Even though a distant PIM may have information that is one, two, or more transduction moments in the past relative to the current dominant PIM, its major representational characteristics will probably be similar.

A collective S-curve map for a single transduction-integration-transmission moment across many PIMs would show a distribution of points (one for each PIM) of effector influence with a tightly focused distribution around the dominant PIM's location, and this point distribution might be skewed to indicate a direction of movement along the curve. That is, the shape of the point cluster would actually indicate the path of behavioral effect, toward either more or less reinforcement or inhibition. Thus, we note that the general background (parallel) activity of the other prefrontal modules would tend to support the effector influence of the dominant PIM. Based on this functional model of sensory influence distribution, we can see that a shift of the dominant focus across a field of PIMs over time, and the resultant shift in behavioral effects, will usually proceed in a smooth fashion, as a result of the statistical inertia of the biophysical systems as they interact with the stimulus context.

This model provides a method of visualizing a functional shifting of the dominant focus from PIM to PIM across neural activity time. In this manner, we can define a reference PIM (like the $R_a t_n$) and discuss the flow of information to and from a PIM and between PIMs across milliseconds of afferent influence. It is thus a relative focus system that creates a *vector of serial information processing* across the prefrontal regions in the dominant modules and in the parallel nondominant areas. It creates a vector of serial information processing by which we can track the past, present, and future of sensory representations in this region (memory input notwithstanding).

It physically defines the past as the corticocortical information that is leaving one dominant focus PIM to enter another.

The past is defined only relative to the selected reference moment of the *now*. The current afferent representations reaching the dominant PIM *now* include the afferent input from all other sensory cortices, memory systems, and other sources and the afferent input from a PIM that was the dominant focus during the previous moment of synaptic zone activity. That PIM processed the *now* one phase before the current *now*, and thus its input is considered the relative past.

As we have indicated, the reference PIM receives the *now* contained in $(R_a t_n, R'_a t_{n-1}, R''_a t_{n-x})$. The biophysical past is the $R'_a t_{n-1}$ factor with respect to the *now* PIM and the $R_a t_n$ input. The more distant past, evoked from a relative frozen, structural memory state, $R''_a t_{n-x}$, is more easily conceptualized. In the dynamic, millisecond-to-millisecond flow across dominant PIMs, the present point representation becomes the past and the future may be predicted to occur in a nearby area. Of course, that physical future-to-be will become the now and then the past in two brief moments of sensory integration and encoding lasting less than a second (as measured in the background reference system of neural activity). This model allows for bookkeeping for the type of information entering a region and the output products of its computational cycle. And while at this time in our science this model is ultimately a heuristic one, we may find that it has a significant basis in the biophysical reality. We will revisit this when we look at the flow of time and experience in consciousness.

Finally, this model of prefrontal structure and function explicitly and implicitly sets limits and constraints that will become important when we examine the grand concept of consciousness as a phenomenon created in this region. By proposing that a dominant focus wave of activity travels between nearby PIMs, the model localizes the synaptic linkage of information flow to short, module-to-module axon terminal regions and synaptic zones. A traveling wave of dominant representational activity will also have limits as to the number of processing cycles (and hence the time) over which it can sustain a coherent focus. When will a given dominant traveling wave of sensory representation reach a biophysical point where it must either restart or repeat a regional path or reset the focus to another dominant wave? Does this differ from species to species? How does this process react to external interruptions of metabolic homeostasis or mechanical force trauma? When the traveling wave is forced to restart, repeat, or reset, what happens to the flow of information (to the flow of time)? With respect to the representational content of prefrontal modular processing, our model indicates significant limits and constraints on the *now* computation. However, our model of PIM structure-function at least provides a material construct that not only demands that we ask such questions, but holds the promise that we may actually be able to search for the answers.

For all its bewildering complexity, $f(R_a t_n, R'_a t_{n-1}, R''_a t_{n-x})$ produces only a millisecond moment of sensory reality. The model predicts that these *now* moments will fade as each processing cycle generates a new present. From synaptic zone to synaptic zone, from modular integration to the next modular integration, the present information is *computationally diluted* into a more distant, fading, past representation, as the $R'_a t_{n-1}$ product entering each successive dominant module contains less and less information about what was its original *now.* And the constraints of this model are such that at some point in the temporal progression, when a present computational moment it is brought back into the prefrontal PIM fields from the recombinant memory system $(R''_a t_{n-x})$, it will contain only information about a distant past. Otherwise, at a critical limit of computational dilution of informational content, the present-that-is-now-past is lost to the prefrontal modules.

The fade of the now becomes a biophysical construct in the model of biological relativity. We must also ask how these limits and constraints affect behavior and learning. Are there differences in the rate or magnitude of the computational dilution of the past across animal species? If so, can we observe the computational differences in corresponding behavioral limits? When we discuss this model with respect to consciousness, we may ask, what do we experience (and what can we not experience) as a result of these limits? To phrase it a little differently, how does it feel to experience a critical point of dominant representational reset, refocus, or the fading of the *now?*

The model of biological relativity and emergent organic evolution states that we may observe the transition from one frame of reference to another. The cell and its metabolic products are the physical systems that propagate the unique 4D existence we call life. We observe the order of life relative to the background biophysical frame of reference. And, while the billions of years of organic evolution have devoured any true protocell lines, we can infer their existence before the dawn of the living cell. The emergence of a new organic frame of reference, which we call consciousness, may be observed relative to the background biophysical field, but it also may be observed against another background frame of reference, the field of general neural activity.

The conceptual model of the PIM in the mammalian brain is our focus for the observed transition from pre-consciousness to consciousness. The pre-consciousness PIM may be conceptualized as the evolutionary analog of the protocell, and the consciousness PIM as a completely functioning cell. The afferent neural activity flowing through any PIM, whether in a brain with consciousness or a brain without consciousness, has an initial informational content and undergoes a biomathematical transformation, and its maximum 3D representational order decays along a temporal function as it is converted into nerve impulse output waves, as we have discussed. All PIMs operate at this time-locked frequency of basic neural processing, wholly dependent upon the flux of afferent synaptic zone activation to perform its functions.

We will now focus on only one of the efferent output connections of the module: that of the corticocortical fibers to an adjacent PIM. The maximum order or representation within a dominant focus PIM per operational cycle, $f(R_at_n, R'_at_{n-1}, R''_at_{n-x})$, begins a decay along a complex curve derived from the biophysical nature of the system. Factors in these unknown equations include the initial order or information contained in the afferent flux; the metabolic state of background cellular systems; the number, type, and arrangement of the efferent axons carrying computational solutions; and the structure of the synaptic zones that they form in the next prefrontal module. We propose that in the pre-consciousness brain, the efferent output projections from a given dominant PIM, in a freeze-frame moment, will contain a *subcritical fraction* (to be defined) of the maximum possible information present during that single operational cycle. Therefore the adjacent PIM, as the next focus module for the *now* computation, will receive only a fragment (contained in R'_at_{n-1}) of the higher-order information of the prior moment's complete point representation $(R_at_n, R'_at_{n-1}, R''_at_{n-x})$. This significant information loss reflects the cost (entropy's bill) of the biocomputational transformation and the transduction to an axon nerve impulse code. This loss of resolution is exactly the same that we have seen at virtually every step of neural processing (e.g., receptive-field enlargement in the associative neocortex).

The progression of sensory information as it moves from dominant module to dominant module in the prefrontal region of a brain with pre-consciousness function is depicted in Figure 6-4. On the vertical axis, we have plotted the degree of information or 3D representational order that may be present in the collective afferent inputs to a focal PIM $(R_at_n, R'_at_{n-1}, R''_at_{n-x})$, and the horizontal axis marks the temporal dimension defined by cellular operations. Thus, the background sinusoidal wave in the figure represents not only the rise and fall of afferent neural activity energy per nerve impulse wavefront, but also, and inseparably, the maximum and minimum amount of order or information present.

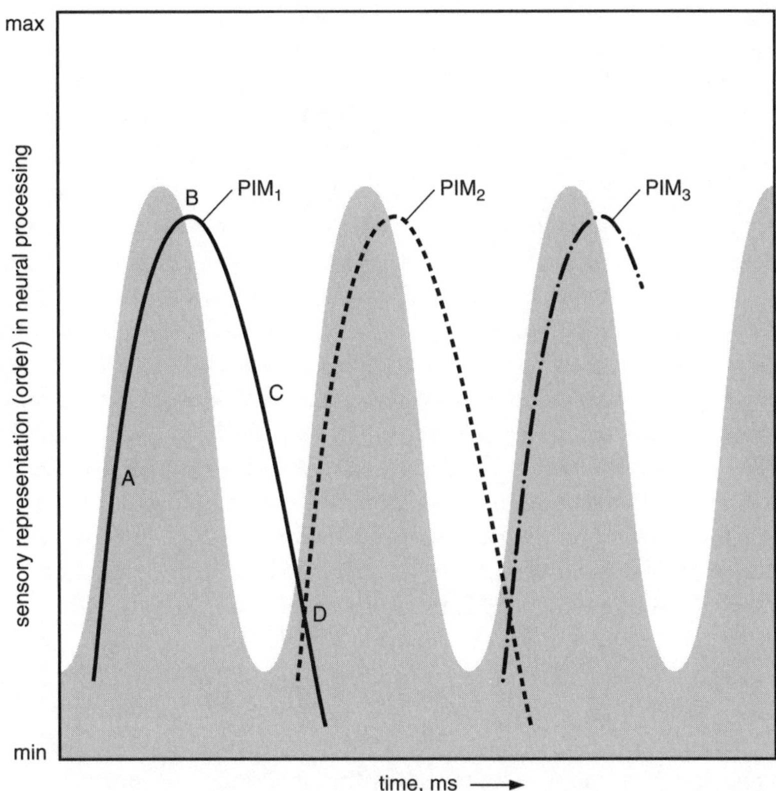

Figure 6-4 Function of the prefrontal integration module (PIM) in the pre-consciousness brain. The rise and fall of sensory representation within PIMs across neural processing cycles is depicted against the background of all information processing (shaded area). Each hypothesized PIM activity curve represents (A) neural transduction of sensory information, (B) integration and conversion of information into efferent impulses, (C) the axonal transmission phase of processing, (D) and the relatively small amount of sensory information about the past moment that enters a PIM to undergo computational analysis with current sensory representations.

This graph of energy and order provides a visual depiction of the biomathematical transformation within the volume of a PIM across a single afferent-efferent cycle. It implies that between afferent stimulus pulses, the energy, order, and thus informational content within a PIM decay to some minimal state. (Of course, the individual maximums and minimums will vary across input moments and prefrontal regions, and with changes in background metabolic or neural activity.) This basic, time-locked, and repetitive sinusoidal wave of order and information is the background neural activity that drives the computational operations of all PIMs.

Now we will designate a reference dominant module (PIM_1) as our starting point from which to track the flow of sensory representations in neural activity, and follow it across a sequence of closely linked dominant modules in serial order (i.e., from PIM_2 to PIM_3, and so on). Each PIM has its own order/time curve plotted against the background flux (Figure 6-4). As we can see in the figure, the steep rise in the curve for each PIM, A, follows the background neural activity trace. This reflects the initial phase of afferent synaptic zone activity within a PIM, indicating the transduction of the totality of information ($R_a t_n$, $R'_a t_{n-1}$, $R''_a t_{n-x}$) by the volume of living tissue within the boundary of the module. The peak region of each PIM curve, B, represents the time of integration and conversion into efferent nerve impulse activity. The cost of this process in terms of a loss in the maximum possible amount of energy and information is indicated by the slightly lower peak curve of the PIM curve relative to the potential maximum information available. The right-side portion of each module's curve, C, the falling phase, illustrates the axon transmission of information from one PIM to the next. The intersecting points, D, indicate the relative level of order or information that may be sent from one dominant PIM to the next module in the corticocortical fibers conveying $R'_a t_{n-1}$. Thus, in PIM_2, designated as the current (*now*) reference module, the $R'_a t_{n-1}$ factor in the ($R_a t_n$, $R'_a t_{n-1}$, $R''_a t_{n-x}$) afferent set comes from PIM_1 and represents the absolute maximum amount of information that PIM_2 may receive about the prior moment in sensory representation. It is the only source of information for the immediate past. We propose that in the pre-consciousness brain, the order or information that leaves PIM_1 will correspond to a point along part C of the curve. We do not know where on the curve (and that point may vary as a function of many biophysical parameters), but we propose that it will be significantly less than (a subcritical fraction of) the maximum potential amount of information available within the transduction-integration cycle. In other words, the information from PIM_1 that becomes available to PIM_2 (D) will be significantly less than the maximum amount within PIM_1. The same relationship also holds from PIM_2 to PIM_3 and for all ipsilateral and contralateral module-to-module connectivity.

The relative loss of order or complexity during the transduction-integration-transmission cycle may be due to physical or metabolic properties of the cellular systems. Factors such as the structural organization of the afferent synaptic zones (e.g., the number of synapses, the number of neurons they innervate, or the relative location of synaptic contacts on dendritic shafts or spines), the biomolecular composition of the cells and tissues involved in the integration process, or the number or organization of the efferent fibers may all affect information processing efficiency. Thus, at the interface of PIMs (D) over serial moments of processing time, only a certain fractional amount of information from one PIM is available for the next computational operations. The flow of information from dominant focus PIM to dominant focus PIM in the pre-consciousness brain will indeed support a wide range of complex behaviors that encompasses nearly all the behaviors that we have discussed. The interface points (D) in the figure are placed low to depict the relative loss of information. There is no number or equation that can begin to provide a measure of this overall reduction; we are limited to a conceptual model.

We may summarize the pre-consciousness state and PIM function as follows: The nervous system functions to bind in time a variety of sensory stimuli from the internal and external worlds. A PIM may receive afferent information containing a high degree of 2D and 3D representations of the current stimulus context, the previous moment of PIM computational analysis, and past experience ($R_a t_n$, $R'_a t_{n-1}$, $R''_a t_{n-x}$). Within the operational cycle of a PIM, an integration is performed on the available information, and the new, novel information is encoded in efferent nerve impulse activity. It is within the PIMs that the most complex representations of the sensory environments may converge. It is also within the PIMs that multimodal and multidimensional information about the past and present may meet. The phase disparity computations in the pre-consciousness PIMs derive some new information about space and time. The efferent outputs to other PIMs, and to all other target regions, serve to influence the ongoing behavior and internal states and to modify the memory systems.

But we hypothesize that the partial transduction, integration, and/or transmission of the maximum information that is perhaps theoretically available to a PIM does not meet a *critical threshold level.* Thus, while a PIM may receive highly ordered information about the current sensory conditions ($R_a t_n$), it may receive only a subthreshold amount of representation of the last sensory moment ($R'_a t_{n-1}$), and therefore of the more distant past ($R''_a t_{n-x}$). Ultimately, therefore, all prefrontal influence on behavior in pre-consciousness may be viewed as a result of a series of discrete computational moments in millisecond time frames, highly complex integrations closely linked in spatial and temporal dimensions.

The prefrontal neocortex in a pre-consciousness brain may be viewed as a massive modular field of flickering electrochemical activity, time-locked to each driving pulse of afferent energy and information, creating novel output products that affect behavior and memory. Each *now* computation contains only a faded fraction of the past, a fraction that cannot provide enough representational order to propagate the past into the next present computational moment. We speculate that through the process of organic evolution, the order and complexity of afferent sensory representations that flow to the prefrontal regions and the efferent output products that move between integration modules continue to increase. Perhaps ever so slightly and seemingly insignificantly, but nevertheless in a progressive climb against the background level of informational entropy in neural representations of the 4D sensory worlds, more of the past flowed into the present. Perhaps a little more order, a little more transduction-integration efficiency, a little more transmission accuracy, or some other variable defined a focal point of the process of evolution in the mammalian nervous system and brought a critical amount of the biophysical past and present together in unique cell-like regions of the prefrontal cortex.

The Emergence of Consciousness as a Frame of Reference in the Prefrontal Neocortex

The pre-consciousness brain that we have been describing meets or exceeds virtually every operational definition of mind or consciousness that one can find in the historical literature or in modern discourse. However, we maintain that there is more to an adequate model of consciousness. On the scale of evolutionary time, we suggest that genetic modifications continued to alter the structure, and thus the function, of the mammalian prefrontal neocortex. The integration modules may have become more complicated or more efficient, and the information that was derived and transmitted became more ordered and more complete. The unknown genetic modifications may have affected the PIM function along one or more parameters.

If we look again at Figure 6-4, depicting pre-consciousness PIM function, we can speculate that evolutionary change may have operated at one of the transition points in the order/time function. With respect to the background order flux, perhaps a more advanced pre-consciousness PIM captured more of the available information, thus elevating the theoretical transduction peak (A) of the curve. Alternatively, a PIM nearer the consciousness threshold may have performed a more efficient integration-transmission operation on the novel computational product, thus changing the slope of the efferent portion of the curve (B-C). These or other modifications could have raised the interface threshold (D) between dominant PIMs in such a manner that more and more of the current and past 3D sensory worlds were being simultaneously represented within a PIM during each operational cycle.

At a moment in evolution, at a stage during development, a new mammalian brain reached a maturational state wherein the nervous system began to create a novel order of biological existence. In that brain, conditions were such that in a dominant PIM, the afferent information from an adjacent module possessed a threshold complexity of 3D representation of the prior moment in sensory experience. When this was integrated with the present influx of multimodal and multidimensional sensory information, a novel product was produced that contained a critical threshold of representational order that now included information about the only remaining sensory world dimension to be derived by disparity computation: time, the fourth sensory world dimension. First one, then several, then a serial field of prefrontal modules began to perform disparity computations for two 3D sensory representations, one representation of the past and one of the present. In millisecond time, across the neural flux through afferent synaptic zones, the only other possible dimensional relationship between moments of sensory experience began to be calculated and then encoded as an efferent product above a critical threshold of order, and thus information.

As the dominant PIM's *now* computation came to include a past that had not faded to subcritical levels, an independent 4D coordinate information system emerged. This threshold change in prefrontal function is graphically depicted in Figure 6-5. The interface between PIMs on the order/time curves (D) reached a critical threshold of shared order and available information. The persistence of this 3D informational order across the moments of neural activity flux, sequentially through module after module, permitted the full limit of dimensional integration between two moments of sensory experience. Time, the final sensory world dimension, was now a biophysical (encoded) factor in the equations of prefrontal synaptic field activity. It was an *internal* time dimension derived from the 3D representational order of the sensory environments. It was an *independent* temporal dimension, as was the third spatial dimension (demonstrated in its derivation from two 2D random dot images). The information was perhaps always theoretically available in the overall flux of mammalian neural activity, but now in this particular brain it became organized into a coordinate system representing three spatial and one temporal dimension, as a consequence of prefrontal neocortex structure and function.

Thus, the new computational time metric was not just a simple function of the background flux of afferent neural activity. It was created by the momentary organization of sensory information within a modular tissue volume. This novel 4D biophysical representation is probably the most complex momentary organization of information in the universe. The prop-

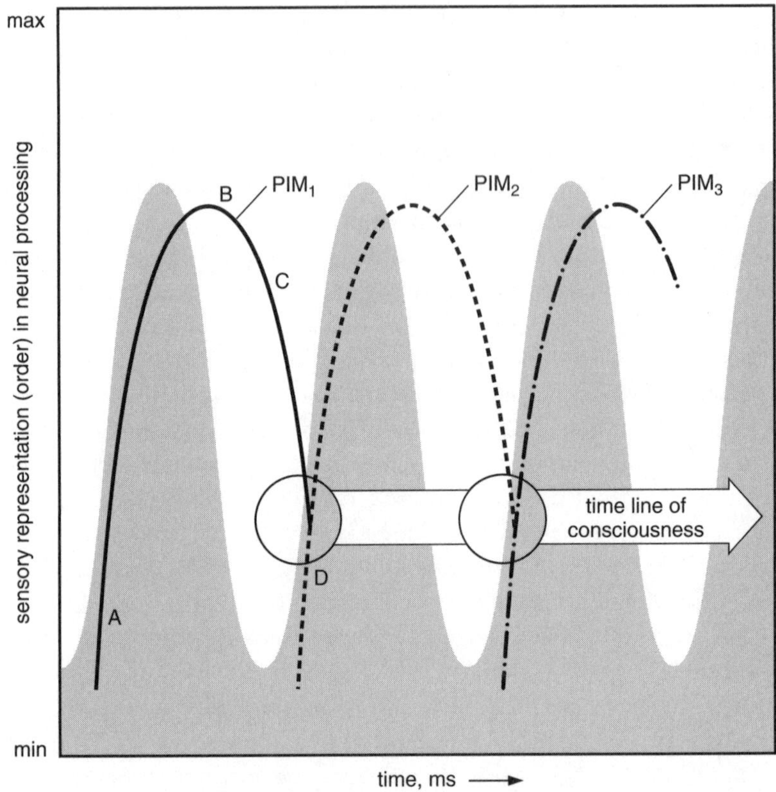

Figure 6-5 Emergence of consciousness as a frame of reference through prefrontal integration module (PIM) activity. The hypothesized evolutionary change in brain function that brought consciousness allowed a threshold amount of sensory representation of the immediate past external and internal 3D worlds to become integrated with similar information about the present moment of sensory representation. The biocomputational processes of the PIMs in a brain with consciousness derive an internal 4D coordinate system that binds the past with the present, and thus a new time line of existence is created. The shaded area and explanations for curve regions A-C are the same as in Figure 6-4. Curve region D indicates the critical fusion of past information with current sensory representations in the PIM.

agation of this threshold level of representational complexity from PIM to PIM created a flow of a new temporal dimension and an emergent 4D system of organic existence. Thus, the referent system we call consciousness emerged from minute, highly organized regions of the cellular field of life, slowly shaped and refined in evolutionary time: the prefrontal integration modules. This seemingly insignificant shift in 3D sensory world representation, the *one small step up an informational energy hill that resulted in a giant leap over a computational hurdle,* brought a change in the products of neural transformational operations. These products and their effect on the nervous system, on behavior, and thus on the world changed everything.

As first presented in Chapter 3, the model of emergence in organic evolution states: *When the evolutionary process creates a sufficiently ordered organic system such that its 3D structure and function possess a threshold temporal dimension relative to the background flux, an independent 4D coordinate system emerges.* This emergent system is defined as a new level of organic existence and functions as an irreducible frame of reference (a unique property thus emerges that may be defined only by referring to the system). We have now described the only two emergent organic referent systems: life and consciousness.

In the flickering of computational activity in the synaptic fields of the pre-consciousness PIMs, time-locked to each pulse of stimulus processing, the present faded in millisecond time into a past lost to further analysis, and thus lost from existence. But then the threshold derivation and fusion of all four-dimensional relationships in sensory representations across the moments of background neural time in a new brain created a novel time line of biochemical existence. We thus again employ the analogy of a flicker/fusion threshold to indicate the essential function of the temporal dimension in the model of emergent evolution and biological relativity. As in the Muybridge galloping horse and in the motion picture projector or the random-dot stereograms, a new dimension arises when similar representations of sufficient order are integrated in neural modules.

The integrated maximal 4D sensory representation created within a dominant PIM functioning above the critical flicker/fusion threshold at each millisecond computational moment is a *thought.* Each operational cycle of these PIMs thus produces a thought, and this thought is encoded in one or more efferent output projections. The individual thought product thus contains a novel 3D informational structure and the inseparable, internally defined temporal dimension. The PIM may therefore be viewed as the basic structural unit, the functional cell, of consciousness. And consciousness, as stated, is the emergent property, the irreducible frame of reference, defined by the creation-propagation sequence of 4D thoughts within a field of integration modules, independent of the momentary temporal flux of background neural activity. The rate of thought generation sets the serial pulse of consciousness, and the unique representational content of the thought function defines the direction for the arrow of *consciousness time* through *propagated 4D information space.*

Thoughts, by the definition of emergent evolution, are indeed wholly dependent on and sustained by the structure and function of the substrate organic nervous system, and thus are generated at the millisecond rate of the computational activity within the PIMs. Each thought is a unique structure that contains information about the sensory worlds in space and in time (the propagation of which creates a unique 4D information space). Therefore, a thought is, in essence, a *novel probability construct*, a 4D event in millisecond time. By this we mean that when the phase difference between two moments of sensory experience is computed, a functional construct about the 4D experience in the intervening moment is the product; it is the biomathematical derivation of the embedded, inseparable temporal dimension. The thought embodies the physical creation of a temporal dimension, a biophysical link, from a threshold level of 3D representation of two sensory moments. It is no different from the disparity computation that derives the third spatial dimension from a threshold level of representation of two 2D stimulus sources or that derives the temporal dimension from the fusion of a series of 2D images that have physically partitioned it. The brain by its very nature binds in time sensory information and derives higher order and dimension. There is no choice in the matter. In the prefrontal regions of certain mammals (humans), this fundamental neural process creates the fourth dimension of our sensory worlds. The propagation of this reference system operationally defines consciousness.

We may look at the function of the PIM above the critical representational flicker/fusion threshold as that of producing both a computational effect (thought) and the emergent property of consciousness. We will examine the computational effect of the thought function on the nervous system, the entire organism, and the environment in more detail in the next chapter. It will become clear why such a seemingly insignificant modification in the representational order of the afferent sources to the prefrontal fields produced profound effects in the manner by which the nervous system operates, affects behavior, and changes the world. Following an exploration of our model of the thought function in evolution and development (Chapters 8 and 9), we will address the emergent property of consciousness (Chapters 10 and 11).

We have followed the development of the human nervous system from the first cell to the emergence of consciousness and the production of thought. This has been an important trek, as it sets up a point of view and a descriptive language that allow us to begin to understand what it means to talk about thought, thinking, remembering, feeling, and wondering—and, equally important, what it does not mean. We have looked at the great capabilities of the nervous system, but we have also taken notice of the limitations and constraints that bind its functions. It will be necessary to refer back to these chapters when we address evolutionary and developmental issues regarding thought and consciousness. And the time we have spent examining the basics of nervous system anatomy and physiology will be of immense value when we present the portion of the model of consciousness that looks at its limitations and constraints. Finally, when biological relativity is compared to other models of consciousness, the foundation laid in these chapters will help to guide us through the murky maze of conceptual and linguistic formulations.

Frames of Reference in Space and Time

Einstein saw space, time, and dimension in the electromagnetic universe as no one else had before. He understood that locations in space, large or small, that could be defined by a 3D spatial coordinate system must also possess a unique temporal dimension, under specific conditions. Thus, a clock could be used to measure the unique time dimension in a given 3D spatial location. All clocks, whether human-made devices or naturally occurring phenomena that have a rhythmic frequency, exist within the overall electromagnetic frame of reference. They may be moved from local system to local system as measuring devices for the time dimension of a particular system. But only when he adopted the relativistic perspective could Einstein see the true relationships between local reference systems. All dimensions are relative to one another, but only as inseparable components of 4D frames of reference. When one 4D local system is observed from the perspective of another, the relative nature of dimension is noticed, and metrics change when one system is accelerating (linear or rotational) with respect to another. Those changes include the temporal dimension. It is no different from the three spatial dimensions in that respect. For the nonorganic local systems described by Einstein, it was necessary to introduce a motion factor to prove the uniqueness of all 4D frames of reference.

We propose that this grand, epochal insight may be extended into a model of biological structure and function across evolutionary time, a biological relativity. We hold that when 3D biological systems possess a function (a complex set of energy equations) that can produce a unique temporal dimension within its boundaries (one that is distinct from the background clock of biophysical energy flux rates either in the extracellular biosphere or in afferent neural activity), then, and only then, this system becomes an individual 4D frame of reference. It becomes a referent system relative to all other biophysical systems, including the sustaining background energy flux (neural activity, biochemical energy, or electromagnetic field). The biological system's functional aspect possesses a natural clock of its own local, unique metric. This is analogous to any nonbiological 4D frame of reference that is accelerating with respect to any other system. There is no single clock marking universal Newtonian time for all systems; there is an individual, unique temporal dimension for every 4D reference system that exists. Perhaps this is also true for unique biological systems.

In our biological relativity model, we have crossed a critical flicker-fusion threshold only twice: first in cells whose systems propagate an independent temporal dimension and thus create a frame of reference that we call life, and second in PIMs whose systems propagate an independent temporal dimension and thus create a frame of reference that we call consciousness. These are the two biological systems that create an internal temporal dimension within their boundaries and propagate that dimension along its own unique line or arrow of existence.

In the life frame of reference, cells propagate a unique temporal dimension in their most complex product, a replication of the system, seen in cell division. The life temporal dimension is thus both embedded in and indivisible from the ongoing cellular function of external energy transduction and organization. In the consciousness frame of reference, PIMs produce thought products, encoded in axon systems that reach other PIMs to propagate a flow of the PIM's own time dimension. The consciousness-temporal dimension is thus both embedded in and indivisible from the representations of the sensory worlds that drive the computational modules. The products of cells, such as molecular oxygen, forever changed the world in a manner unique to life. The products of PIMs, the nearly infinite variations of thought, also forever changed the world in a manner unique to consciousness.

There was a reason why we began with Einstein, time, dimension, relativity, and life as an emergent reference system in biological evolution. The temporal dimension computed in the prefrontal modules is not *just* time. A clock is not *just* a clock. In inorganic relativity, a clock become an integral, indivisible part of all 4D local systems of matter. As our measuring technology becomes more sensitive, we continue to see that virtually any 3D structural organization of space, relative to another, creates its own unique clock or temporal dimension—a dimension as real as any of the three spatial dimensions.

Human thought and memory, as products created in the 4D reference system of consciousness, may contain and utilize information about the two unique temporal dimensions contained in the reference systems from which they are produced: life in cells and the inorganic universe of space-time.

7
The Thought Effect

The cell and the prefrontal integration modules are the two reference systems that we present in this formulation of organic evolution. These two 4D systems are fundamentally equivalent in that they are both essentially collectives of organic metabolic pathways. The cell and the prefrontal integration module (PIM) perform the basic functions of transduction and organization of complex energy flows within a 3D volume that is thermodynamically bounded with respect to the background system. The cell boundary is the semipermeable, bilayered phospholipid and protein membrane, and the PIM boundary is demarcated by afferent synaptic zones and nonsynaptic cellular relationships.

The concepts of information, entropy, and order as they apply to the cell and the PIM may likewise be viewed as embodiments of a common phenomenon, observed at different levels of organic system analysis (as articulated in the theories of Shannon and Weaver, and others). As you may recall, Gibbs's free energy equation ($\Delta G = \Delta H - T\Delta S$) accounts for the total energy of a system and provides a quantitative approach for comparing the order of one system with respect to another or to the background (entropic) state. The potential information contained in one reaction at a particular moment in time, or in one organic system of reactions, and thus in one independent organic referent system, is related to the ΔG factor in Gibbs's equation. In theory, the principles of information, entropy, order, and Gibbs's free energy must apply to all individual chemical reactions and to all coordinated reactions within distinct cellular and neural systems, including those that create sensory representation and thought generation. Because our model of biological relativity provides an approach to quantifying the energy activity and thereby the information contained within the cell and the PIM, it points logically to the quantification of thought. We are currently a long way from achieving this, however, since the multitude of simultaneous and nonlinear reaction pathways in the simplest cell and in the smallest neural module present a computational problem that we cannot begin to solve.

The collective integration of all energy states and metabolic processes, including the sensory information content of neural activity, manifests as the rise and fall of the background order, and thus the information that flows through each semiclosed system of the cell or PIM. These maximal and minimal states of energy/order/information may be expressed simply as the sinusoidal curves of entropy shown in Chapters 3 and 6. We have proposed that at unique thresholds in organic evolution, the structure and function of the protocell and the proto-PIM were modified in such a way that the downward slope of the internal entropic curve was moved *just enough* to the right (i.e., a level of order inside the system was maintained for a little more time) or the curve peak was elevated *just enough* (i.e., the maximal order achieved inside the system reached a slightly higher negative entropy state) relative to the temporal flux of energy, order, and information in the background supporting system.

In the living cell and the thought-generating PIM, a sufficient amount of internal order is maintained across the minimal state of background entropy to permit the transduction and integration of new energy/order/information from each subsequent influx of background energies. In this way a threshold level is reached that sustains an internal 4D coordinate system. This novel internal state thus produces a thermodynamic or informational *disconnect* from the background system by generating an intrasystem temporal dimension that is unique to each cell and PIM. The cell and the PIM ultimately remain tied to the cascading entropy curves of the background system, whether that of the biosphere or of the neural and metabolic activity, but within their respective 4D reference systems, each produces unique products that are *impossible* to create anywhere else in all of nature (e.g., DNA or thoughts). Cells that lose the threshold internal order cannot create their unique products and return to the background entropic state (life is lost). PIMs that lose the threshold internal order cannot create their unique products, and consciousness is lost.

Sustaining internal order in each 4D system comes at a cost to the background entropic state. The cell reorganizes energy to produce a completely new cell as its most complex product. The PIM likewise reorganizes energy to create thought. In all multicellular plants and animals, some of the energy needed to drive metabolic processes in one location must come from the cellular activity of other regions. For example, the brain appropriates an enormous percentage of the body's energy, including about 20 percent of available metabolic oxygen. Even within a single cell, we see that each neuron dedicates at least 40 percent of its energy-rich ATP to maintaining the resting membrane potential, without which it could not generate a nerve impulse. Thus, the production of thought by PIMs (the ultimate organization of energy) may come at a cost in terms of the resolution of sensory representation along a dimension of potentially available information in visual, auditory, and all other stimulus transduction pathways. In a universe of relative entropic exchange, there is no difference between potential energy and potential information.

Metabolic Pathways, Products, Thoughts, and Memory

Organic products of cellular systems are created when collective chemical reaction energy hills are successfully overcome—that is, when activation energy requirements are met at each reaction step. In the amazing interdependent pathways of cellular metabolic sequences, enzymes and other substrates (or cofactors) are critical components that achieve a lowering of activation energy hills in many reactions. The chemical reactants undergo changes and then relax into stable, novel 3D arrangements, such as peptides, proteins, and carbohydrates. The new chemical order *must* persist in time, and a duration of existence of even a picosecond is sufficient to define a new product in the world of chemical reactions.

The application of the biological relativity model here forces a radical concept: Metabolic pathways of cascading chemical reactions within the single cell may be viewed as analogous to the between-cell functions of multicellular systems. Each is an organic process that represents a sequence of steps of nanosecond to millisecond duration that, over a specific time frame, effect a change in some aspect of the cell or organism, respectively. Large-scale outcomes or changes within a cell or within an organism actually represent piecemeal metabolic work, linked together across time. There is no qualitative biological difference between the cellular product of insulin and a lung's production of respiration. The only difference lies in the level of organization that is imposed by the human observer.

The evolution of organic systems is very much the story of metabolic chemical products, and, of course, this includes the creation of the helices of DNA. Novel organic products are the *building blocks of the evolutionary progression*. Each new product, however slightly modified from its precursor, represents a major achievement of local systems defying the entropic curve to provide more order and more information within 3D arrangements of matter and energy. This cannot be stressed enough. The evolutionary viewpoint of biological relativity brings an equality of nature to each step in the changing biosphere: the first enzyme, the first organelle, the first DNA sequence, the first living cell, the first multicellular organism, the first neuron, the first central nervous system, and the first thought in consciousness. Each is equivalent as an evolutionary masterpiece of negative entropy. Within single cells, novel products become organelles (specialized structures), and within multicellular organisms, entire cell lines become the novel products (specialized cells) created in evolutionary time. And just as intracellular organelles can exist only within the environment maintained by the single cell, specialized cells can exist only within the extracellular environment maintained by the organism. The settings change, but the evolutionary process remains the same. One particular specialized cell type, the nerve cell, produced novel products of its own, including neuroactive compounds, their receptors, and synaptic systems.

In the single nerve cell and the multiple synaptic systems it forms or in brain nuclei, the metabolic pathways that underlie the transduction-integration-transmission of sensory energy achieve unique output products: information encoded in axonal systems. The informational products of computational activity may be converted into a long-lasting structural formation called *memory* through processes utilizing other compounds, which include proteins, enzymes, and other molecules. The brilliant physiologist Donald Hebb hypothesized that structural changes occur in neurons and neural networks following their functional stimulation.[1] It is believed that these long-term changes to the physical structure of the cell serve to increase the probability that the neuron or network will produce nerve impulses when a similar (or partial) stimulation happens again in the future. This basic interpretation of the Hebbian synapse theory indicates that under certain conditions, spatial and temporal patterns of nerve impulse activity induce changes in cells and networks of cells that, in effect, represent the original information. And, most importantly, the structurally embedded or stored representation is available in the future to affect the behavior of the system, and thus of the organism.

The trace of sensory information that endures in structural modifications to brain tissues served as the basis for Hebb's theory of memory as a physical construct. In this theory, memory is not a disembodied, psychological entity with no basis in the biophysics of organic systems; it is an acquired structure that changes through experience. Hebb's theory also challenged the belief that we are born with our memories (perhaps as part of a genetic or spiritual endowment).

The search for the elusive memory trace or *engram* continues today. Eric Kandel and colleagues have done seminal work in defining how nervous systems physically change: in behavioral paradigms of response extinction and habituation, for example. Yet with all our formulations based on various Hebbian synapse theories and the current multidisciplinary neuroscience of genetic, molecular, cellular, and system research into memory, we have still not achieved a full understanding of the way neural systems convert information into long-lasting structures that may be used again and again.[2] For the purposes of this book, however, we can state that the effects of memories may be observed in the many changes that neurons and neural groups undergo following exposure to certain patterns of sensory stimuli. We can also study the process of memory by noting changes in the behavior of the entire animal. Thus, the term *memory* is used in behavioral analysis to infer neuronal changes that may underlie observed large-scale changes at the system level.

Learning and memory can be observed in the nervous system of every animal, from flatworms to humans. Since all nervous systems appear to be capable of forming memories, we suspect that some of the biophysical mechanisms that create memories have been conserved in evolution. Perhaps the manner in which the brain converts or consolidates sensory information into long-term structural representations is similar, if not identical, for all mammalian brains. Thus, when we discuss memory in animals with thought and in those without thought (and thus without consciousness), the relative difference in the way memory affects behavior may not reflect an evolutionary modification to the memory system *per se*; instead, it may indicate a change in the *information* that is being processed. The novel computational product of the prefrontal modules in brains that achieve the frame of reference of consciousness may move through the forebrain memory system in the very same way as any pre-consciousness informational product generated in the brain's neural networks. Based on these considerations, memory may be further operationally defined in all mammals as a *partial* structural representation of an afferent informational wavefront that persists beyond the initial nerve impulse-related event. We further propose that the memory consolidation process (which may involve hundreds of individual metabolic pathways) may preferentially occur within specialized modules or networks in the forebrain memory system. Memory thus is defined as a long-term, dynamic information store.

The dynamic nature of the memory information store may reflect an updating function that matches past information with related, but newer, input to produce a change in the long-term structural component (the trace). In a pattern of recurrent, reiterative processing, new afferent sensory information may enter specialized memory modules in the forebrain that have related, but older, information embedded in the stabilized structure of the cells and tissues of the module. The computational cycle of these modules may then perform the disparity analysis that causes the specialized metabolic processes to alter the information that will remain as part of the module. Incoming afferent representations will be matched with stored ones, and only novel information will create new, long-lasting changes. A representation that was already stored within the memory system does not have to be recreated each time the same sensory stimulus patterns reenter the nervous system. The forebrain memory system will be in a constant state of initiating metabolic processes of consolidation that lead to long-term structural changes, while at the same time performing biocomputational operations at each cycle of afferent sensory flux. Thus, this system may be the single most flexible, dynamic, *noisy*, and energy-consuming aspect of brain function.

It appears that specific afferent input evokes stored memory patterns that have some common informational content, and thus have a reinforcing effect on long-term changes in the memory system. Thus, the efferent output of a memory module that has been stimulated by related sensory afferent flow might have a more significant effect upon the next modular processing region or on motor effector systems (e.g., making a learned action occur more quickly or with less variability). The relational factors or common attributes of the new sensory input and the stored memory may be subtle, but there must be a threshold of sensory information that initiates a linking of representations. The memory efferent outflow from the specialized modules is also constrained to the biophysics of nervous system function, and thus may impart its informational content only in millisecond patterns of axon activity. A long behavioral sequence lasting for several seconds (e.g., reaching out with a hand to choose a food reward in a delayed memory task) is remembered (projected out through effector pathways) only through hundreds of linked millisecond components. We will soon discuss the manner in which the memory system may alter the collective forebrain information library over time and function, and how this may profoundly affect behavior.

Drawing Lines: Pre-Thought, Thought, and Memory

Biological relativity is a model of limits, constraints, and thresholds. The threshold to thought and consciousness, in our model, is to be found in the prefrontal neocortex of certain mammals, the result of an apparent subtle evolutionary modification along the long, long path of increasing order in local multicellular systems. The momentary integration of information sources in PIMs reached a critical limit that produced new local systems, referent systems that maintained internal 4D structures of the sensory world for a threshold time, and propagated this order above the background neural activity flux. Prior to this flicker-fusion threshold of information, the prefrontal neocortex, in concert with the nervous system-generated behavior, learned and remembered quite well with only pre-thought production. Thus, in the brain with consciousness, the thought products are generated only from the PIMs, and all other computational products are of pre-thought order.

The basic neuroanatomy and functional processes in nervous systems without thought are nearly identical to those in nervous systems with thought. The general information flow from PIM to adjacent PIM (by corticocortical short afferent projections), and its output effects on other regions of the nervous system, including the forebrain memory system, is the same in pre-thought and in thought. With respect to the effector systems, both pre-thought and thought effects project onto the same S-curve function presented in the last chapter, relating their general role in the inhibition or reinforcement of ongoing behavior. The operative term here is *ongoing behavior*, because we will see very different behavior in animals with thought.

The major pathways between the PIMs and the forebrain memory system are diagramed in Figure 7-1. There are important timing factors in the flow of sensory representation within the prefrontal region, within the memory system, and between the two. These relationships are illustrated on a time line of neural activity in Figure 7-2. We set the time it takes for a PIM to perform a single cycle of sensory representation processing at about 200 milliseconds (ms). The variables that affect this determination include the afferent synaptic zone activity, intramodular synaptic functions, the internal capacitancelike properties of the entire tissue volume and their role in the informational convergence, and the output flow of nerve impulse activity. Thus, the biophysics of ion flux; nerve impulse generation; neuroactive compound release; transduction by postsynaptic receptors on dendrites, cell bodies, and axonal segments; the cascade of bioelectric and biochemical forces through the tissue volume of the module; and the encoding process of nerve impulses in axon arrays must all be considered when analyzing the operational cycle of a brain region. We do not know enough detail about biomathematical computations by neural tissue to say

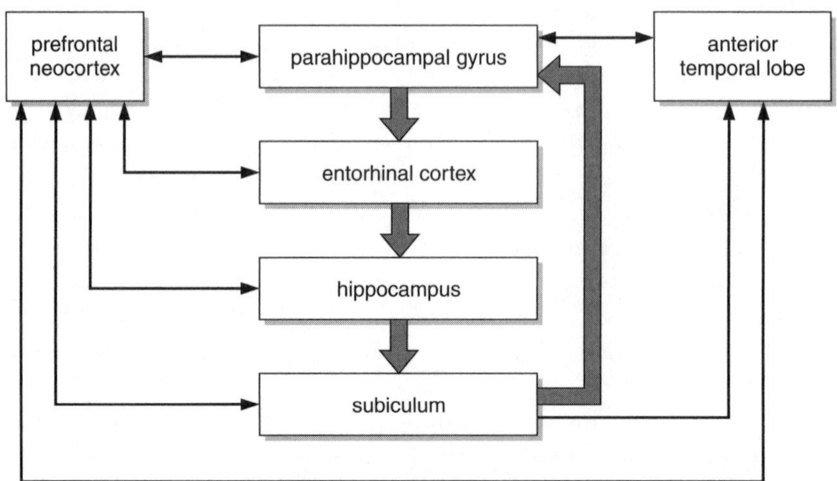

Figure 7-1 Schematic representation of some key forebrain memory system nuclei and their connections with the prefrontal neocortex. The temporal flow of past and present sensory information may be traced through these neural loops. The thick arrows indicate a higher degree of synaptic connection between the brain regions.

whether 200 ms is an accurate estimate, but we will revisit our choice of this time range in a later chapter and explain why we think it is a reasonable estimate. Each modular computational moment therefore results in an efferent output to the adjacent PIMs, the memory system, and all other target regions, affecting their activity at the same rate. The PIM input to the memory system merges with that from other afferent sources (various cortical areas), reaching these same regions across a variety of frequency rates. For the presentation of this model, we will depict the processing of PIM output into the memory system at the same 200-ms time rate, but it should be noted that within the memory system, information might be integrated through its modular regions at other rates.

If we look at the time line in Figure 7-2, we see the PIM-to-PIM, corticocortical processing sequence. Each module marks an integration operation of 200 ms along the horizontal axis. Thus, five modules equal 1 second (s) of sensory representation processing. The efferent output of each module to the memory system is also shown. Memory system integration steps are shown as 200-ms processes, as mentioned. The output of the memory system back to the prefrontal modules is also illustrated. As the time line proceeds (time measured in local background system units of milliseconds), we can track the PIM-to-PIM representation afferent flow $(R'_a t_{n-1})$, the output to the memory system $(R_e t_n)$, the within-memory-system processing, and the afferent contribution of the memory system to a PIM $(R''_a t_{n-x})$. At each prefrontal module location, we note that the reference (*now*) sensory afferent source $(R_a t_n)$ is initiating the integration cycle and that each module is regarded as the dominant PIM during its operation cycle, relative to the next module in the sequence. We can select any module as the time reference and assess the status of the information flow relative to it in a freeze-frame moment.

The forebrain memory system provides a link between the past, the present, and the future for an animal with or without thought. Looking at Figure 7-1, we see the pathways that form a within-system loop: parahippocampal gyrus to entorhinal cortex, to hippocampus, to subiculum, and then back to the beginning. The input from the prefrontal cortex enters this system at many places, but we will consider the parahippocampal/entorhinal

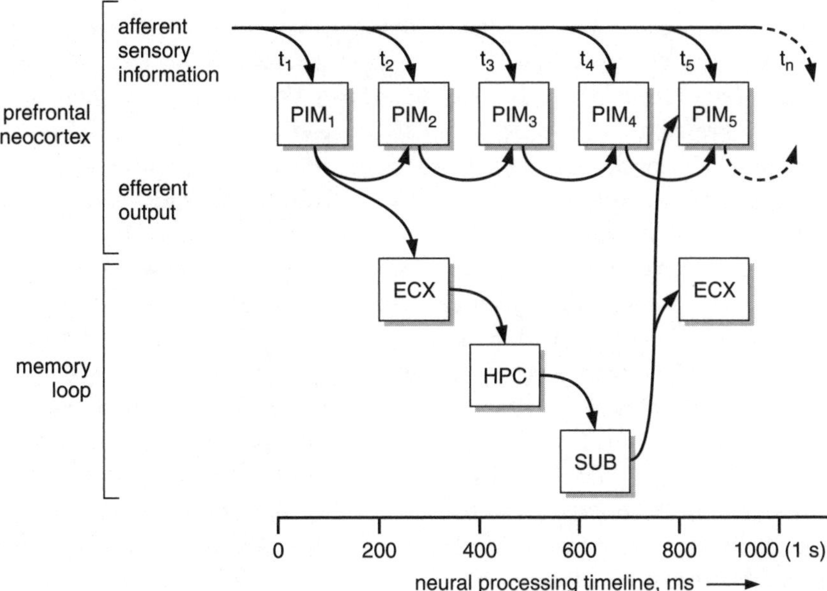

Figure 7-2 Detailed trace of sensory information as it flows through the prefrontal integration modules (PIMs) into the memory system and back again to the prefrontal regions. ECX = parahippocampal entorhinal cortex; HPC = hippocampus; SUB = subiculum. A complex representation of the external and internal sensory worlds may take nearly a second to reenter the prefrontal modules from the memory loop.

region as its primary synaptic region for each focal PIM output moment. The prefrontal modules provide the highest order of sensory representation to this multisynaptic circuit. Recall that this interconnected region of nearly completely multimodal cortex contains information that is already highly processed and that is funneled into the hippocampal spatial location generator by the one-way projection from the entorhinal cortex.

Let us choose this afferent projection into the hippocampal formation as our reference starting point, and follow an informational flow through the processing loop. All sensory information reaching the entorhinal cortex is multimodal, including that from the prefrontal modules. PIM 1 (Figure 7-2) thus sends its *now* output to the entorhinal cortex as a memory system projection. This information is integrated within the entorhinal cortex during that processing moment. That moment would also correspond, in sensory processing time, to PIM 2 as the *now* dominant focus of afferent representation. At the next processing moment (PIM 3), the entorhinal output reaches the dentate gyrus granule cells in the hippocampal formation. It is here that the sensory information that originally came from PIM 1 is projected into the real-time 3D spatial place mapping function. Recall that the locations in the spatial environment may also contain information regarding learned multisensory attributes of a relative positive or negative nature. The output of the hippocampal formation reaches the subiculum and the prefrontal cortex at the next processing cycle (PIM 4). We are regarding the intrahippocampal processing as occurring within the time frame of one modular moment. Finally, the subiculum sends its output to the prefrontal regions (at PIM 5) and to the multimodal areas of the parahippocampal/entorhinal cortex. Information that is integrated through each stage of the memory system recurrent loop begins its conversion into a structural memory of the long-term store. Exactly how, when, where, and what is actually stored is not yet known.

In our diagram of the time line of information flow, we show that the contribution of PIM 1 to the memory system may reenter the prefrontal modules at around PIM 5, or nearly one full second in background time after its derivation. From the perspective of PIM 5 (the current *now* point representation), $R'_a t_{n-1}$, comes from PIM 4, the prior moment, and $R''_a t_{n-4}$, the memory afferent, may contain a partial representation of the *now* as it was at PIM 1. Although perhaps degraded in information and combined with other related sensory representations from the memory system (of perhaps days or years in the past), $R''_a t_{n-4}$ links the current *now*, at PIM 5, with the immediate prior moment ($R'_a t_{n-1}$, from PIM 4), reinforcing a temporal sequence or continuity. In the previous chapter we noted that within the information of PIMs 2, 3, and 4 are some remnants of PIM 1, although at

PIM 5 they have passed through four cycles of computational dilution. Our model proposes that in pre-thought the integration operation within PIM 5 cannot derive the internal temporal relationships between the sensory representations, as they have lost a critical amount of order. However, an incredible repertoire of complex behavior that requires the memory system and prefrontal modules does proceed without thought or consciousness.

The key to understanding complex behavior that depends upon the prefrontal and memory systems, and the link between the hippocampal spatial map and the prefrontal PIMs, lies in the *multimodal 3D spatial environment* in which most behavior is conducted. *In the pre-thought brain, the external 3D multimodal sensory world, as it is transduced by the nervous system, provides the temporal dimension for all complex, learned behavior that must be performed over long time frames.* As behavior is learned and thus transduced into an enduring structural sequence in forebrain memory, the temporal dimension of the external world provides the continuity between the moments of sensory processing. No pre-thought learning can take place otherwise, even with intact prefrontal and memory systems. If, for example, half-second (or second, or ten-second) moments in a behavioral sequence to be learned were in some manner partitioned and the sequence was mixed up in temporal order, no learning of the entire sequence could take place. Learning is produced along a temporally consistent dimension created by the background sensory environment, the local space-time system. This may sound obvious because we take it for granted and do not even notice the structure of our moment-to-moment sensory processing that the environment, the *context*, provides.

Ivan Pavlov demonstrated the key role of the temporal dimension for the simplest of learning tasks that needed a memory system but not a prefrontal cortex.[3] In his conditional learning experiments, he demonstrated that a dog could be taught to salivate in response to the sound of a bell by ringing the bell shortly before giving food to the dog. After several trials of this paired stimulus presentation, he discovered that the sound alone would cause salivation—a simple, but truly remarkable, demonstration of what learning is all about. If the temporal dimension of this learning situation is disrupted—that is, if the food is presented before the bell—no learning takes place. No association is made between the two stimuli; no integration is performed in the memory system that produces the structure of a learned behavior. All other spatial dimensional constructs remained intact; only time was altered. This classical conditioning paradigm holds that in pre-thought, in any complex learning situation that requires a sequence of conditions, procedures, choices, and rewards, it is only when the proper temporal alignment of learning procedures are presented that learning can take place.

For another example, let's imagine that a healthy adult male chimp was to be trained to do the following task: (1) Keep a blank video screen in his visual field for several seconds without looking away, (2) remain still while a single light comes on and goes off, (3) wait until a different (*go*) light in the middle of the screen comes on, (4) and then reach out and touch the place on the screen where the first light appeared. The chimp can learn this delayed-matching-to-sample (DMTS) type of procedure, although it may take hundreds of sessions to shape the behavior into a sequence. At each teaching step, a paired stimulus and reward must be used to guide the learning and memory toward the final, linked, complicated behavioral sequence. If the food reward is given before the desired behavior during any part of the learning of this sequence, the chimp will not be able to learn the procedure—ever. Or, if the chimp has previously been taught to touch the screen when a light goes off but now is put in front of the screen and given no reward until after the entire sequence of light-delay-*go* light, the chimp will not be able to learn the procedure—ever. If on one day the *go* light comes on before the signal light, and on the next day the order is reversed, the chimp will never be able to learn the procedure. If a reward is given after the signal light, but before the *go* light, the chimp will not be able to learn the behavioral sequence. And so on.

We might ask, why could the chimp not eventually figure it out, especially if he sometimes got food after the correct temporal sequence, and especially if he already knew about touching the screen after a light goes out? Perhaps we could just have him watch another chimp perform the correct task. But that does not work either. Even the simpler task, in which the chimp reaches out to touch the place where the light has just gone out, cannot be learned if during the early training phase we sometimes gave the reward before the light went out. The task is always too difficult if the temporal sequence is not strictly maintained and if the pairing of stimulus and reward is not used at each segmented behavioral point along the complex sequence during the training sessions. This has always been the case in animal and infant human learning and memory. From Pavlov's dog to the brightest nonhuman primate, there are strict limits to what can be remembered when the temporal sequence of a procedure is altered. The examination of task difficulty, stimulus saliency or adequacy, and other parameters of experimental learning and memory studies are always important considerations and must be carefully addressed; as should be the considerations of what exactly is being taught, learned, and remembered.

Paradoxically, the radial-arm maze experiment described in the last chapter would appear to contradict the importance of a strict temporal sequence for pre-thought learning. In the standard eight-arm radial maze design, a rat or mouse will effortlessly learn to forage for food in each arm without making a repeat visit. Even when considerable delays or distractions are imposed between the choices, the rats or mice perform at a high level of accuracy. This is equivalent to a delayed-nonmatching-to-sample (DNMTS) task, and rodents do it with very little shaping. Let us step back and look at the entire context of the experiment, the room, the open maze, and the animal as it moves along its paths.

As we watch the animal move through the behavioral sequence, we can see that all the sensory information by which it conducts its movements is always there and that this information remains stable over the entire time of the task. Not only is it there, but it is there in a constant 4D arrangement. Let us juxtapose this setting with another that was used in many memory experiments during the decades prior to the invention of the radial-arm spatial maze. It was always known that a rodent, a dog, a cat, or a monkey could not keep a list of choices in its mind during memory tasks; thus, these animals were seen as having limited intellectual capacity. In many standard linear maze settings of the time, a behavioral choice made at point A, usually a go-left or go-right choice, had to be remembered at the subsequent choice points B, C, and so on in order for the animal to efficiently gain the reward at the end of the correct path. It was found that animals could learn to perform a series of left, left, left, or right, right, right, choices fairly well, but that when the sequence was set up with any more complexity, such as left, left, right, left, and if any delay was imposed, no animal could learn the task.

What was the difference? In the linear sequence maze tasks and many other memory test settings, the information at choice point A is not externally, spatiotemporally available at choice point B; the information at neither choice point A nor that at B is present at choice point C; and so on. No rat, dog, cat, or monkey can take the 4D sensory context along with it: Each stimulus setting disappeared as the animal moved ahead in the maze. The *now* faded by the time the next choice point came along. But all of a sudden, rats in Olton's maze were displaying comparatively genius-level memory work! Because Olton's maze was radial and not linear, it provided a context in which the 4D sensory environment, and all choice points or places within it, did not fade in the nervous system and hippocampal spatial map; the entire maze was always there to drive and update the system's function.

In settings where a 4D sensory environment, or several of them, is present for the duration of the memory task (even when delays are imposed), the full power of the prefrontal-hippocampal memory system may be allowed to exhibit itself. Simple one- or two-choice actions can be accomplished quickly, without a delay of more than a second or so; but in any behavioral sequence in which one moment of behavior is needed to guide the next, the temporal dimension between the two must be provided by the external 4D sensory environment. If the 4D setting is not available to provide an enduring temporal dimension to the nervous system, behavioral learning is limited to the immediate *now*, which fades in seconds as the animal either moves beyond a local 4D system or is removed by the experimental procedure. The information that is provided by the external context fades rapidly in the pre-thought brain when it is removed. In the pre-thought world, the past may be used in the present to form decisions, but much of what the past is (that is, the 4D sensory environment) must exist in the present as an informational force that provides the link between moments of behavior.

We can follow this progression in Figure 7-2. From the memory system, the output of the spatial map generator reaches the prefrontal cortex, and together they can keep a behavior flowing smoothly along its learned sequence. As long as the external sensory environment provides the information to generate a real-time internal representation, learned comparisons about locations in the environment, or choices, may be computationally possible. No discrete, independent, memory-generated lists of locations or of the steps in a long behavioral sequence and no memory of where one has been or what one has been doing need to be maintained in the prefrontal cortex or memory system. Most of this information, along with the temporal dimension linking the moments of behavior, is present in the 4D sensory world: *The context determines the behavior*. When the context is removed, or when the 3D spatial arrangement is radically altered, the ability to maintain the information fades rapidly within the nervous system of the pre-thought brain. The nervous system, including the prefrontal and memory regions, cannot keep the past alive long enough to help it decide what to do in the present; the fade of the *now* is too rapid. (There is more to this story, and we will return to it in Chapter 8.)

Now we will cross our threshold line and discuss what happens in the brain with thought and consciousness. Again, we can follow the temporal flow of information between prefrontal modules and the memory system in Figure 7-2. We propose that the prefrontal modules create, maintain, and integrate a level of order and information about two sequential moments of the 3D sensory worlds by including the unique internal temporal dimension. As this order of information, now a 4D sensory representation, is propagated across the prefrontal modules and into the memory system, the past is retained above a critical threshold, and a fusion of moments in full 4D endures as the referent system of consciousness. Therefore, unlike in the pre-thought brain, the past in all its dimensions is internally available in the present, and the integration of the two may produce thought products related to behavior sequences that now do not necessarily depend upon the local 4D spatiotemporal context. They certainly can take computational advantage of it, as it makes nearly all complex behavior easier to conduct. Again, this is usually the type of environment within which we naturally function. It is the context within which all cellular life evolved. We just do not pay attention to this fact in our daily moment-to-moment existence, and we ignore it far too often in our scientific and philosophical endeavors.

In thought and consciousness, the ongoing fusion of complex sensory information about the current state of the external and internal worlds with the thought-memory of the past defines a new order of computational possibilities. The products of PIM function, thoughts, may contain full 4D sensory constructs that do not wholly depend upon the current 4D environment. These thoughts also affect behavior and the memory system. The thought effect may be context-independent in the consciousness frame of reference.

The temporal dimension, which provides the critical link between moments of computational activity and thus behavioral sequences, is internally derived from the integration of two or more moments of 3D sensory information. In consciousness, a new context—an internal one—is produced that now may move with the individual in space and time. From one external context to another, from one moment to the next, the internally created 4D sensory worlds do not fade as quickly in the absence of the just-past local external environment.

We have now begun to introduce the power of thought and its effect on computation and behavior. An evolutionary modification brought a threshold organic order that generated novel 4D local systems (thoughts) that are linked by ongoing nervous system activity to produce an independent propagated frame of reference called consciousness. This evolutionary modification produced a computational disconnect between the nervous system and its background sensory context, as did the modification that brought a thermodynamic disconnect between the cell and its complex energy background. They are one and the same, from a perspective of relative entropy, order, and information in local organic systems.

Drawing Lines: A Finger in a Pool of Mud

In Chapter 4 we followed the development of the human fetus and described the little girl who was born. She developed normally, and we last saw her playing near a pool of mud. Our focus was on her index finger, as she dipped it and then moved it in the muddy liquid. We noted that the external observation of large-scale movements in her hand and finger was actually an illusion based on a multitude of millisecond-scale nervous system functions performed by billions of cells. Now that we have moved through the development of this child's nervous system, from below the brain to the cerebral cortex and to the prefrontal integration modules forming thoughts in the referent system of consciousness, we will add to the account the full complement of sensory experience, memory, and computational ability.

The child's little finger moves along a path in the pool of mud. Each 4D multisensory moment is fused with the next in the prefrontal cortical modules, and the thought products flow into the next dominant focal PIM and to the memory system (Figure 7-2 again shows the timing of the information flow). Within this stable four-dimensional external context, the real-time spatial map system may continue to update the location of the finger and its relationship to the body (parietal function), the mud (visual and multimodal), and other local places (hippocampal and multimodal). The ongoing change in finger position and its effect on the mud are present in the fused moments of thought, together with the prefrontal multimodal function. In 200-ms moments of the PIM-memory-PIM flow of an internally derived 4D sensory experience and context analysis, a world of relationships between each movement and the resultant change in the mud become computational information.

The point in the mud where the finger began its current movement, the past, is now computationally maintained and integrated with each successive (≈ 200-ms) change, and these integrated moments of thought enter into the memory system's loop of reiterative activity. As the child continues to move her finger, a line begins to grow in each of two overlapping sensory domains of thought: the integrated vector of motion in the somatosensory and viscerosensory informational flow to the brain, and the integrated changes in the surface of the mud. This visually dominant information (when vision is possible), fused in moments of thought and then thought-memory, grows along the vector of motion. The line in the mud has dimensions of length, depth, and width that the nervous system may now compute in updated moments of time. The entire 4D structure of the line is now a computational entity in the thought-memory system of the child's brain. The individual moments were not lost between PIM computational cycles, as they would have been in the pre-thought brain, but they were fused in the ongoing internal representation of the 4D sensory worlds.

The young child takes her finger out of the mud. The deformation she created in the shallow pool quickly dries in the heat of the afternoon sun and becomes an enduring part of the surface structure. She looks at her work, her art, her construction. A line becomes both a computational construct in thought-memory and a visual entity as well. The two are stored and recombined in the dynamic memory system. When the demands of the current environment and homeostasis allow, the computational fields of prefrontal modules may again experience these moments, perhaps when the child views another line in another setting. The similar memories that are evoked may be integrated with the current sensory context in the PIM regions. This is where one line may be computationally compared to another line, where one and one may become two. Perhaps it is also where the one line, as an expression of the child's ability to change the world, is paired with a representation of her own self as her personal mark in memory.

The Beginning of the Thought Effect

No longer bound to the tides of momentary sensory experience, the past and present may be brought together in a thought and then recombined with a future moment in a future place. In memory, the dynamic additions and reorganization of each thought product bring an additional, explosive effect. The reiterative, recombinant function of the memory system on each linked moment of thought produced by the prefrontal modules brings about astronomical computational possibilities for this information. The only limits are the representational content of each thought and the time it takes to interrelate the thoughts.

Over decades of experience, an enormous amount of novel information may be created, stored, and used in thought activity. Moreover, the nervous system does not *care* what direction the internal information flow follows. Thus, when conditions permit, thought-memories may dominate the PIM activity and the past may become more heavily weighted in the real-time computations of sensory experience. Furthermore, the integration of two or more moments in PIM activity may produce a novel thought product that has few or no correlates in the current sensory worlds. The internally generated 4D system of thought, as propagated across time, has its own independent temporal flow that is determined by the sequence of information content entering into the dominant computational modules. Under certain conditions, the internal arrow of computational time may flow into the past or along an informational stream never experienced in the external sensory environment. It is an internally created world of brief, fused moments. It remains dependent upon the background reference systems to some extent, however, and it is the external and visceral internal stimulus environments that usually dominate and drive the vast majority of thought content.

The foundations of the powerful thought effect can be seen in the imagined thoughts of our young girl playing in pools of mud and comparing dried lines. It is the effect of thought in the reference system of consciousness that generates all math, music, language, art, tools, technology, and science. The thought effect is at once a computational effect in the prefrontal modules and the memory system, and a behavioral effect on other living systems and the larger referent system of the biophysical universe. The computational effect serves to link moments of sensory experience so that the gains of the past are not lost as the changing context of the future arrives. The memory system builds lasting internal structures from these context-independent, moment-to-moment gains. The behavioral effect serves to link moments of effector actions on the background referent systems so that the gains of the past actions are not lost as the changing context of the future arrives. The behavioral effect builds lasting external structures from a series of context-independent actions that are linked along their own, unique temporal dimension.

We can finally begin to imagine where in the nervous system lies not only the letter A, the word FIRE, a pencil, or a face, but also an emotion, a sense of time, math, music, art, science, and a sense of beauty, truth, and love. We also can imagine the potential for genius and creativity and the horror of insanity as a disorder of the thought effect. What were impossible computations and behaviors below the flicker-fusion threshold are now the building blocks of development of thought and consciousness. Besides the little girl in our example, who else crosses the threshold to thought in nervous system activity and behavior? When does thought begin during brain development? What are the limits and constraints of the thought effect? We may now begin to answer each of these overarching questions.

Context Is Everything

Biological relativity is a model of limits, constraints, and thresholds. Now we have enough tools to explicitly draw some lines that will further separate our model from nearly every other formulation of thought, mind, and consciousness. We will also endeavor to use basic terminology organized into useful operational definitions. Our purpose in doing this is to be able to easily compare the definitions produced by the model with sources of experimental data, with our daily experience of life and consciousness, and with all other models and definitions. In this way, we can determine whether our model has utility and validity.

The biological relativity model postulates that there are no partial frames of reference in nature—not in the electromagnetic field, not in cells, and not in the nervous system. Thus, it follows that there are no partially living cells and no partial thought or consciousness. Either a cell produces novel products by metabolic processes or it does not. Either a PIM produces novel thoughts by computational processes or it does not. Only cellular function defines the 4D referent system of life, and only PIM function defines the 4D referent system of consciousness. For better or worse, when we use our model to make comparisons to others, we do not have to equivocate on these points.

Thought is a novel product of specialized prefrontal integration modules that contain a 4D sensory representation derived from the momentary integration of afferent information sources: $f(R_a t_n, R'_a t_{n-1}, R''_a t_{n-x} 0)$. Each thought is limited in informational content and time duration, but contains an internally derived temporal dimension that is indivisible from the three spatial dimensions contained in its informational structure. Only when a specialized PIM integrates a threshold order between 3D sensory representations may it generate an internal 4D product, the thought. Each thought is a novel construct, and thus the brain produces an unimaginable (but finite) number of different thought products over a lifetime. The propagation of these novel 4D sensory representations across prefrontal modules binds these moments into an internally generated, ongoing temporal dimension of experience.

Thinking is the process of thought propagation and integration between prefrontal modules and the memory system. *Mind* is the description of the current 4D informational space, the internally generated sensory world as it is expressed in real time. It is the currently available knowledge base of thought. *Consciousness* is the collective properties of the propagation of thought in time. It is the name of the irreducible 4D frame of reference that emerges from the operations of PIMs generating the product of thought. We will describe consciousness and the language of its emergent properties in Chapters 10 and 11.

Part Four

THRESHOLDS OF THOUGHT IN EVOLUTION AND DEVELOPMENT

8
Insect Thoughts and Animal Minds

To look for evidence of thought and consciousness in the animal world, we must understand and operationally define the ubiquitous concept of behavior. Behavior can be simply defined as a process of actions and reactions. Behavior reflects the changing relationships, or the changing order, in a temporal sequence of linked actions and reactions. All descriptions of behavior depend upon both the individual units of matter involved in the actions and the surrounding 4D space-time context.

The connection between the smallest particles of inorganic matter and the most complex actions of human behavior begins to unfold when we adopt this operational definition of behavior. The process of behavior is defined by the 4D context within which it occurs. There is no fundamental, qualitative difference in behavior across all organizations of nature; only the context and organizations of matter and energies change. This conceptualization of behavior logically follows from the operational definitions of energy, order, and information as manifestations of the general process of entropy.

To illustrate the operational definition of behavior as the process of changing order in time, we may look at a metabolic process inside mitochondria known as the citric acid cycle (or Krebs cycle). The paths that molecules take through the Krebs cycle are depicted in Figure 8-1. This complex sequence of mitochondrial metabolic reactions ultimately produces the energetic compound ATP, which is indispensable in sustaining life. If we imagine ourselves standing among all the incredible activity of energy exchange and chemical bond formation occurring at the nanometer scale of organic organization, we will easily acknowledge that this is indeed a behaving system.

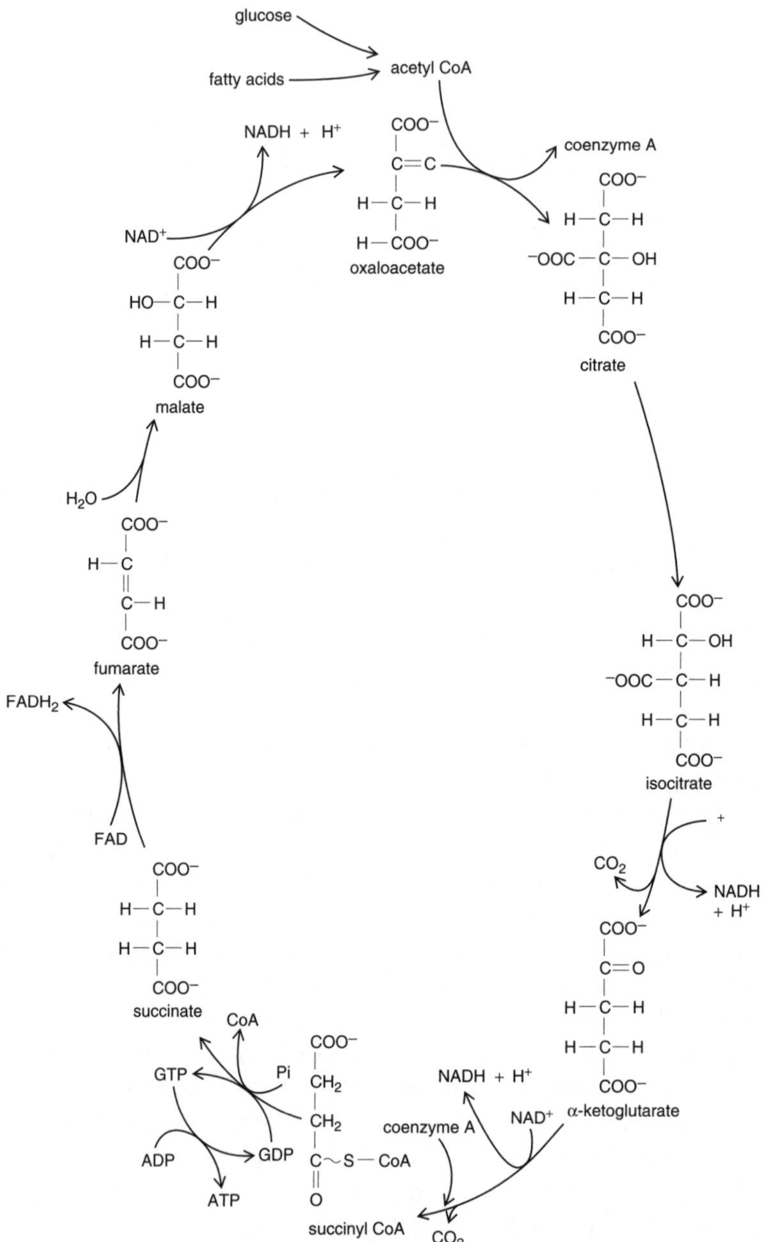

Figure 8-1 Citric acid cycle. Biochemical pathways in living cells demonstrate the complex behaviors of molecules. The citric acid cycle depicted occurs in the mitochondria and produces life-sustaining energetic compounds. (*From The Encyclopedia of Science and Technology, 8th ed., McGraw-Hill, 1997, vol. 3, p. 732; reproduced by permission of The McGraw-Hill Companies.*)

We can observe the process of behavior in multicellular systems on the millimeter scale of organization and context. The basic circulatory system found in air-breathing animals involves hemoglobin molecules picking up oxygen in the lungs and transporting it to all peripheral tissues, then bringing carbon dioxide from the cells back to the lungs in an exchange cycle. In this relatively large-scale context of matter and energy, we observe the complex behavior of hemoglobin as it rides around in red blood cells performing its function of oxygen exchange and sustaining the life of the entire animal. We observe the changing, dynamic relationships of cells in a temporal sequence that takes place within the larger context of the circulatory system, which, in turn, functions within the larger organism. At this same scale of organization, the nervous system also evolved its own repertoire of behavioral sequences.

We cannot divorce any of the aforementioned pathways of changing relationships and order from their local contexts. In evolutionary time or in real-time behavior, each inorganic, organic, cellular, or multicellular system is inexplicably tied to its environment for description and understanding. *The context determines the behavior* that we, the observers, classify into temporal sequences and then name. As mentioned in the last chapter, we just tend not to notice the local 4D context system because it is always present. Thus, when we select just one collective pathway for study—e.g., the Krebs cycle, the production of a neuropeptide or urine, the process of respiration, an eye blink, or the galloping of a horse—we tend to ignore the importance and determining influence of the local context. We must do this in part to reduce the informational load when we look at a complex pathway or behavior. But our tendency to focus on one pathway to the exclusion of the larger environmental influences may lead to an illusion of context independence for certain classes of behaviors.

We must recognize that along the long road of organic evolution that produced living cellular systems, the genetic code has been slowly shaped and molded by the local external context. The results of these evolutionary modifications are cells and organisms that can exist, and thus behave, only within a particular niche (regardless of how big a niche it may be). As we now begin to look at behavior in animals (on several scales of organization) for evidence of thought and consciousness, we must remain acutely aware of the importance of the local 4D context when we impose any particular scheme of behavior partitioning upon nature's ongoing and interdependent organic existence. For, if we define a particular time-limited sequence of organic actions and reactions as a behavior but fail to include the influence of the surrounding 4D niche, we may create the illusion of an action that is disconnected from its environment. When this happens, we may erroneously infer that all the information and energy for the particular behavior was generated from within the animal, when, in reality, the conditions of the context influenced the sequence of actions to a significant extent.

Is all behavior at every level of organization explicitly tied to the local 4D reference system? We can imagine that each atom in a long fusion chain reaction that is building a more complex element does not have any choice in the matter (pun intended). In cellular life, we can imagine that each enzyme in the citric acid cycle is under the full control of the surrounding cellular system. We can imagine that a red blood cell traveling its course around the body, bringing oxygen to each and every cell, does not have any options available to it. However, when we observe a single-celled organism, a plant, a jellyfish, or another more complicated animal that moves around its niche by the action of a nervous system, does our story change? In the life referent system, when is an animal's behavior not a consequence of the immediately present local systems interacting with its genetic-based functional systems? In the terminology of biological relativity, when does a nervous system generate a thought product that propagates an internal 4D frame of reference—consciousness—that liberates the animal from the strict millisecond moment-to-moment stimulus-response control of the local context?

Does it take more than one neuron to generate thought and consciousness? If so, then we can imagine that animals with very few neurons do not generate thought, and therefore that each of their computational moments, such as they are, is driven by the real-time sensory environment, and that each effector output (reaction) is related to these conditions. We must note, however, that a certain amount of learning and thus memory, expressed as enduring changes in certain behavioral responses that come with experience, is found in virtually every nervous system studied.

The threshold of thought and consciousness in animal nervous systems is found where the past is computationally available in the present at a critical order and dimension that allows the internal derivation and propagation of an ongoing unique 4D existence. We propose that the evolutionary transition to this emergent frame of reference can be observed in large-scale behaviors expressed through effector output pathways of the memory and motor systems.

In the following sections, we will examine large-scale or multisystem animal behavior and decide if and where such actions may indicate the crossing of the flicker-fusion threshold into thought and consciousness. Four examples will provide a broad view of animal behavior and at the same time reinforce the fundamental processes of behavior in context that relates them all. We will first describe particular behaviors in the language that is typically employed in nearly all descriptive accounts, which we have termed anthropomorphic lexicology. Following the descriptive passages, we will analyze the behavior in context and apply our formulations.

Caste in Mud: African Termite Cities

Rising out of a hot, flat terrain covered with patches of wild grass and isolated groves of small, bushlike trees, we see several towers of reddish brown clay. Each tower, or mound, tapers up from a large base to a narrow, open, cylinder-shaped peak. One of these towers is about 5 feet high; another is more than 10 feet from base to top. In the quiet, dry heat of the day, these towers hide bustling communities of life. These odd mud mounds are the constructions of the African termite, one of about 2,500 species of insects of the order *Isoptera* and a distant relative of the cockroach.

Termite cities begin when a male and female pair, direct descendants of a king and queen, fly away from their birth colony. Upon landing and losing their wings, they create a wedding chamber in the mud, mate, and then begin to give birth to their own subjects. The reproductive couple is now at once entombed in their wedding site, their mating chamber, their delivery room, and their grave. They will not leave this chamber, and the queen may live for more than a decade. As this royal pair gives birth to the first of their young, they will cannibalize many of these offspring for nourishment. As the growing number of young larvae begin to develop into infant termites, they are put to work taking care of their parents.

The genetic code in each larva can produce a royal termite, but local environmental conditions alter its complete expression to produce one of three classes of insect. The growing colony has a strict caste system of royals, workers, and soldiers. Once a young worker termite is born into a caste, it cannot ever hope to be anything other than what it is. Each worker has antennae, but is a blind, wingless, pale subject about 5 to 6 millimeters (mm) in length, with a lifespan of 3 or more years. The soldier termite is much like the worker, but it is slightly larger, has a harder covering on its head, and has larger pinching jaws. The soldier is also blind and wingless. The queen begins to produce more and more eggs each day. She grows in size to a grotesque length of up to 10 centimeters (cm). She is virtually immobile and must be groomed and fed by the attendant king and workers. In her peak productive years, she may produce literally thousands of eggs each day, and millions in her lifetime.

The workers begin to build the city with dirt, spit, and feces. It is hard work, with long days and little time for rest or reflection. The workers carry a heavy load. They must build and repair the city, gather food and water, feed and groom the queen, make all roadways through the mound and special chambers, and feed and groom every soldier termite. The soldiers' only function is to react to intruders and to give their lives to stop invasions. They cannot see, they cannot feed or care for themselves, and they can never reproduce or leave to set out on their own. When their archenemies, the ants, come near, they attack and will fight to the death to defend the queen. If a hungry anteater should arrive and begin to destroy the city walls in its foraging, the soldier termites will not run or retreat, but will engage in a futile battle with the furry giant. They do not waver from their duty, their singular purpose in life.

The worker termites construct an amazing metropolis, the likes of which are not seen among the constructions of any other insect, bird, or nonhuman mammal on the planet. Within the unassuming mud towers, the workers create a nursery for the young larvae, roadways for travel and removal of waste products, and a ventilation system that maintains temperature and humidity within a narrow range. Perhaps even more mind-boggling are the fungus gardens that the workers build, seed, tend, and harvest to provide food for all. The crowning achievement of the termite city occurs when the atmospheric conditions of temperature and humidity reach a critical threshold. Pairs of young royals lift off in flight to cast their fate to the wind; if they are fortunate, they fall to the ground to begin their own kingdoms.

Should we now begin to discuss the emotional and cognitive life of the members of this incredibly complex society? Should we empathetically imagine the horror of eating one's firstborn, and the emotional scar that it must leave on the ruling couple for the remainder of their reign? Does the young worker termite lament its sterile, blind, wingless status and dream of ascending to the throne? Does the colony experience an unimaginable fear as an anteater crushes hundreds of its members? Have soldiers ever rebelled, led by a termite Spartacus? Does the queen care about her subjects? Does she hear their cries? What are the termites' thoughts, their memories, and their experience in consciousness?

If our descriptive presentation of termite life is valid to some degree, then perhaps our model and our operational definitions of thought, mind, and consciousness are too restrictive and are limited to a nervous system of far too much complexity. It may be that other operational definitions and models of thought, mind, and consciousness that would accept some or all of the above passages are reflective of the reality of life. Under a more generous model, the termite nervous system might produce thoughts and have consciousness of some type. If this is the case, the threshold between pre-thought and pre-consciousness, on the one hand, and thought and consciousness, on the other, might be found somewhere else along the evolutionary pathway of nervous system modification; we should then be focusing on the ants, the worms, the jellyfish, or the hydra to locate the threshold of thought and mind. If an adequate and sufficient conceptualization of thought, mind, and consciousness, of choice, will, intent, the past, the present, the future, and societies in common purpose, is present in the termites' city of mud, then we need go no further. If this is the case, the historical and current debates in human society about consciousness have been a needless exercise. If this is the case, an adequate theory of consciousness merely needs to state that if a neuron or a network of neurons exists, there is thought and consciousness. However, if termite behavior indicates thought and consciousness, is this the same as canine or primate thought and consciousness? Ultimately, if there exists a different type of consciousness for each and every nervous system, then there is little need for the term.

All single cells, their intracellular behavior, and their reactive behavior relative to the background context can be fully described and understood within the biophysical parameters of the life field, as the collective behaviors of multicellular animals must also be. It is just far more difficult and time-consuming to describe large-scale behavior without resorting to terminology that reflects our human experience in the consciousness field. If any single cell or any termite generated thought in some manner, and thus functioned within the consciousness frame of reference, it would have an internally derived 4D informational space that would grow in size and complexity over time. As its experience accumulated, its behavioral repertoire would grow. The expansion of its repertoire of behaviors from an inborn, inherited, genetically coded set of predispositions and internal cycles to more complex epigenetic or novel actions would be observable by their effect on the organism and the local environment.

Thus, if termites generated thought, as defined by our model, a member of any caste would be able to modify its routine, based on past information, in the present context. Some behavior would not be explicitly tied to the totality of 4D sensory information supplied by the immediate, millisecond context. Something would change; variations would arise, and new patterns would develop. This is the developmental process that we so carefully monitor in human infants, children, and adults. Thought and memory combine to produce a progression of informational, and thus behavioral, change. We do not find a termite Spartacus or Gandhi inciting a working-class revolt, or a queen that grows tired of giving birth and longs for the independence of her youth. The past in termite time is lost as each moment of nervous system computational activity brings the next wavefront of sensory information to the association regions of the termite's tiny brain. Wide variations in behavioral repertoires, or a developmental progression of significant behavioral change, might not work for this system of living organisms. The process of evolution molded the colony, and that encompasses how each multicellular member interacts with the local surround.

The termite brain contains several hundred thousand nerve cells and other tissues. The neurons are like those found in all other brains, and they are arranged in a nervous system that contains receptors and peripheral and central or associative regions. The specific distribution of types, numbers, and locations of receptors is unique to the termite, but these receptors are mechanical, thermal, chemical, and photon energy transducers (of course, only the royals have functional eyes). The genes that code the complete protein library in each termite have been shaped in evolutionary time. The nervous system in the termite, like the nonneural cells and systems, functions in moments of metabolic time, and this time scale is basically one of milliseconds.

Each behavior that we observe, categorize, and name is, as we will continue to state, a collection of millisecond moments for every nervous system. In freeze-frame, stepwise sequences, a termite behaves within its local 4D context of sensory influences. The sensory environment that surrounds each larva—the chemical, thermal, and perhaps mechanical forces—determines whether a reproductive, worker, or soldier termite will develop. The determination is complete in the interaction between the genetic products and the environment. There is no partial worker, no half-blind royal with one wing who gathers food and grooms other termites. Each product of developmental pathways, each caste of termite, has a behavioral repertoire that was built little by little over an immense number of generations. The common branch of cockroachlike insect diverged around 200 million years ago.

Thus, at each moment in the local environment of sensory forces, the all-encompassing context determines what the termite will do at the next moment, millisecond to millisecond. If we looked at a freeze-frame sequence of the context-behavioral dance at the millisecond rate, we would see that the coordinated movements of a termite are guided by changes in the sensory surround. At millisecond moments, the termite brain binds in time as much of the sensory world as can be transmitted to it, performs computational operations, and sends efferent output to effector systems.

For example, an approaching ant would be preceded by its chemical identification, a wave of pheromone molecules that would stimulate the receptors on the soldier termites. This stimulation would initiate an internal motor sequence that would move the termites along the chemical gradient, and thus toward the source of the stimulation, and cause their jaws to open. The closing of the soldier termites' jaws would occur when a mechanical force, like a hard object, stimulated them. As long as the pheromone chemical gradient is above a threshold stimulating concentration, the soldier termites will fight. Even the ultimate product of colony behavior, the flight of the reproductive pairs, is determined by the local environment of temperature, humidity, and other factors that stimulate the pattern of behavior that opens the wings and leads to an airborne exit from the mound. The couples do not just decide to go off and build a new home.

If the grand complexity of the termite world does not (in fact, cannot) depend on the presence of thought and consciousness, what does that tell us? It reinforces what we have been showing at every level of organization in living cells and cellular systems: that when we observe systems over time, we the observers are compelled to describe these systems in terms that impart to them aspects of our experience in thought and consciousness. We make the termites thoughtful and mindful. We see them making choices, tending gardens, protecting the colony, grooming other termites, and designing cities. We infer that they have a growing informational system that includes concepts such as architecture, gardening, and war. Termites are not able to step back and observe (or remember) their ongoing behavior on such a long time scale of minutes, hours, or years. Their world is composed of chemical, temperature, and moisture gradients that stimulate simple, repetitive motor sequences that may be modified to some extent by learning mechanisms. They behave to the full extent of their genetic expression within the confines of their environment, and that is all. It is we who make them so thoughtful, so mindful, and so clever.

Love Is Blind: Clever Hans

The much-told story of the horse named Hans, its owner Wilhelm Von Osten, and the scientist who studied them, Oskar Pfungst, retains its importance today for several reasons.[1] First, it has great historical significance as a tale of how uncritical acceptance of staged performances may influence how we think about mind and consciousness. Second, it marked an important moment in the science of behavior, as it was one of the first formal studies of animal intelligence. Finally, the story of Hans serves to highlight how information in the local context determines ongoing behavior, but, if disguised or ignored, can lead to dramatic illusions about the source of intelligence.

Turn of the century Germany produced a phenomenon called Hans, the amazing horse. Hans and his teacher, Wilhelm, toured Europe demonstrating Hans's remarkable intellect and thinking abilities. Hans, as Wilhelm had discovered, could count. It turned out that not only could Hans count, but he could add, subtract, multiply, divide, and analyze complex formulas written on a blackboard, including calculus. Beyond math, Hans could spell people's names. Hans, not surprisingly, was popular.

When Wilhelm held up a number on a card or asked Hans to count to a certain number, Hans would begin to stomp his front hoof and then stop at the correct number. Sometimes he would make a mistake. He used only his front hoof to communicate his mathematical abilities, and he did not make vocal noises that corresponded to individual counts or to specific numbers. He did not wag his tail in a manner that would communicate that he was counting, nor did he take a piece of chalk in his mouth and write on a chalkboard. He did not blink his eyes to relate the solutions to equations. He only stomped his front hoof. When spelling, Hans stomped once for A, twice for B, and so forth. He would pause between letters (it may be assumed that he was never asked to spell long words or words with x, y, or z in them!). Of course, hoof stomping is a natural motor pattern in horses and other animals. Doing it in special situations, in numerical sequences that correspond to a number, a letter, or a solution to an equation, is the unique talent Hans exhibited.

Oskar Pfungst was skeptical. Why Hans? Why math? Why not a horse that draws a picture of his teacher or of his stable? Why not a horse that speaks in Morse code by varying the rate and duration of its sounds? That would be a lot more efficient than stomping a hoof to communicate. Pfungst observed the setting in which the human-horse interaction was taking place. He saw a stable 4D local environment and determined what information was available to Hans at each moment of neural processing and subsequent behavioral expression.

Pfungst understood the reality behind the illusion, and he brought the show to a close by working with Von Osten to study Hans and find the source of his intelligence. Pfungst determined, by creating controlled studies, that when Wilhelm, or any other teacher, held up a number that he or she could not see, or when an equation was presented without Wilhelm being present, Hans failed. Hans was completely unable to recognize and relate the simplest of numbers accurately under these "blind" conditions. Was he really just stupid? Should we look upon Hans as a failure? Did he lose some psychic power to read human minds (as was actually hypothesized at that time)? Of course not. Hans was as smart as any other horse; he was a great success as a horse, and he had a long, loving relationship with Wilhelm. It is these special relationships between humans and animals that from time to time bring out special abilities in public attractions. Our loving relationships with our pets, in our homes, on a daily basis lead us to remark on their unique abilities and special talents.

Hans's brain was processing sensory stimuli as best it could, on a millisecond time scale. As Pfungst showed, Hans had his eyes fixed on the teacher, at first his owner Wilhelm and later anyone who assumed Wilhelm's role. To Hans, these teachers all looked the same with respect to this particular task. Hans learned to begin hoof stomping at a signal, whether it was a verbal command, the raising of the card, or some other initiating stimulus. He also learned to cease stomping when a teacher made a change in facial expression or head movement (such as a nod), or perhaps some other visible change in body position or overall state of muscular tension. Hans learned well. He was indeed clever. Even when the teachers tried to restrain themselves from giving Hans the stop clue, they sometimes could not help it, and Hans would stop at the correct number.

From Hans's perspective, there were no numbers, no letters, no equations, no math, no spelling, and no communication. There was go, stop, and food. All the information he needed was present in the external 4D stable environment. Nothing had to be computed in the mind of Hans; nothing about simple addition or long division or integrals had to be remembered from past learning: Such learning did not exist. There were early clues to the fact that Hans's intelligence was an illusion, as he could solve an equation just as fast as he could recognize a single number. He did not appear to need even the normal processing time that a human would require (hence, the conjectured psychic connection).

We will not beat this dead horse, as we have much more to discuss. The following factors are critical in formulating an approach to the study of large-scale behavior and assessing where the informational components exist and when they are present.

Context Is Everything

A full appreciation of the information available in the local 4D environment is vital in making any distinction among types of behaviors and the neural processes underlying them. It is just the basic bookkeeping that any scientific endeavor demands. It is not always easy or apparent, but the 4D stimulus context always contains information, and all of this information must be accounted for and placed in the external-information column before any information may be regarded as being internally generated by computational activity that involves the memory system and an informational store. If we miss some critical information that the context provides, then we are fooling ourselves and we are mistaken about where the information comes from and what level of behavior we are observing. (This mistake in informational bookkeeping is deliberately created in magic acts and con games.) When we ignore external information, the books are not balanced, and we give the animal, person, or even inanimate object under observation too much informational currency. In other words, we anthropomorphize. More important, we err in our attempt to reduce the probability that we are fooling ourselves and others and that we are working on illusions. Such errors can be tragic, or at least wasteful, in science and medicine. We will speak to this point in every remaining chapter.

Intramodal Transfer of Behavioral Expression

This is an important concept that we will introduce formally here, although we have alluded to it on several occasions. Intramodal transfer is just an association made in the brain nuclei that leads to there being more than one output pathway for a learned motor behavior—a transfer from one pathway to another. Examples of this include a transfer from hand (or hoof) to another limb, to the mouth, to tail movement, to an eye blink, to vocalization, or to any other efferent motor output system. The vast majority of ongoing behavior is conducted by efferent fibers stimulating striate and smooth muscle cells. Any computational activity in the association regions of the neocortex, including the prefrontal areas, has output to most motor pathways. In many animals we observe intramodal transfer in their normal routines on a daily basis. For example, if a domesticated dog or cat wants to go out, it may scratch at the door with its front paw; if that doesn't work, it may alternate between its front paws, or it may try a back paw, its mouth, head butts, or even barking or meowing. The transfer of a motor sequence between many effector systems, even vocal motor ones, is natural.

So why didn't Hans use another motor system to express his so-called counting behavior? If he was computationally performing the actual act of number recognition and relating it to the motor output of hoof stomping, the transfer to any other motor output fiber pathway should not have been much of a problem. As we noted, hoof stomping is a natural act for a horse, but so is tail waving, eye blinking, or even vocal sounds. If the computational activity in the brain is deriving information that then is expressed behaviorally through output motor systems, the intramodal transfer between motor systems should be readily available, especially if the motor output is naturally used in daily activities. A computational product that is representative of a higher-order multisensory construct, such as a number or letter, is entered into the internal 4D informational space, where it is available in thought and consciousness. The particular motor system by which that piece of information is expressed is nearly irrelevant.

In our human example of the young girl who made a line with her finger in the mud, we can imagine that she makes five of these lines to represent the written symbol 5 or the written word FIVE. She may blink her eyes five times if her hands are held still, or she may use her toes to draw the lines. She may make five noises from her vocal motor system, and eventually she may learn to collapse the concepts to the single spoken word "five." She may learn to write the symbol 5 in the mud as an equivalent representative mark, thus integrating the comparative informational constructs performed in the prefrontal modules. If she has no speech abilities, she may learn to make a sign with her hand that represents the number 5 or the word five. She might just stick her tongue out five times. All these things and more are easily performed in the consciousness referent system with thought and memory.

In pre-thought behavior, there is another general class of readily observed actions that cause many to infer that a thinking mind must be involved. We will refer to these actions as *reflective* behaviors and note that we may observe them in most animals. If a similar animal or human moves in certain rhythmic fashions in an animal's real-time visual field, the animal will *reflect* or *mirror* that action with its own paw, head, or body. Sparring animals like deer or fish demonstrate this readily in specific settings. And, especially in certain birds, an acoustic stimulus will elicit a reflective vocal output; this is demonstrated in the impressive mimicking abilities of parrots. While there are limits to this behavioral expression, it is nevertheless an interesting natural ability that has been shaped in evolutionary time.

When we as humans try to elicit reflective behaviors in our pet cat or dog, we find that more subtle motions, such as eye blinks, lip movements, or finger flexion, usually do not work. The animal's genetic-based motor reactions are not tuned to that level of sensory stimulation. It typically takes large-scale movements to entrain or elicit the reflective action. Eye-to-eye contact among certain animals can cause a reflective freezing of a body position, or a matching of head movements as the eyes are locked. It can also elicit defensive and offensive postures (crouching), sounds (growls), and movements (attacks); it can elicit equally interesting behaviors from a human participant (e.g., screams and retreats). These are complex behaviors that involve the real-time interaction of the animal with its local context and are determined to some degree by the millions of years of genetic shaping of behavioral predispositions. A visual-motor stimulus, an acoustic stimulus, or a visual-to-visual stimulus may elicit a reflective behavioral sequence. The entrainment of actions by visual-motor or acoustic stimuli in the local setting is an interesting phenomenon that will come back into our discussions.

Special Relationships between Animals and Humans

Throughout history, there are many examples of nonhuman animals performing amazing feats. Invariably, this occurs in the context of a special relationship formed between the special animal and its caring human teacher. We will always love and care for our animals, and we will always form special relationships with them (see Chapter 13). However, whenever we hear of one special animal, unlike any other of its species, that can perform humanlike tasks, we must take a careful look with our information ledger book wide open. With Wilhelm and Hans, the behavior was not specific to Hans. Many other animals could have been cared for by Wilhelm, and could have learned the same, simple tasks. Hans may have been a good subject, with good visual acuity and a temperament that allowed him to perform for the masses. But he was not a freak of nature. He did not have magical powers. It was the context, not the specific players in it, that determined his performance.

In isolated cases, in specific behavioral sequences, we can shape, mold, train, teach, and thus program animals to do things that look like something only humans can do. But we are the ones who are doing the training, the shaping, and the programming. We have an endpoint already in mind, and little by little we move the animal closer to an approximation of it. It is significant that in the entire history of mankind shaping animal behavior, we have only these occasional stories and sideshow acts as evidence of humanlike abilities in animals. Our model of biological relativity is an attempt to identify some lines in nature across which some animals may never venture, regardless of their loving teachers. We are getting closer to the point in evolution and phylogeny where we see that threshold, where we can draw a line.

What Does Polly Really Want? Clever Alex

We have examined termite and horse brains and behavior. Before we move on to the primate brain, we will look at the bird brain and its behavior. Birds may process sensory information in a manner unlike that of mammals, and they may be able to produce bird thought and bird consciousness. The *avian* evolutionary branch does indeed contain animals that are unlike any others. They fly, they build nests, and they may travel across vast distances in their daily or seasonal behavioral routines. Ostriches have been observed to pick up rocks and drop them onto eggs to break the eggs open. The brains of birds are much like those of mammals, but they have distinct organizational differences. There is a small cortex of sensory association areas, an apparent forebrain memory system, and a highly developed spatial mapping system. However, birds do not have true binocular vision, as their eyes are positioned along the lateral aspects of their heads. Thus, they map two distinct visual fields when their heads are in one position. They appear to learn and remember as well as most mammals.

A special relationship between an African gray parrot, Alex, and his teacher, Dr. Irene Pepperberg, has resulted in observations and publications about humanlike information processing by this bird.[2] It has become a celebrated case of one bird doing what no other has ever been noted to do before. This may be the result of many years of devoted, brilliant, and caring shaping, molding, teaching, and programming of the bird by his human owner. Let us begin to examine the surrounding context in which these behaviors take place. With our ledger book, we must account for the information present at any given time and apply our standards for the presence of thought, which include context-independent behavior, and intramodal transfer of computational solutions, in the 4D informational space of consciousness.

After many years of teaching, Alex was reported to be able to make sounds that are the human words for shapes, colors, numbers, and other aspects of objects and their arrangements. A generalized routine might include a question-and-answer session in which Alex was presented with a plate containing two blue cubes and three red cubes, and then was asked by a trainer, "How many blue cubes?" Alex would respond with "Two." In response to the question, "What color?" he would say, "Blue." If he was asked, "What shape?" he would respond, "Blocks." Many iterations on this basic theme were performed with a reasonably high accuracy rate of response. There were limits to what Alex could identify and how high he could count.

In other settings, Alex might be presented with a plate containing a mixed set of 3D objects, such as blocks, pyramids, and balls. After a delay, the trainer would present another plate with either the same arrangement or a different one; this is similar to a delayed-matching task. When Alex was asked, as he viewed the plate, "What's different?" he might respond "None." This would be correct if the stimulus objects were identical. If he was asked, "What's same?" he might again answer "None." And, this would be correct if the objects had changed. He also performed tasks that asked him to differentiate between large and small or between over and under. At other times, it was noted that Alex could discuss objects that were not in the present environment. One example was the exchange, "What color corn?" to which he would respond, "Yellow." There is much more that has been published about this parrot, but we have presented the basic design of the studies and the context in which they took place.

Acoustic Reflective Behavior and Context

As we have mentioned, reflective behavior is an interesting real-time response that elicits basic motor programs that mirror some aspects of the external stimuli. Parrots have a highly developed natural ability to reflect acoustic stimuli through their vocal motor output. More importantly, they have a great ability to remember these motor sequences, and to repeat them in the future. In many households for many centuries, this talent has been exploited by programming the birds with specific words, phrases, or sounds. Parrots may reflect and remember the sounds of bells, meows, barks, telephones, blenders, sirens, musical notes and short melodies, clicks, buzzes, snaps, crackles, and pops.

Nevertheless, all the information a mimicking parrot needs is provided by the local context as it flows through the parrot's real-time internal neural processing and effector output systems. The bird's forebrain memory system can store many of these patterns, and they may be recalled in an input-output linkage within a real-time stable context. "Polly want a cracker?" "Cracker," says Polly. Polly says "cracker," but is that what Polly is thinking about? Is a cracker what Polly really wants? If no cracker comes Polly's way, does she get angry? Does she know what is going on, and does she care? Who is supplying the concepts of *cracker* and *want*? It is the loving owner, the instigator, the programmer.

With effort and reward for behavior, Polly could in time be slowly shaped toward a slightly different behavioral outcome: to respond with "cracker" when asked, "Does Polly want a *lacker*?" or, "Does Polly want to *eat*?" She could further be shaped to say "cracker" in response to "What does Polly want to eat?" When this paired stimulus-response behavior is accomplished, do we say that we have established a new level of communication? Polly has never seen or tasted a cracker. Polly doesn't know what we are asking; she doesn't even know *that* we are asking a question. It is a compelling illusion. We hear the question, and we know what it means. Because Polly's vocal response is in the class of answers that fit the question, we think that she understood it and is giving us an answer. We are fooling ourselves.

"What color corn?" "Yellow." We can take a step back and ask if there is any informational relationship between the acoustic sequence of stimuli that make up the chained sounds of what-color-corn and the motor vocal output of the sound yellow. Who is supplying the information that creates a context in which, when a question about a vegetable and its color is posed, Alex selects an answer from an internal database that contains information about corn, other vegetables, the color spectrum, and the fact that corn is usually yellow (although it is sometimes brown or white)? Where is the information coming from? If we ask, "What *mother* corn?" Alex might continue to answer, "Yellow." If we gave him reinforcement over time, we could program him to answer "yellow" to the question, "What time corn?" or, "What time *born*?" Then "yellow" wouldn't work anymore, and a visitor might think that poor Alex had dementia or psychosis. This is our human illusion, our construction, our bookkeeping error. As a carnival sideshow, it is entertaining. As a scientific or medical study, it is unacceptable.

Context-Independent Behavior

It really does not matter whether the words a parrot says are true or not. The information that is being created and utilized within the neural tissues is the important factor. A person who cannot speak can still create and use information and express it as intelligently as those with speech. The sounds that Alex makes are almost irrelevant, however cute and humanlike they may be. If when Alex surveys a plate of objects he is really determining that there is or is not a difference compared to the plate with which he was just presented, then he must be comparing a lost past, through memory, with the real-time sensory world and deriving the internal solution. He then should be able to express that information—that computational solution—not only with an immediate noise, but if need be in other ways. Because he has generated this novel information internally in his memory and real-time integration modules, he should be able to be removed from that particular stimulus context and express his knowledge by pecking (a natural behavior) a button on the left for no change or a button on the right for change. And no human should need to be anywhere nearby! The internal 4D information space generated within Alex should be able to travel with him, in time and location. The behavior should be independent of the current context. There are many other experimental settings that would test whether Alex is internally generating information about the present that is explicitly dependent upon a distant past whose information is not also contained somewhere in the present context.

If this bird is calculating a number or responding to a color and is linking those sensory constructs with a stored vocal motor pattern that they represent, then he must be able to link the concept of green blocks with a green light in another room, removed from the current context information (green blocks) and all human assistants. He must also be able to link his internal concept of a number to a similar number in another room, away from any human possessing the information. There are many situations that would adequately test for context-independent information expression, and they all must be performed without the presence of a human observer with the information.

Intramodal Transfer and Context

In the prefrontal modules of humans, the intramodal transfer of information occurs all the time. If a person has no voice, either from birth or even temporarily, he or she may use his or her hands, his or her feet, or many other motor output systems to communicate. Birds certainly can tap their feet. Can Alex tap his foot (like Hans), or tap his beak, or flap his wings, or shake his head to express the internally derived information? All of these are quite normal behavioral actions that a bird can easily perform. If he cannot, we must ask why. Is his voice just a shaped response without a 4D informational relationship to the internal representation of the contextual stimuli (as in thought and consciousness)?

In thought and consciousness, the relationships among objects—their properties, colors, textures, shapes, numbers, or arrangements—may be linked to complex auditory sequences that are uniquely tied, in memory, to each property. If Alex were producing thought, he should be able to touch each stimulus object with his beak and say whether a particular object is rough or smooth, how many are rough, whether the arrangement was the same as or different from a prior one, or whether an object is larger or smaller than another, *with his eyes covered*! This is a multimodal computational solution, and the visual input is not necessary in thought and an internal 4D information space.

Finally, if we look at the higher-order concepts of quantity, more, less, over, or under, we note that they must involve memory and real-time processing to produce a solution. This integrative disparity computation of past and present must then be transmitted in efferent axons to effector motor systems to communicate it. The critical issue is that all this must be done without anyone else who knows the information being present! Otherwise, it may be another illusion resulting from misplaced information. The concepts of more or less, bigger or smaller, and same or different all reduce to simple yes or no situations, whose answer can be unknowingly contained in the way the verbal question is asked, in eye movements, or in facial and body muscle movements. This class of yes or no (and "how many?") questions must be asked after the subtraction of all potential information in the current context. If this is not done, any information expressed by the bird may be our illusion and poor bookkeeping. If we imagine a meeting between Hans and Alex, if Hans tapped his hoof five times, would Alex say "five"? Or, if Alex looked at Hans and said, "five," would Hans tap his hoof the correct number of times? No, and no.

Near the Threshold of Thought: Apes and the Life Field

The order of primates contains the four great apes: gibbons, orangutans, gorillas, and chimpanzees. The most extensively studied are the gorillas and chimpanzees, and among the chimps (*Pan troglodytes*), the pigmy chimp (*Pan paniscus*) or *bonobo* has received considerable attention. These apes are as close a relative to *Homo sapiens* as the living world provides. The DNA of chimps is about 1 to 3 percent different (we will use the midrange estimate of 2 percent) in its basic sequence homology from that of humans. Thus, there must be great similarities in the exact number of genes and their nucleotide sequences (we won't know this for some time), the types of proteins produced, the metabolic pathways created, and the structure and function of cellular systems, including the nervous system. Like humans, the apes have opposable thumbs, have five fingers and toes, walk in a semi-erect manner, have binocular vision, and have a large prefrontal neocortex. The chimp is the most human-looking of the great apes, and the bonobo may show the greatest flexibility in its behavioral repertoire. After the major evolutionary branching point around four to ten million years ago (we will again use the midrange estimate of five million years) that sent modern apes and modern humans along their own evolutionary paths, any other closer link to the human is missing. Thus, this is as close as we can get to a potentially thinking, mindful animal other than the human. We can look to see if apes produce thought and consciousness by our model of neural function and behavioral expression. It is here that we will stand at the threshold of thought, and draw a line.

The study of apes in their natural habitats has a long, respected history, and it has provided many important insights into complex animal behavior. Moreover, much of this important work reminds us of our responsibility to the animals of this world. The detailed accounts by Goodall and others have shown how close certain ape actions are to human behavior.[3] As mentioned in Chapter 6, the genetic change that brought thought and consciousness to the brain was probably a subtle modification; so any animal just below the flicker-fusion threshold may be very similar to those on the other side of that line. It is the informational content in the dynamic memory system that brings the great dividing changes in behavior.

Apes (primarily chimps) will engage in such higher-order, humanlike activities as using sticks to gather termites, to obtain honey in combs, to hit bees, or to beat each other. They have been observed to pick up a stick, push it into an ant tunnel, pull it out covered with ants, and then either put it in their mouths or wipe the ants off with their hand and eat them. They use tree leaves to gather insects or to crush them, as a blanket to sit upon, as a fan, and sometimes to rub against the body or on a wound. Sometimes they hit nuts and other hard food with pieces of wood or rocks in a variety of manners. Many chimps have been observed to dance in the rain, and some apes throw rocks and other objects, sometimes with good aim. Most, but not all, of these behaviors are related to procuring food.

There is wide variation among the appearance of these behaviors across groups of chimps. Some are seen regularly in only one or a few groups, and others are not seen at all in many groups. Other behaviors are detected, but are not part of a typical pattern within the group. It has been suggested repeatedly that these variations are an expression of the uniqueness of local ape culture, and that they are thus an indication of local social awareness and thought. But if the same methods of detailed behavioral analysis were applied to other animal cultures, similar results would most likely be reported. For example, each group of beavers probably has its own variation on the process of building dams. Each bee colony may have its own unique (however subtle relative to the big mammals) methods of creating a hive. Each bird species may use sticks, mud, and other materials to build nests in a manner that is *culture-specific.* Interestingly, in ape culture, we do not have reliable reports of the building of dwellings, dams, or gardens, and there is certainly no writing, drawing of basic pictures, or development of songs or musical instruments.

The study of apes in human cultural settings, such as research centers, zoos, or homes, has produced an equally significant body of knowledge about our nearest relative. Truly heroic attempts have been made to enrich the daily context of apes to determine if any one of them could respond by changing its behavior in a way that made it more humanlike. Other, more systematic attempts to shape or program chimps to behave like humans have also been conducted in decades of quality, caring, and dedicated research. Patterson and her gorilla Koko have received great publicity for their relationship and for her attempts to teach the ape sign language.[4] The research team of the Gardners brought the chimp Washoe into their home and taught American Sign Language (ASL) to her over many years.[5] Herbert Terrace taught his chimp, Nim Chimsky, ASL as well.[6] Project LANA, initiated by Rumbaugh and colleagues, used a special button array, a large keyboardlike device on a wall, to teach chimps to use symbolic language.[7] A most important pioneer in the field of primate research, David Premack, used 3D objects to teach symbolic language to chimps.[8] The bonobo chimp Kanzi, born and reared in a laboratory setting, has been the subject of much attention for his proclivity with ASL and keyboards, under the direction of Savage-Rumbaugh and her colleagues.[9] The behavior of all apes in front of mirrors has been thoroughly investigated, first by Gallup, and now by many other scientists.[10]

Many of these formal studies and teaching attempts began in this country in the late 1960s and 1970s, and they continue today. A detailed examination of the theories, methodologies, data collection and analysis, and conclusions would require a book in itself. However, the critical basic conclusion that can be drawn from them is that to date, there has been no ape or group of apes that can communicate with sounds, symbols, drawings, or other motor movements at anywhere near the level of an adult human. As with observations in the natural field setting, it may be what we do *not* see and what we *cannot* make an ape do that provide the greatest insight into the evolution of thought and consciousness. Many researchers and other observers place the behavior of apes as equivalent to that of human children around the age of two years. Perhaps they are quite correct in their assessments.

We must address a few aspects of human-ape interaction that are remarkably avoided in most literature. Apes, along with other mammals, have been living among humans for hundreds of years in circuses. In very close human relationships, apes have been fed, trained, and loved on a daily basis by thousands of humans. If any one ape, or elephant, dolphin, or tiger, for that matter, could have been shown to be humanlike along any one of many behavioral dimensions (singing, talking, drawing, tool using, or doing mathematics), it would have been a star (like Hans or Alex). This would have brought attention and fame, and thus financial success, to the circus, and many other animals would have been taught the behaviors. That is to say, the motivation to find or create a more humanlike ape or elephant has always been great, regardless of the setting.

Furthermore, in more recent decades, the training of skilled animals for the television and movie industry has been a lucrative field for a few talented trainers. It would bring one of these dedicated professionals a windfall of attention and success if he or she could actually teach an ape to be more humanlike. But this has not occurred. On a longer time scale, we must also note that apes and humans have lived together for thousands, if not millions, of years in many parts of the world. The zones of interface between groups of humans and apes, at the edges of villages, towns, or cities, has not produced a cooperative arrangement in which ape and human develop common behaviors and communication that benefit both. In distinct contradiction, any human, no matter how foreign a culture he or she may come from, no matter how different his or her language and routines, will always be able to communicate with another group of humans and develop a functional interface. The only Rosetta stone we have was made by humans and was used by humans. Throughout history, there has been a line between ape and human; perhaps we can identify it in nervous system function and behavioral expression.

Developmental Curves

Let us now apply a conceptual organization to the behavior of apes relative to that of their human relatives. In the course of human events, the 4D informational space grows and changes from onset to dying moment. Novel combinations of thoughts expressed through many effector output systems lead to more novel thoughts and behaviors. The temporal path through this informational progression defines the developmental curves of the human lifespan. In verbal language, tools, drawing, writing, building, and cooperative endeavors like games, business, and science, there is an identifiable change in the behavior of each individual over time. The critical point is that many of these changes involve the integration of earlier information with new information in an ongoing reiterative, recombinant manner. This is the forge of thought and thought-memory, in the referent system of consciousness.

In the history of the individual ape or ape groups, we do not detect anything approaching these information-based developmental curves. Behaviors may be learned and modified, and new ones may be added, but the expansion of the behavioral repertoire in a progression based on daily experience is very limited. Sticks for ants, leaves for rubbing, rocks for pounding, key pressing, finger positioning (ASL), and many other natural or taught behaviors do not progress along significant developmental curves as a result of daily experience. The term *arrested development* has been applied many times to indicate the relative limits to this process in apes, which keep them at about the level of human two-year-olds. Perhaps they are halted by an evolutionary roadblock.

Behavior in the Field of Life

All cellular life expresses its entire behavioral repertoire in the local environment. The process of evolution is one of shaping through interaction. On the time scale of cellular evolution, in a manner of casual speaking, insects and animals do the best they can with what they have, and if they could do better, they would. What they have is a 4D environmental context that provides sensory energy information on a millisecond time scale and a habitat-specific distribution of organic and inorganic materials upon which to act, to live. Furthermore, when we take an insect or animal out of the niche in which it has evolved, it will continue to exhibit the set of actions that it is capable of performing, even when (from our human perspective) those behaviors are terribly inappropriate or inadequate to the new context. Many times an animal is incapable of processing new patterns of sensory information or expressing behaviors that utilize the materials of a new environment in a context-appropriate manner. For example, apes have not been able to use toilets even after years of exposure to humans using them. It may be said that you can take the boy out of the farm, but you can't take the farm out of the boy. But the truth is that, because a boy is human and possesses thought, he will be able to adapt, change, and integrate the new patterns of sensory information into his existing informational store, and to create context-appropriate behaviors to an extent unlike that of any other animal in nature.

Animals and insects display an amazing diversity of behaviors within their local habitats. The behaviors that tend to draw our attention are the ones that appear to be humanlike and acceptable in human society. It is, of course, not surprising that individual or group behaviors in animals that reflect our best human behaviors interest us. However, when we project our human rules of conduct onto the larger living world, we tend to ignore the majority of the daily behaviors in which most animals engage. Parasitism, cannibalism, matricide, patricide, infanticide, incest, promiscuity, metamorphosis, mass suicide, and a multitude of other equally complex and amazing behavioral sequences tend to be less interesting to most humans, but they all must be included in the equation of cell-environment interactions that define behavior in the reference system of life. The life field moves through time without judgment as to whether actions are good, bad, or indifferent. Only human behavior is influenced by these concepts. The point is that we must be aware that we tend to focus on a very small part of the behavioral repertoire of nature when we discuss animals and their humanlike qualities and actions.

A short list of the interesting behaviors that involve changes made to the local environment by animals contains such achievements as the hexagon-based honeycombs of bees and the honey they produce; the dwellings constructed by ants, termites, and wasps; the trap-door homes of desert spiders; the many nests built by birds; and the dams assembled by beavers. All these represent long-term, stable reorganizations of local materials through repetitive behavioral patterns expressed in millisecond-to-millisecond steps elicited by the momentary internal and external sensory contexts.

The archer fish is named for its ability to eject a stream of water out of its mouth to knock an insect out of the sky. Frogs may do the same with their long tongues. Ostriches have regularly been noted to pick up rocks and drop them onto eggs to crack them open. California sea otters are known for using rocks to pound open mussel shells that they lay on their stomachs while they are floating on their backs. Raccoons and some apes in the northern islands of Japan put their food in water before eating it. Cats are typically seen cupping their paws and dipping them into a cup or glass to withdraw the liquid to drink. Young cats regularly treat their reflections in mirrors as another cat and take aggressive postures or attack the image. Some cats are very prone to repeatedly throwing a mouse or other small object into the air, only to catch it as it falls. Squirrels and other mammals collect food and store it in their dwellings. They also tend to collect nonedible objects along with the food. Birds and whales are known for their melodic sound repertoires, which may change with learning. The honeybee may impart information to other bees by performing a series of movements that we call a dance. Insects, reptiles, birds, and mammals all perform many behaviors to keep their young alive. And many insects and animals, from termites to apes, live in groups and interact regularly with one another in a manner that tends to benefit the entire group. When we compare this list of behaviors to those listed for the apes, it does not make the apes look that much more intelligent or thoughtful than the remainder of the animal kingdom. Their behavior may fit well within the life field, without exception.

Context and Behavior

As many people who conduct research with apes know, it is the context-independent behavior that holds the key to a division between ape and human. The model of biological relativity formalizes this point of view, giving a neurobiological structure and function to the concept. It is also a model of thresholds, and for ape behavior to express a computational crossing of the flicker-fusion threshold to thought, it must show the internal generation of a 4D information space that may be expressed independent of the real-time context. Over months and years, and thousands of learning trials, we may be able to program a chimp to perform a lengthy series of button presses or hand signs that will result in a food reward. At some point in the process, we might stand back and say, "Oh, my, isn't that behavior clever and thoughtful." But on closer inspection, and with the use of our freeze-frame, millisecond-by-millisecond method of viewing the nervous system activity, we see an incredible number of (well-learned) small behaviors that are tied inextricably to the guiding information in the local 4D context at each learning moment. The trainers induce the chaining or shaping of the behavior sequences to create an action that lasts for several seconds of background time. The training program has the entire sequence and endpoint as the *a priori* goal. The small learning steps in the training program create the illusion of an internally derived temporal dimension that links the moments of neural integration.

From the point of view of the ape's nervous system and our model, each complex sensory integration cycle of the prefrontal modules generates a complex product, but a subcritical amount of representational information is then present at the following computational moment in the next dominant PIM. The ape can learn all the pieces of a behavioral sequence (with very severe limits), but the higher-order information that is represented in the entire sequence, the 4D information that includes the linking temporal dimension, is not available to the ape. The sequence must be performed in a stable local 4D environment that provides the linking information to keep the sequence moving along its moment-to-moment learned segments. As we discussed in Chapter 7, disruptions of the temporal sequence in learning and memory procedures can result in poor learning or poor recall performance. If the higher-order (what our model considers thought-dependent) information of the entire program—the rules of the game—were available to the ape, it could build on this base, in time, and could develop novel iterations and combinations, expand the sequences in length, and use them in many settings. To date, all quality research has found strict limitations on the ape's ability to learn and use, in a context-independent manner, any form of human communication.

The intriguing behaviors that have been reported for adult orangutans and chimps when they have regular access to mirrors are worth noting in this section. The behavior is indeed context-dependent, in that all behaviors are expressed in one stable 4D setting. Cats, dogs, and birds are also regularly noted to engage the image in a mirror. These behaviors may be classed with the reflective actions that we observe between animals, where one animal mimics an action being performed by another in its visual field. However, chimps go beyond the simple reflective behaviors and appear to be aware that they are looking at their own reflection, as some will touch places on their own bodies as they view their image in the mirror. They may turn around and touch places that they could not ordinarily see without a mirror. The mirror and the context are providing all the information needed to behave in this manner. The chimps are acting in a manner that they naturally do, inspecting, picking, and grooming themselves with their hands. They are just doing it with their visual image entrained in an exact duplication of themselves, present in a stable, 4D image moment to moment through the function of the mirror. They do not appear to do this around water ponds in their natural settings. If the chimps were processing higher-order sensory information that included an internal integration of a stored self-image and the external image, and the resultant disparity computations were entered into working or long-term memory, they would be able to do many more things.

We must wonder, with respect to the self-concept, whether in a split-screen presentation where one-half of the screen is a mirror and the other half is a film projection of the same chimp at a different time, the chimp would recognize itself in both images. We do not know if this observation has been made. However, Gallup did perform an ingenious set of experiments with chimps and mirrors.[11] Under anesthesia, a red odorless dot was placed on a chimp's forehead. During the next mirror session, it was noted that some chimps would touch the dot as they looked in the mirror. Perhaps, it was thought, this is a reflection of self-awareness. We must note that B. F. Skinner and colleagues published a report that showed that a pigeon could be taught to peck at a red dot on its own chest when it viewed itself in a mirror[12]—an equally ingenious study. If the chimps are processing a level of sensory information that includes the self-image and the painted dots, then this information should be entering into working and long-term memory. They should be observed touching the dots when the context-dependent information provided by the mirror is removed. If the reflective image is gone, does the behavior disappear along with it into a lost past moment?

Finally, the internally derived information about the dot on a self-image should be available for use in the near future, at least. Let us imagine that a chimp is first trained in the simple task of pressing a button with a dot on it, or a star, a square, and so on, when such a button is presented on a video screen, for a reward. He is trained to do this to the best of his ability, with the longest delay possible between stimulus presentation and button-pressing response. Now, while the chimp is engaged in mirror behavior, one of the stimulus images is projected onto his forehead with a laser light and a shape filter. The chimp can see the shape of the stimulus only by looking at his self-image in the mirror. Next, the chimp is taken to a room where he performs the reward task and is given a choice of a picture of his face with the shape, the face of another chimp with the shape, and another pair of these faces with an incorrect shape on them. Will the chimp select the self-image with the correct shape on it? If he is just choosing his own face, he has a 50-50 chance of getting the wrong shape, and the same probability holds if he is choosing just the shape. Can he hold the self-image and the shape in mind? There are many variations that could test whether the self-image of the chimp, as seen in a mirror, is one that exists in the brain as useful information once the mirror image is out of sight. Or does out of sight mean out of mind for the chimp?

Intramodal Transfer of Behavioral Expression

If a 4D information space is being generated by the prefrontal modules and forebrain memory systems of apes, then the output of the computational solutions should be available for use in many effector motor systems, even if only to get a piece of food or a drink of juice. We consider that a sequence of finger movements represents a letter or phrase in ASL. The internal representation of the letter or phrase in informational space may be linked, through learning, to other forms of motor expression. Morse code represents the same letters and phrases in series of short and long sounds or marks. The chaining of simple motor vocal sounds, such as "oooh" "oooh" "ooooooh," may be associated with a letter or phrase, since it exists as a computational entity in neural activity. Chimps should be able to speak in Morse code as they can speak in ASL, and they should be able to move between the two in intramodal transfer. Likewise, a series of eye blinks, foot stomps, or lip smacks may also represent a letter, phrase, or number. Finally, the self-image is also a multimodal construct in the prefrontal modules, as they integrate sensory maps of the body from all receptor energy classes. It is in the parietal multimodal neocortex and the prefrontal modules that the associations of the visual self-image and the somatosensory and viscerosensory impulses converge. Can a chimp that studies himself in a mirror recognize his self-image by touching a 3D replicated model of his face or full figure? If so, would changes made to the model cause the chimp to examine his own face? This tactile mirror test would look at intramodal transfer of internal representations.

Special Relationships

We must include the factor of special relationships because it is very important to keep in mind. The vast majority of research into ape intelligence has set the standards for conducting difficult investigations on animals while maintaining a caring, humane relationship with the subjects of the study. The few instances of a special relationship, where unique abilities were claimed but were also confined to the interaction of the ape and its teacher, have not had great effect, except among the popular press and television. In part, this is due to the fact that there have now been several decades of superior research, and there are knowledgeable specialists who can immediately investigate and comment on the behaviors being claimed. Also, the general public is much more aware of the need for the application of the scientific method to reduce the chance of being tricked, even if only by a case of blind love.

Five million years and 2 percent of the genetic code separate the chimp and the human. If apes have not crossed the threshold to thought and consciousness, then what is it about their behavior that reflects a position near the critical level of sensory representational order that must be attained in the prefrontal modules? They have great manual dexterity and many sensory receptors on their fingers, as well as superb visual acuity and full binocular vision. Their size is roughly equivalent to ours, and thus their relative spatial perspective of the external environment might be similar to humans'. Their internal sensory world is also similar in structure and function to that of humans. Thus, the relative distribution of all sensory receptor classes, the number of receptors, and the transduction-transmission processes of the peripheral nervous system of the ape may be very similar to ours.

The representation of the sensory worlds in the ape brain may also be near their representation in ours in type and acuity. The receptive fields for the internal and external maps of the ape homunculus and the final projections to all multimodal association regions and the prefrontal neocortex may also be humanlike. In the prefrontal integration modules, the convergence of all sensory information, the momentary point representation, may have a very similar receptive field for the totality of the afferent information. This point representation sets the viewpoint of the animal with respect to the external and internal context. The computational viewpoints of the ape and the human may be very similar. The model proposes that the differences lie in the critical level of representational order that is available to the next dominant PIM from the computational moment past (approximately 200 ms). The $R'_a t_{n-1}$ may not bring a critical threshold 3D representation that permits the integration of the past moment with the *now* computation, and if this is the case, there is likewise no adequate level of sensory information in the $R''_a t_{n-x}$ afferent from the forebrain memory system.

Nevertheless, the basic receptive field of each PIM at each moment may be very similar in the ape and the human. This near-human sensory representation map integrates its afferent information and the output affects behavior in the manner depicted on the S-curve projection of Chapter 6. If the subcortical processing and genetic-based behaviors are also closely related, then the overall moment-to-moment movements and some sequences of behavior would be quite close to those of humans. The contexts in which apes can survive and adapt are thus also very similar to the human ones. Important to our sense of kinship, the general flow of behavior between apes and between parent and infant are likewise reflective of the human condition. The genetics, the neurobiology, and thus the sensory viewpoint of the internal and external worlds and behavior of apes are indeed very humanlike. But our model holds that the threshold to thought and consciousness is to be found exclusively in the human brain.

A Reverence for Life

Complex pathways of changing order in living systems relative to the immediate environment: This is the behavior of life as perceived from our point of view in consciousness. From a single cell to the great apes, all this behavior can be included in the frame of reference of life, when we acknowledge the process of evolution in shaping intracellular and extracellular pathways of interaction. We have not seen a behavior or pattern of behaviors that must be described in a different level of language. We may use anthropomorphic lexicology to impart our sense of kinship and caring or to make descriptions of animal actions more interesting; but such language does not reflect any real similarity between animal behaviors and higher-order human ones. Many of us may not like these conclusions and this point of view. It may not feel right. The current *zeitgeist* may tell us to not even think that this may be so (this is nothing new for almost any scientific process). Biological relativity still contains a larger, overarching perspective, yet to be discussed, that will place these considerations of ape thought in a context that may or may not be more palatable.

If all of the actions and learning across the entire field of life, from a cell to a chimp, do not require thought and consciousness, then the onset of thought and consciousness must bring very impressive changes. Near the threshold of thought, the chimps are only five million years and 2 percent in genetic code away. Compared to the human brain, that of the chimp has less prefrontal neocortex relative to cortex volume, less synaptic density, and less total dendrite length; and perhaps there are other differences as well. There may be different enzymes, or metabolic pathway functions, or other intracellular or extracellular changes from ape to human. What small step in evolution, what critical increase in order, brought the changes that allowed the integration of two moments of sensory information to derive a 4D internal representation, and the propagation of it to create the emergent frame of reference of consciousness? The realization that we are the products of such a modest modification in the genetic code may instill a reverence for life and a sense of responsibility to our nearest relative and to all species.

Perhaps the most important conclusion about ape behavior that has been articulated over and over again is that apes are like 2-year-old humans. This is typically invoked as a statement of equality to humans, but perhaps it tells us something much deeper, much more revealing about complex behavior and thought and consciousness. Perhaps the comparison is correct. Perhaps we have identified the crucial difference between the two species. Perhaps there is an equality of behavior near the computational threshold of thought in one species and at the dawning of thought in the other.

9

Human Thought and the Emergent Twos

The human prefrontal cortex (in concert with the entire organism) is the only place in the biophysical world where thought is produced and propagated in the consciousness frame of reference. This is the threshold to thought and mind postulated by the model of biological relativity. Now that we have drawn this line in evolution, it forces the following important questions: When in human development is the emergent threshold surpassed? That is, when does sensory representation flicker fusion occur? Is this event observable by an effect on the behavior and memory of the person in which it has occurred? We may also ask if the brain immediately maintains a stable emergent consciousness frame of reference, or if it has starts and stops, repeated moments of flicker and fusion, as it attains a functional state. How would that manifest itself in thought, thought-memory, and behavior?

We walked (some may say suffered) through the development of the human nervous system so that we can now stand at the threshold of thought and understand precisely what it is that we will witness as flickers of discrete sensory moments become a fused flow of 4D continuity in the human brain. We followed the path of our young girl in development, from the moment of conception to the first differentiated nerve cell, to a fully functioning cerebral cortex deriving all the dimensions of space and time in its modular disparity computations. We saw how the coordinated biological organization of information produced fascinating behavior as she played in pools of mud and reflective water. But was her play thoughtful and mindful? If so, exactly when did her thought function begin? Was it when the first neuron began to generate action potentials, or when the first brain nucleus began to operate? Was her thought generated *in utero,* upon birth, in the first day, week, or year?

Biological relativity compels us to search for answers to these questions. For, if thought is a quantifiable product of neural processes (forged in the consciousness frame of reference), then its existence must be detectable. And even if the exact biocomputational processes are, for the moment, beyond our knowledge, we should be able to observe the effect of thought on system-level neural function, and thus upon the behavior of the individual producing it. We postulate that the emergence threshold is crossed well after an infant is born, since our model considers thought and consciousness to be dependent upon the highest order of sensory representation in the prefrontal neocortex (the last region to mature in postnatal life). Therefore, a threshold in the time line of human development is predicted and indeed anticipated, as it was in the time line of nervous system evolution that created the first brain with thought. Each human child entering into thought and consciousness is thus recapitulating a wondrous evolutionary accomplishment. The time of human emergence into thought should be a revered moment in development. We predict that the transition into consciousness for every child may become celebrated as the *emergent twos.*

We have to this point refrained from the anecdotal reports of amazing behaviors that always seem to begin with phrases like, "Well, my dog once . . . !" or "Well, I saw a dolphin on TV that . . . !" or "Well, I read that chimps . . . !" and even "Well, yesterday my baby . . . !". We have avoided most of the stories about incredible cases of plant, insect, animal, and even human behavior that fill human history. We have placed strict parameters on how we will go about observing the behavior of life, utilizing a hypothetical ledger book to keep track of the origin of all available information and influences that drive behavior. We must always determine whether information that drives behavior belongs in the external-origin bookkeeping column of the explicit sensory world, or if it goes in the internal-origin bookkeeping column. We have also attempted to stay cognizant of our descriptive words when we define a nerve impulse or a complex motor behavior, and to avoid the anthropomorphic lexicology that astonishingly plagues even recent attempts to explain how minds think or how the brain works. It is even more vital at this juncture to remain aware of the illusions that we, from our point of view in consciousness, are so prone to create when we impose our experience on other animals or try to program them to be more humanlike. We must be able to explicitly understand the circumstances in which we provide the thought-generated information to a learning and memory situation, and thus program other animals to act like us. We must be able to step back and account for the history of information that exists in the present, even in the most special of human relationships.

The last half-century of naturalistic observation and laboratory research on apes has ignited an overwhelmingly productive discourse on the limits of chimp behavior and the interface of ape and human intellectual abilities.[1] This stimulated a new round of conceptual redefinition and refinement of methodological procedures for both ape and human behavior research that continues today. The last 25 years have seen a number of investigations and reviews of the literature that explore the degree to which a chimp is like a human child, and what behavioral developments begin to separate the two.[2] Evolution, as time and entropy, has created a biological chasm between the chimp and human. The behavioral differences that emerge between the chimp and the growing human infant reach a critical point at which the human child will dramatically and permanently leave the chimp behind. Our model proposes that it is precisely at this moment in development that the human child begins to generate thought in the reference system of consciousness. The point of departure between human child and chimp would reflect a function of the five million years (time) and 2 percent of the genetic code (entropy) that separates the species.

Developmental Curves, Threshold Leaps, and the Dawn of Thought

We must always remain acutely aware of the tremendous growth activity that is taking place in all cellular systems, including the nervous system, during the first 2 years of life and beyond. Several measures of human brain development correlate with the time frame for the emergence of thought as we have proposed it. There is an incredible growth in the size and connectivity of the neural cells until about 18 to 24 months, after which cell growth and new synaptic formation activities begin to taper.[3] Cells grow in size and express larger, longer, and more complex dendritic processes upon which axospinous synaptic zones will form. Again, an explosive growth curve along these parameters begins to level off in the second year of life.[4] The prefrontal neocortex undergoes a dramatic maturational process during the first two years of postnatal development.[5] Schore (1994) concluded that the first 18 months of human life is the critical period for the maturation of the prefrontal cortex.[6]

In a recent study, Thompson and colleagues (2000) found that there was rapid growth in the frontal neocortical regions from 3 to 6 years of age, as mathematically derived from serial MRI brain scans.[7] Functional studies of the brain bioelectrical properties measured in complex electroencephalograms (EEG), conducted by Thatcher (1992), demonstrated cyclical changes that span many years of development, and included changes that indicated a maturation of the corticocortical connectivity between frontal and other regions of the left cerebral hemisphere over the ages of 1.5 to 3.0 years.[8] Metabolic studies of brain activity using PET in infants have been interpreted as indicating a significant increase in synaptic activity in the frontal and other neocortical regions occurring up to 18 months of life.[9]

Now that we have entered the realm of human behavior, and only now, we must introduce concepts such as language, math, music, drawing, writing, technology, science, and imagination and self. For any one of these categories, discussions of onset and development always include the eternal question of whether the ability to internally represent an object or idea and communicate it, generally placed under the large umbrella of language, must come prior to any other complex human behavioral development. In other words, is it possible to create math, art, drawing, tools, technology, and imagination and self without some type of substrate language scaffolding? For the moment, we will avoid the ultimately important concept of genetically coded predispositions and abilities as it relates to these classifications. It must be reiterated that our model describes a fundamental biophysical process of the brain that operates on any afferent sensory information entering into the prefrontal modules. The integration of the various sources of past and present sensory information is performed and the output solutions are encoded into efferent axon arrays regardless of the specific intrinsic information contained in the afferent wavefronts. Higher-order concepts, language included, are generated only after the thought-generating brain has developed them as processes in the 4D reference system of consciousness.

Biological relativity is about the threshold onset of the function of an organic system, either in the cell or in the prefrontal integration module (PIM). It reveals the engine of evolution that produces 4D referent systems. The unique and novel products of such a system—peptides, enzymes, or thoughts—may exist only because each emergent system creates an internal 4D space that is propagated in time. Within the human nervous system, the physical products that are born in, inhabit, and modify that space—thoughts—may have an action back on the brain as memories and through effector output systems. In the forebrain memory system, and its recurrent interactions with the prefrontal modules, the onset of thought begins to alter the structural properties of the information store. In a reiterative, recombinant manner, this 4D information space may grow and develop along many specific dynamic representational pathways that include all those that are classified as language, math, music, art, technology, science, and imagination and self. The biophysical system doesn't make judgments about the background energy flux of the electromagnetic spectrum in all its forms; it just generates an internal 4D frame of reference through which these energies flow and become reorganized, integrated, and maintained across critical thresholds of 3D order and 1D time. In the human child, we propose that the brain achieves this ability to derive an internal 4D order from the waves of sensory representation, which thus begins the thought effect, at 16 to 24 months of age.

Schore (1994) published a monumental volume that brings together several fields of research and observation into a brilliant model of the changes that occur in the early years of human life.[10] He postulates that a *practicing period* ends at about 18 months, and that this correlates with the onset of an internal world of thoughts, emotions, and experience that marks a qualitative shift in human behavior. Jerome Kagan, Joaquin Fuster, Stanley Greenspan, A. N. Meltzoff, and their colleagues have produced seminal contributions regarding the early behavioral experiences of children, across a wide variety of research areas.[11] They and others have written with great eloquence and understanding about the importance of this period in the life of a human child with respect to the development of complex behavior, an internal representation of the world, and emotional growth. The enormous amount of interest in this period of human life only reinforces our view as to its relationship to the model being presented.

The language abilities of children between the ages of 2 and 3 years undergo a dramatic change. From simple word combinations and learned associations linked to current contextual situations, we see the onset of the ability to form longer sequences that express complex questions about current, past, and potential future situations.[12] Greenspan and Benderly (1998) write, "At the end of the second year of life, as communication for communication's sake begins to overtake communication merely to meet a need, the child embarks on a course he will continue throughout life."[13]

While many studies differ on what word use means, children at 1 year generally speak about 3 words that are linked to real-time responses; at 15 months they have about 19 words in their vocabulary; and they have 22 words at 18 months.[14] After about 18 months, there is a truly astonishing shift with respect to language as a child begins to expand her or his vocabulary, form longer sentences, ask questions, and describe things and situations that are not in the local context. The pairing of internal states and external objects and situations begins to be observed in the actions of children at about this age, and these internally derived associations become expressed in verbal language shortly thereafter.[15]

By 18 to 20 months, a child begins to acquire an internally derived understanding of the larger context of his or her interactions with other people, and thus becomes able to regulate the expression of emotions such as anger and happiness.[16] The child can hold an internal image of a parent across longer distances and thus durations. "Consciousness at this stage consists of a greater awareness of feelings, behavior, and actions—the patterns that are the foundations of the sense of self,"[17] writes Kagan. In psychoanalytic literature, we can find some agreement that a unique internal representation, generally called the ego ideal, may be constructed only after around 18 months of age. Some behavioral manifestations of this construct include a sense of external time and delayed actions.[18] Other complex conceptual behaviors, which can have many interpretations, are those of morality, empathy, or altruism.[19]

Across the board, in almost any area where a child's behavior may be observed or measured, there appears to be a major discontinuity in the development of mental abilities at about 18 months.[20] Meltzoff (1990, 1999) describes a "watershed transformation" in the ability of children, beginning at about 18 months, to hypothesize about future possibilities, and thus demonstrate an internally generated "theory of mind."[21] So many have said and written this in a variety of ways. Across history, societies, and professional specialties such as ape research, child development, language studies, education, social research, neuroscience and behavior research, and medicine and nursing, the idea that *something big is going on* during this phase of development has resonated. Within this consensus, there will continue to be energetic debate regarding the underlying theories that have guided research and thus the conclusions made with respect to infant, toddler, and childhood learning, memory, and behavior.

All modern theories of infant and child development in the areas of higher-brain function, thought, and consciousness stem directly from (or must acknowledge their relationship to) the profound formulation published by Jean Piaget in the 1950s.[22] His major treatise, *The Child's Construction of Reality* (1954), followed 30 years of working with children and attempting to understand their developing vision of the universe. To date, we know of no deeper insight that has produced such a collective, worldwide body of knowledge about human thought and its development.

The principles derived by Piaget have solidly withstood the test of time, no matter how hard some have tried to modify or deconstruct them. More recent research on the developing nervous system and its processing of sensory information has gone a long way toward integrating modern neuroscience with Piaget's principles to form a more complete theoretical model. Though there are many details still to be worked out, Piaget's conceptual framework remains a cornerstone of our knowledge, and it should be respected as penetrating wisdom about the progression of information growth in the human child's brain as daily, monthly, and yearly experience modifies, recombines, and reorganizes it to bring new levels of understanding and functioning. From the standpoint of biological relativity, Piaget in effect provided the first systematic assessment of the threshold emergence of thought and consciousness.

The Piagetian Progression

Piaget's background included work with Alfred Binet in Paris on children's intelligence testing, and with Manfred Bleuler, who provided the first systematic investigation and description of psychotic thought disorders. Across 30 years of working with children, Piaget observed, tested, and recorded his findings. He found that certain basic internal computational manipulations of sensory information (mental operations) appeared in the repertoire of children along a sequential pathway through development. More interestingly, he discovered that mental operations that appeared later in adolescence could not be taught to or programmed into children younger than a certain age range, no matter how hard or how long one tried. Perhaps even more fascinating was his finding that a child could not proceed to the next level of operational information unless she or he first attained the previous level of mental function. He was able to group these observations into stages of development that held for any child, anywhere, under almost any learning conditions. His human intellectual growth curve was unlike anything seen before or since. Despite decades of further studies worldwide and serious attempts to disprove his observations, only minor modifications in the most basic and fundamental aspects of Piaget's progression may be claimed. It was not that Piaget had conceptualized all of brain function and the development of informational systems, but he had penetrated deeply into basic neurobiological functions by observing children behaving and derived an important series of maturational and informational stages that are reached only in certain years of human development.

The *sensorimotor* period of intellectual development may last until around 2 years of age. Piaget was well aware that genetic and environmental factors would lead to variations in his time frames. However, for most healthy children, his age ranges hold. In this period of life, the infant and then the young child functions with its inborn reflexes and other basic behaviors. The period can be divided into six stages, marked by progressive behavioral flexibility and learning. In stages 2, 3, and 4, children begin increasingly to interact with the local environment and the people in it, and learn basic stimulus-reward associations. In the final stages of this period (stages 5 and 6), as their behavior becomes more exploratory and interactive, children will begin to manipulate objects in the local environment. The critical behavior that Piaget observed and defined as the end of this period was that of *object permanence.* The basic interpretation of this concept is simply reflected in the old adage *out of sight, out of mind.* Prior to reaching object permanence, a child will not be able to locate an object, even a highly attractive one, when it is covered by another object (e.g., candy under a blanket or a doll behind a pillow). After a certain point in a child's neurobiological maturation, he or she can perform this task. This is a threshold function that cannot be taught or programmed into a child before he or she has matured to the point where he or she has the functional capability. From the perspective of our model (and others), this is a spatial memory function that requires an operating temporal lobe and hippocampal place mapping system. In earlier chapters, we discuss the radial-arm maze and the place behavior of rats and mice. Rats and mice could keep a place in local 3D space in a short-lived working memory, and this would allow them to find a food reward without revisiting foraged places. When the hippocampus or its primary connections were damaged, place behavior was lost. There is also a developmental onset to the place learning abilities in animals, before which they cannot learn the task. Both abilities may relate to the postnatal maturation of the hippocampus and its synaptic connectivity.

Piaget's *preoperational* period lasts generally from 2 to 7 years of age. This is the time of profound change that is unmatched in all other animal life. Language, drawing, symbolic expressions, delayed behavior and imitation, and imagination all appear at this stage. Children begin to ask questions about the world and about space and time, and to gather information from the answers. This is the period when Piaget stated that a child forms a representation within the mind, one that is not based on direct perception. We will return to this period shortly.

The *concrete operations* period usually is seen between the ages of 7 and 11. During these years, Piaget discovered, children begin to understand concepts of the physical world, concepts derived from internal informational reorganization. The operations in this period include the famous conservation concepts. Children in this age range (and not before) can understand, and express verbally or in other ways, that a quantity or mass remains the same even if it changes shape, and that the length of an object does not change with its relative position in space. The basic laws of our physical existence are now computational possibilities in the child's internal world.

The *formal operations* period is the last in the Piagetian progression, beginning around 11 to 12 years of age and extending through adolescence. It is described as a time when children and adolescents begin to *think about their thoughts*; they become more reflective and construct ideals and possible futures. The ability to assume another perspective or point of view begins to appear during these years. Metaphors have meaning when the formal operations period is reached. Hypotheses may be generated, and inductive and deductive reasoning may be applied to problems. In mathematical expressions, a child performing formal operations can derive the solution that $X > Z$ when told that $X > Y$ and $Y > Z$. Or, if $A + B = D$, and $B + C = D$, then $A = C$, and so forth.

Object Permanence, Preoperational Representation, and the Threshold to Thought

Let us examine the threshold that Piaget defined between the sensorimotor and preoperational periods. It is here, early in the second year of life, that a child has attained the ability for object permanence behavior and the ability to represent the world internally! From our perspective, the child has moved from pre-thought to thought and into the emergent consciousness frame of reference. The representation that Piaget described would correspond to the internal 4D sensory representation derived in the prefrontal modules through disparity computation. Piaget proposed that a child could not move into the preoperational period until the critical level of functioning in the sensorimotor stage was attained. This is *not* a semantic or learning threshold. What Piaget showed—where his fundamental insight lies—is that regardless of the information, the teaching, or the training, the nervous system *cannot* perform the operations that underlie language, symbolic gestures, drawing, artistic expression, internal imagery, or anything else that a child, an adolescent, and an adult may do until the brain reaches a stage of functioning that produces object permanence behavior! It is a *barrier in nature* that Piaget observed in the behavior of children! If for some unfortunate reason of genetics, trauma, or disease a child could not generate object permanence behavior, he or she could not continue on in the development of higher-brain operations. What a fundamental statement!

From the perspective of biological relativity, the onset of object permanence signifies at least a functional temporal lobe, hippocampal place, and working memory system. Recall that the hippocampus undergoes significant postnatal neurogenesis, synaptic connectivity, and myelination until around 15 months of life. This occurs in parallel to the rapid maturation of the neocortex, including the prefrontal region, which is the last to reach a full structural and functional state.

We propose that simultaneously with or within a few months after the development of a fully functioning hippocampal place and working memory system, the prefrontal integration modules begin to generate thought and propagate it across the modular fields. The forebrain memory system provides the afferent projections that bring both the sensory representation of the past and the real-time spatial representation of the local environment to the prefrontal modules. This critical information source would then be operational before or at least at the threshold of prefrontal emergent function. The efferent output of the prefrontal integration modules (thought) may then enter an operational forebrain memory system to begin the reiterative, recombinant process of creating a dynamic 4D informational source for a lifetime of experience.

When the 4D informational space comes into existence, it begins to fill with all the thoughts produced by the afferent sensory representations. As thoughts begin to accumulate into organized structures in the forebrain memory system, behavior may become independent of the local context. As many have observed, and as Piaget discovered, children over 2 years of age can take the world with them and use the information in other settings. In the easily testable and quantifiable behaviors of children over 2, we see new abilities gradually appearing that allow them to compare, juxtapose, rotate, combine, integrate, change perspective, and reshuffle just about any sensory information that has entered into the thought-memory system and reemerged into the real-time disparity computation modules of the prefrontal neocortex. The internal 4D world grows and becomes more refined, and it has an independence from the local context in many behavioral activities that may be expressed as a lifelong developing repertoire that is unparalleled in nature. Piaget recognized how long it takes the human mind to accumulate and reorganize information to produce new levels of computational solutions. The underlying biophysical and biomathematical computations remain the same; it is the order, the information, and the mind's internal dimensionality that changes.

When we reflect on the limited abilities of Hans, Alex, and the chimps, the power and flexibility of the human biophysical reality is striking. As the internal 4D representations develop in the human child beyond the threshold of thought, the effector output to nearly any motor system becomes a computational possibility. A melody that was learned by silently reading a sheet of music may later be sung or played upon any of a number of musical instruments in a completely different setting! A foot may perform the function usually done by the hand; this is computationally accomplished by the juxtaposition of the two representations in the real-time 4D prefrontal modular system and the transmission of the efferent output solution from one to the other. Thus, if the context creates a situation in which the hands are not available to perform a task, the computational possibility that a foot may be able to do the same task becomes an option. As the internal representation of the body, its parts, and their actions and limitations all become interchangeable pieces in the informational space, the transfer between motor systems may occur.

The developmental progression of human behavior after the onset of thought and consciousness is radically different from that of any other animal. In many types of behavioral measures, the pre-thought-to-thought state change produces a nearly vertical rise in the complexity and flexibility of the actions that the child may perform. The second year of life sees an explosion of novel behaviors such as word use, sentence structure, question upon question, the reproduction of behaviors that were experienced in other settings, the use of objects as tools, a growing self-awareness, more complex interactions with others, expression of emotional states, and others. These are the *terrible twos* that are so familiar to any parent. The onset of a 4D information space in thought and consciousness, and its growing and changing structure through memory, enables the child to express his or her dynamic, internal existence to the world, for better or for worse. If these behavioral changes indeed do mark the onset of the thought and thought-memory function, then from this point on the unique information structure will increase, and the child's behavior will become more complicated and intricate as each month and year goes by. This is the progression of complex internal thought processes mapped by Piaget.

During this critical phase of maturation, the prefrontal cortex may undergo periods of stops and starts—flicker and fusion moments—until a stable relaxation of the system maintains the generation and propagation of internal 4D representations. Memories in thought, as in pre-thought, are the millisecond moments of neural information that cause a cascade of metabolic and structural events leading to more permanent effects on selected neural pathways in the forebrain system. As thought products are generated in the prefrontal modules and sent into this memory system, at the approximate rate of five per minute, they modify the memory structure of thought and pre-thought information. Until the emergence of thought, all human learning and memory is of a pre-thought quality and cannot contain the information produced in thought computations. Thus, any memories of the self within a particular past environment (context-independent) and of several moments of ongoing experience may be produced only by a prefrontal cortex that is generating thought. The recall or real-time experiencing of such memories would likewise be possible only in a prefrontal cortex functioning above the emergent threshold.

Childhood reports of consistent memories (single images or sequences of the past) typically begin around the third or fourth year of life. There are reported cases, however, where a particular single moment or a few events in time that occurred in the second year of life appear to have generated a full 4D thought-memory.[23] What is interesting about these cases, and the only reason they are being mentioned, is that these thought-memories usually are of a strong sensory nature, such as a crisis situation involving illness or the birth of a sibling. These memories may, of course, simply be the only ones that remain from that time, perhaps because they are the most sensorily powerful; or it may be that the thought-memory system of the very young child recorded only those moments that had a certain stimulus weight. In any event, it is fascinating to speculate that these cases may describe a flicker-fusion moment, driven by a high-energy, high-stimulation context, that in effect drove the system into thought for a brief duration of time before relaxing back into pre-thought function as the extraordinary stimulation declined. It would certainly not be surprising if the developmental transition into a stable mode of thought generation involved moments of threshold function followed by others in a pre-thought state.

Now that we have established a model for a human-only thought function and a consciousness point of view, what does it mean? How do we process the 4D information from real time, the moment past, and distant memory? What are the limits, constraints, and illusions within which the system operates as the 4D information space grows in size, detail, and resolution by the reiterative, recombinant cycles of processing moments? What does it mean for us in the reference system of consciousness?

Only now can we begin to look at the specific information of both sensory worlds (external and internal), and the information's transformation in the forebrain memory system as patterns of 3D neural activity enter the PIMs to produce novel thoughts— novel products that exert their force on the other brain computational regions, on effector systems, and back into the memory structural information regions. We only glimpsed the representation-specific thought effect when we looked at a young girl playing in pools of mud and water, liberated from the temporal flux of the background environment. As we walked through the animal world, we did not see thought, thought-memory, consciousness, or the fundamental behavior changes that follow from their emergence. We tried to speculate on what it would be like if termites, horses, parrots, or apes did have minds, but we could not see the basic structure of behavior—the interactions in time—that would be present irrespective of the information or the effector system used to express it if they did. Now we have localized the threshold to thought and consciousness in the human child. Piaget and many others have documented the astonishing changes in behavior that occur once this threshold is surpassed.

In the next chapter, we continue to present the underlying principles of the biological production of thought and consciousness, expressed in the language of emergent, organic, referent systems. These fundamental concepts must be discussed without regard to the intrinsic information (the subject matter, as it were) encoded in the patterns of afferent energy wavefronts. We will examine the principles of neurobiological structure and function that underlie this phenomenon as a model, as best we can, before we analyze the specific sensory information, its effects, and what it means with respect to human development, illness, knowledge, limitations, and our individual and collective abilities to observe, measure, and think about the universe.

We have drawn another line and proposed that the emergence of thought and consciousness occurs sometime around 16 to 24 months. This exclusively human event that occurs near or in the second year of life should be cause for splendid expectancy and celebration. The terrible twos could be affectionately renamed the emergent twos in honor of an exclusive moment in all of nature and the human family.

Part Five

INFINITE REFLECTION

10

Reference Systems of Consciousness I: Constraints of Structure and Function

Consciousness is the propagated 4D frame of reference that emerges from human prefrontal module activity, and life is the propagated 4D frame of reference that emerges from cellular activity. These are the two biological systems of evolution that internally generate a unique temporal dimension within their respective dynamic boundaries. And, as local systems emerging from the surrounding background of the electromagnetic field, each has quantifiable limitations related to its physical structure and metabolic function.

The demarcation and delineation of biophysical boundaries and constraints actually provide a focus and clarity to the context within which life and consciousness may exist. By illuminating the processes of evolution that generated emergent systems, we may better view what lies on each side of nature's thermodynamic thresholds of biological order and information. Biological relativity provides a set of guidelines to refer to as we explore our existence through daily experience, science, and medicine.

A quantitative model that operationalizes thought as an informational product generated in moments of human neural activity demands that we reformulate how we *think* about thought. We must reexamine the ways in which illness, disease, and trauma affect the nervous system, and the manner in which they alter or eliminate thought and the flow of consciousness. We must redesign our scientific approach to the investigation of thinking, mind, and consciousness in animals other than humans. The model of biological relativity forces a radical restructuring of the way in which most scientists and physicians have been taught to regard thought and mind. We may likewise need to radically alter the diagnosis and care of patients with central nervous system disorders. Biological relativity may enable us to predict and anticipate the loss of thought production in certain disruptions of brain processes and to determine when and if they may be restored.

The threshold of consciousness, as proposed, reveals the truly gossamer nature of its thermodynamic disconnect from the background of all neural activity. The internal 4D representations that have liberated us from our environment are nevertheless still bound to the enveloping worlds of energy and matter and the information they provide. The subtlety of the evolutionary threshold that separates humanity from other primates, and the developmental threshold each of us crosses at around 2 years of age, may serve to humble us. Thought and consciousness do not give us unlimited control.

An analysis of the limiting parameters and constraints of the consciousness frame of reference will provide us with insight into the unique individual nature of our exclusively human experience of reality and will provide a focus for the application of science and medicine to understanding the ultimate molecular processes and disruptions of nature's most ordered biophysical system.

Structural Parameters

The prefrontal integration module (PIM) is presented as an interlaced, repeating structure that exists in each cerebral hemisphere and receives an array of multimodal topographic information that forms the most complex sensory representation of the internal and external environments in the present moment, the recent past, and the more distant past from memory. Individual cortical cylinders may be up to several hundred microns in diameter, and a PIM may consist of one or more of these anatomically and physiologically defined structures. This is ultimately a theoretical construct, so we do not know what the exact dimensions of these modules would be or the spatial arrangements they would take in the functional brain. At each successive 200-ms computational cycle of afferent information flow through a module, the formula $f(R_a t_n, R'_a t_{n-1}, R''_a t_{n-x})$ represents the entire content of representations that undergo a biomathematical transformation.

We consider this prefrontal modular structure and basic function to be essentially equivalent in all mammals with this brain modification. In both pre-thought associative learning (where the temporal dimension linking each computational product is provided only by the external context) and thought (where the sequences of association are contained in internally derived temporal dimensions), the prefrontal modular structure processes the incoming information and produces an efferent output back to the brain nuclei, the memory system, and effector motor systems. Across the thermodynamic divide between pre-thought and thought (in evolutionary and developmental thresholds), we propose that the basic structure-function design and operation of the brain has not been significantly changed. The prefrontal effect on either side of the thought threshold is one of inhibition or reinforcement of ongoing behavior. Either in thought sequences (with the added power of context-independent learned sequences that may enter into the real-time computational equation and have a weighting function) or in pre-thought sequences (associative relationships tied to the real-time context), the momentary actions of the behaving animal may be influenced only within quantifiable parameters. Only the sensory information, its order, and the internal temporal dimension were added in human thought; the basic input-output structure of the system remained the same.

In addition to the neuroanatomical and neurophysiological considerations that lead us to propose the similarity between prefrontal structure and function in all mammalian brains, we noted that studies of the particular behaviors that appear to be affected by damage to this region in nonhuman primates and humans also show a great deal of similarity. The descriptive, and sometimes quantitative, classifications of behaviors that are impaired by prefrontal structural damage include those of decision making, abstract intelligence, attention, awareness, cognition, choice, will, self, thinking, and consciousness. Virtually all reported cases of human behavioral changes resulting from prefrontal lesions involve partial damage to one or both cerebral hemispheres, and they provide us with a method of localizing (mapping) regional or hemispheric specialization of function. Luria, Hebb, Penfield, Sperry, Gazzaniga, Milner, Weiskrantz, Levin, and many other physicians, scientists, and scientist-physicians have derived great insights into the role of the human prefrontal regions by carefully and compassionately studying changes in behavior following a wide variety of brain insults to patients from trauma, disease, stroke, epilepsy, and surgical intervention.[1] A large literature on a few interesting patients, their particular lesions, and the resultant behavioral changes has developed, and secular fascination with these cases has grown. In general, it may be stated that lesions to human prefrontal cortex appear to cause conditions such as distractibility, impaired future planning, personality change, memory disturbance, speech problems, apathy and loss of will, depression, hypersexuality, immorality, paranoia, decreased awareness of self, and thus general impairment of our most human executive abilities and deeply personal characteristics.

However, we completely lack an understanding of what functional behavioral deficits would arise in human patients whose entire prefrontal cortex (orbitomedial and dorsolateral) in both cerebral hemispheres was completely destroyed or excised. The primary reason for this lack of information is obvious: Such an extreme extent of damage would most likely result in the loss of life. Even the surgical prefrontal lobotomies and leucotomies that were performed on thousands of patients diagnosed with intractable mental illness during the 1930s, 1940s, and 1950s, in the failed hope of curing psychosis, did not produce that complete degree of damage, at least not in those who survived and who were reported on in the literature.

Biological relativity proposes a new way to look at thought and consciousness: as an exclusive product and property of the mature human prefrontal neocortex. A direct postulate states that it would be theoretically possible to eliminate thought and consciousness if a critical amount of prefrontal tissue were damaged or removed. Thus, it is predicted that there is a minimum necessary and sufficient structural condition for the production of thought and consciousness in the prefrontal modules. Indeed, if the basic prefrontal integration module is on the order of several hundred microns in diameter, a very small amount of brain tissue (on the order of cubic millimeters) with structural integrity may be sufficient to generate a limited thought function and propagate consciousness. How a limited faculty to generate thought products and produce a consciousness field would affect an individual's experience of reality and observable behavior is unknown, but it is a hypothetical state of being in our model.

The final conclusion and statement of constraint, from this presentation, is that a complete resection of the prefrontal region, or of those specific portions that contain the PIMs (unknown at this time), will eliminate thought and thus consciousness from the human brain. This would be an extreme condition involving the loss of up to 30 percent of each cerebral cortex. We again note that our model proposes that a thought function is produced in each cerebral hemisphere and that these functions are unified by the axon connections across the corpus callosum. The much-publicized and ground-breaking research performed on patients with surgically separated cerebral hemispheres (the "split-brain" condition) by Sperry and Gazzaniga and the continued cutting-edge work by Gazzaniga and colleagues indicate that each cerebral hemisphere has at least some type of independent high-order information processing.[2] The level of behavioral performance generated by each semi-independent hemisphere appears to reflect the production of thought and consciousness. We might ask, then, what would the result be if all the sensory input to healthy prefrontal modules involved in thought production were effectively blocked? In this case, could a thought be generated? And, if not all the afferent input was blocked, what would happen if one, two, or more major sensory pathways could not reach the PIMs? At what point would a degraded afferent source of information drop below a critical threshold order and fail to sufficiently drive the thought-generating computational operations of structurally intact prefrontal modules? Do cases of a type of *informational* lesion exist, wherein patients possess a healthy and intact structure of prefrontal cortex, but live without thought and consciousness? Obtaining the answers to these questions requires that we examine the key functional parameters of the prefrontal modules.

Functional Parameters

Sensory Representation

The major afferent projections to the prefrontal regions include the primary sensory representations of the visual, auditory, somatosensory, viscerosensory, vestibular, gustatory, and olfactory systems. In the normal development of the human nervous system, the thought-generating process would be able to integrate information from all these sensory systems as they presented in unimodal and multimodal representation to the prefrontal modules. The quantitative model of biological relativity leads us to consider the hypothetical limits on the amount of information that is necessary for the intact system to function. As we asked, if the prefrontal region is structurally intact, what informational input is needed to drive the computational activity and integrate two moments of sensory experience to derive the temporal dimension?

We can imagine that if all sensory information were stopped at the brainstem level, thought and consciousness would cease. The loss of specific external sensory information through focal brain damage could hypothetically be evaluated to determine whether the functional removal of one or more primary sensory modalities is sufficient to prevent the prefrontal modules from generating thought and consciousness. The loss of internal sensory information from the visceral-autonomic afferent sources may also significantly affect thought and consciousness. However, conditions such as blindness, deafness, partial tactile loss, loss of smell (anosmia), and loss of taste do not appear to lower the informational threshold of afferent input to the prefrontal modules below that necessary for thought and consciousness. Thus, the function of the PIMs is robust to at least the loss of one major sensory modality. While we do not know the minimal requirements for sensory information needed to drive thought and consciousness, we may learn about how the brain develops without more than one major sensory modality. The life and development of Helen Keller stands as a testament to the resiliency of the human brain, and to her extraordinary sense of nature and human compassion.

Helen Keller was born on June 27, 1880, in the state of Alabama. As far as we know, she developed in a normal manner until her illness attacked. At the critical age of 19 months, in the dead of winter, she suffered what was reported as "acute congestion of the stomach and brain," accompanied by high fever. Perhaps a meningitis infection, it affected her for several months and left her without sight or hearing. The accounts of Helen's life following her amazing survival from such a ferocious infection are quite fascinating.[3] From the perspective of human development and our model, Helen was struck down right at the time when the threshold of thought, thought-memory, and consciousness might have been occurring.

With the gracious and grateful perspective that fills her prose and poetry, Helen wrote about her first 19 months. "I had caught glimpses of broad, green fields, a luminous sky, trees and flowers which the darkness that followed could not wholly blot out. If we have once seen, 'the day is ours, and what the day has shown.'" These sentences, albeit *post hoc* and reflective, appear to indicate that she had formed a few memories from a thought-generating process: 4D computational moments resided in her memory as glimpses of the sensory world right around the time of her entry into the Emergent Twos.

We mentioned reports of early, brief memories of highly emotional situations that take place near the second year of life and how they might represent the first flickers of thought and consciousness. Helen may have been reporting something of the same nature in the sentences above. In the following years, she wrote clearly of her awareness, her thoughts, and her complex attempts to communicate and interpret her world, however cruelly diminished. Without the primary sensory modalities of sight and sound, and without the benefit of a formally taught language, Helen appeared to produce thoughts that provided detailed information about her external and internal 4D environments, and these were entered quite well into her forebrain memory system.

Helen developed her own signs for objects, acting a scene to communicate her message and meaning. If she wanted bread, "I would imitate the acts of cutting slices and buttering them," she wrote. "If I wanted my mother to make ice-cream for dinner, I made the sign for working the freezer and shivered, indicating cold." She learned all these actions by touching people as they performed the behaviors, integrating what she sensed in thought and memory, and then expressing the 4D information through her own motor systems at the right time and in the proper context: Clearly this is context-independent behavior, with the intramodal transfer that is indicative of thought in the frame of reference of consciousness.

Helen wrote of knowing what her mother and others wanted and what they were implying with their touch, their movements, and even the particular type of clothes they wore, yet she was frustrated by her inability to communicate more fully. She explained, "Sometimes I stood between two persons who were conversing and touched their lips. I could not understand, and was vexed. I moved my lips and gesticulated frantically without results. This made me so angry at times that I kicked and screamed until I was exhausted." Helen was a smart and driven young girl! Her life was nevertheless a rich one, as she learned many things, solved many problems, and formed many memories about her experience in time and place.

Then, when she was 6, everything changed. Her parents took her to meet Dr. Alexander Graham Bell, known then as an educator who specialized in teaching the blind and deaf. Helen expressed the powerful impact of their first encounter on all her senses. "He understood my signs, and I knew it and loved him at once." At the suggestion of Dr. Bell, Anne Mansfield Sullivan arrived at the Keller residence in March of 1887, when Helen was 7. In just about 3 months, under Ms. Sullivan's determined guidance, Helen made an association that marked a change in her young life. The moment portrayed in so many theatrical productions was that of the day Ms. Sullivan took Helen out to the well house and held one of her hands under the running water from the pump, while simultaneously signing W-A-T-E-R in her other palm.

Let us apply the model of prefrontal integration module function to this crossroads in Helen's life. In that pivotal moment, Helen was simultaneously integrating the sensory representation of the cold, flowing, forceful water and the sequence of signs that made up the word. This moment, lasting perhaps a few minutes, was being integrated in 200-ms PIM computational cycles; two distinct sensorimotor events were being integrated and thus bound in time. As the process continued and the *now*, the immediate past, and the delayed past of seconds ago (reentering from the memory system) became compared in 4D disparity computations, the information from the two patterns formed a novel construct, a new connection. The internal sensory world provided strong positive feedback for the new information, as Helen recalled. "Suddenly I felt a misty consciousness as of something forgotten—a thrill of returning thought. . . . I knew then that 'w-a-t-e-r' meant the wonderful cool something that was flowing over my hand."

Helen had been signing and communicating with only limited effectiveness for several years prior to this event, but in only 3 months, Ms. Sullivan's more formal approach and dedicated efforts were successful. After this moment, Helen's learning rate grew exponentially. She had already been producing thought for many years, and she now had a new tool layered upon them. The language of formal signing, and all the power and fulfillment that it brought to Helen's life, came after her emergence into thought and consciousness, as evidenced by the written accounts of her memories long before Ms. Sullivan's arrival. Helen graduated with honors from Radcliffe, and among her writings she recounted the joy of attending the 1893 World's Fair together with Ms. Sullivan and her admitted first love, Dr. Bell.

We find in the story of Helen Keller that thought and consciousness are not related to any specific sensory modality, and that thought functions with a minimum of primary sensory information. In terms of the developmental aspect of her case, Helen probably benefited greatly by having normal growth during her first 19 months of life. She may have just crossed into thought computation before she contracted her illness. It may be more difficult for those who have never experienced any stimulation from vision and hearing sensory systems. However, we do not yet know the absolute minimum amount of sensory information that is required to drive the system across the threshold of thought in structurally sound prefrontal modules. Theoretically, one could lose visual, auditory, somatosensory, and perhaps more sensory afferents and still generate thought. What the content and scope of these computations might be, and how they would be expressed in memory and through behavior, has not been systematically investigated. Perhaps, with biological relativity as a guide, we may formulate an approach to this critical concern.

Memory Function

Our quantitative approach to the production of thought predicts many limitations on the integration of external and internal sensory information. A single thought is a construct created on a millisecond scale; it cannot contain more information than is derived within this limiting variable. Furthermore, as each thought is transduced and transmitted to other brain regions, it decays in informational strength; it is computationally diluted by newer sensory information. Even in thought, the present fades into the past. It is the function of the forebrain memory system continually to bring representations of the past into the present, where they may influence ongoing neural computations and behavioral events. How, then, are thought and consciousness affected when the forebrain memory system is functionally destroyed? Can the consciousness frame of reference be propagated without the past reentering from memory? Let's take another look at the case of H.M., this time within the framework of our model.[4]

H.M. lived a strange existence following his surgery. Without the hippocampi and anterior temporal lobes, his forebrain memory system was severely compromised. From the point of view of our model, his well-documented behavior in real time indicated that he was producing thought and that it was being propagated across his intact prefrontal neocortex; thus he was in consciousness. His momentary awareness, assessment of the sensory context of the internal and external worlds, and recall of appropriate presurgical memories appeared to be reasonably normal. However, virtually nothing he experienced in real-time thought entered into structural memory (with important exceptions previously noted).

If we follow the temporal flow of information through H.M.'s impaired functional system, we can see how his experience in consciousness may be formulated. The hypothetical timing of thought as it is generated and transmitted in the normal brain is depicted in Figure 7-2. We see that in the dominant *now* PIM, a novel thought is produced in ≈ 200 ms. That thought product is sent to the next module as the immediate past ($R'_a t_{n-1}$), and then goes into the memory system. After about a second of prefrontal activity (and about five steps of PIM-to-PIM thought propagation), the *now* computation will contain very diluted information, as it will be only a fraction of the newer information entering from the immediate past moment ($R'_a t_{n-1}$). At around this same time, some of that initial moment of information, along with other related representations, may reenter the *now* computational equation from the intact memory system. From here, it may function to refresh and extend the serial flow of time in the prefrontal modules and bring related behavioral sequences from the memory store into consideration.

In H.M.'s brain (from our theoretical perspective), we can watch the *now* fade over a few seconds as it is computationally degraded in each modular cycle and efferent output. The new sensory representations impinging upon the modules overtake the past moments of representation, and the immediate past no longer reenters the PIM system from the memory loop. All thought generated is lost to memory as a result of the extensive damage to H.M.'s hippocampi and temporal lobes. The fading of the *now* timeline in H.M.'s brain gives us insight into the propagation potential of thought in the prefrontal modules without the benefit of the forebrain memory refresh rate and without conversion into a long-term structural information base. H.M.'s perception of real time, as expressed in his ability to remember the past moments, has been relegated to the span of a few seconds by the effects of his surgery. We cannot be certain if this is an exact expression of the prefrontal system alone, as there are some remnants of his hippocampal system in place, along with other regions of the forebrain memory structures. Nevertheless, it is an intriguing temporal decay of the internal 4D flow of experience in thought and consciousness.

The past was not entirely lost to H.M. He had produced twenty-some years worth of thoughts and thought memories prior to his operation. Most of that 4D information space remained in the portions of his temporal lobe that were spared during his surgery, stored in structural memory. Thus, as his prefrontal modules continued to generate thoughts and propagate them across the modular fields, old memories were elicited by stimuli in the real-time sensory wavefronts and then entered into prefrontal computations as the $R''_a t_{n-x}$ component. The external chronological date of each of H.M.'s memory sequences extends back to the years *prior* to his surgery, so the minimal x value in the expression is now more than 40 years, as his surgery took place in 1956. H.M. is living and thinking in real time, but he is locked into the memories of the ever-receding past. He is locked into a consciousness that extends over a few seconds of *now* and years of distant *then*.

What would one's thoughts, behavior, and experience in consciousness be like if one was without the forebrain memory system from the very beginning, from the *onset* of thought? A person with such a disability would theoretically experience the few moments of the *now* in consciousness, but would never be able to build a knowledge base in the 4D information space; for this person, the now would fade from existence as each computational moment brought the next sensory representation of the present. How would such a person present in a clinical examination? How would he or she develop a language, complex behavior of any type, or a self, in time? Infants who are not yet producing thought and do not yet have a fully developed hippocampal place system still can learn basic associations with a partially mature memory system. But there may be children with genetic or acquired disease who do not develop the capacity for object permanence and yet begin to generate thought in the prefrontal system. This combination of function and dysfunction would result in some progression of associative learning, but not the robust progression seen in thought combined with thought-memory. H.M.'s advantage is that he has a 20-year 4D information space library that is available to influence his ongoing verbal and other motor behavior. It is precisely due to his past structure of thought that under casual observation he appears to be a normal adult. There is an

H.M. *past* that is providing a temporal consistency to complex behavior performed by the H.M *now*—flickers in experienced moments of fading thoughts and pulsating consciousness.

Metabolic Function

The metabolic activity in each individual cell and the collective activity of cellular systems provide the energy for the resting membrane potentials, ion channel operation, neurotransmitter receptor function, and nerve impulse generation. The basic metabolic processes support all transduction, transformation, encoding, and transmission of sensory representations that reach the prefrontal modules. All thought and consciousness are thus exquisitely sensitive to the metabolic parameters within every cell.

We hypothesized that early thought-dependent memories in children may be created as a result of increased metabolic activity during highly stressful moments. Novel situations and personal traumas that increase the autonomic tone of the sympathetic system will result in increased heart rate, blood pressure, oxygen consumption, and glucose metabolism. This metabolic upregulation in each cell affects every step of sensory processing, including the biocomputational functions in neocortical modules. We speculated that during the maturational phase, when the structural and functional parameters of the PIMs may be approaching the critical threshold for the production of thought and consciousness, brief periods of heightened metabolic activity may push the system beyond the threshold into an operational state. The thoughts generated and the internal temporal dimension would then enter into memory and be recalled later as discrete memories of places and situations at a time prior to a consistent memory of the flow of personal space and time that comes from ongoing thought in consciousness.

It is difficult to examine the specific effects of altered metabolic parameters on thought and consciousness, as any significant effect on cellular functions tends to alter the processes in all cell types and in all regions of the body and brain. However, some specificity of sensitivity to metabolic parameters does exist in certain cell lines, and these include the highly specialized nerve cells.

The bioenergetic processes that create and maintain the resting membrane potential, generate the nerve impulse, and operate synaptic zone activity place a high demand on the metabolic pathways within each nerve cell, and these may be disrupted more readily than those in other types of cells. Since we do not yet have a quantitative measure of real-time thought production, we have to look at relative changes in this process by observing complex behaviors that depend upon the presence of thought production and looking for memory phenomena that may reflect lapses or distortions in the 4D flow of sensory experience in consciousness. When a patient can perform a complex behavioral sequence (like opening a door), but appears to be unaware of his or her current environment or may be unable to communicate with others in the setting, and later has no memory of the events, we may infer that disruption of nerve cell function related to thought generation may have occurred. We propose that in these moments, complex behavior may proceed (with great limitations) through pre-thought brain functioning that is responding to local contextual stimuli. The patient may not be processing these moments in thought, and this is why he or she can't comment on the ongoing situation, modify the typically *robotlike* sequence of behavior, or recall his or her actions later.

The tenuous state of thought and consciousness in the human brain may be immediately and completely lost with only mild head trauma, intracranial bleeding, intracranial pressure from tumors or fluid cysts, ingested substances like alcohol and other drugs, and the onset of generalized seizure activity. Fortunately, in many cases, this loss of consciousness is transient, and consciousness returns following amelioration of the insult. Even more indicative of the delicacy of our consciousness referent system is the fact that if the molecular oxygen flow to the prefrontal region is reduced below a critical threshold for even a few seconds, consciousness is lost. Furthermore, if the other primary source of energy to the nerve cell, glucose as supplied by the circulatory system, is reduced to very low levels for only a few minutes, the brain cannot support the generation of thought. The genetics of the nerve cell have not allowed for a large internal energy store, and the shift to the metabolism of intracellular energy sources such as ketone molecules may last for only a brief time. High-energy compounds must be continually supplied by the supporting systems of life.

Our study of the development of the nervous system in the context of the growing human (Chapter 4) includes the comment that the evolution of multicellular life began the process of producing novel intercellular environments that did not previously exist on Earth and that these unique biochemical *milieux* led to the further specialization of cells through genetic modification. Thus the nerve cell, as one example, cannot live in the extra-organismal biosphere, but must be surrounded by a specific extracellular solution and have its oxygen and glucose supplied by blood flow. Narrow concentration values of critical ions such as sodium, chloride, potassium, and calcium and the relative acid-base balance or pH must be maintained in an adequate volume of hydrating fluid; otherwise nerve cell processes become disrupted and may eventually be irreparably damaged or even extinguished. Pressure and temperature are also critical homeostatic variables. A body temperature above 40°C or below 30°C is not compatible with nervous system activity. Bacterial infections and toxic substances, including medications, alcohol, and other drugs, may interfere with the local availability of important metabolites or may have a directly deleterious effect on the cell. Direct effects on nerve cells may include increasing or decreasing the ease with which a nerve impulse is generated or how much neurotransmitter is released and remains in the extracellular space to influence other cells.

Depending on many factors related to the type of metabolic insult, the duration and magnitude of its effect, and the ability of the body to reestablish homeostasis, a variety of changes in the generation of thought and consciousness may be observed upon clinical examination. At one extreme of a continuum of consciousness, we may see a patient with a high metabolic rate. This person may have an infection with fever or may have ingested a substance that has caused his nerve cells to consume energy compounds at a high rate. The autonomic system may be overactive, and nerve cell activity may be in a relative state of excitation. The patient's tendon reflexes may be brisk, his behavioral reactions may be quick, and he may talk at a fast rate of speed. The patient appears jerky or agitated. He may report being extra sensitive to all sensory stimuli, such as touch, hearing, smell, and taste. At some extreme, we may also observe that his thought process is affected and that he is making errors in his assessment of the current context. Real-time situations, the immediate past, and distant memories may get mixed up in the integrated moments of the present setting. We may diagnose such a person as being distractible, confused, or, with more extreme behavioral disruption, delirious or psychotic.

If the metabolic disturbances that drive this state continue long enough or if the effects reach a magnitude that is at or beyond the limits of cellular or system function, the disordered thought process may start to enter a declining curve where thought, mind, and awareness begin to fade toward the flicker-fusion threshold. On the way to this relative position on the functional continuum, the patient may appear to be thinking and behaving in slow motion. The patient's own report may be that he is not able to think at a normal rate, that his sense of reality is slipping, and that he can't keep track of what is going on. He may reach a state of stupor, in which it appears that he is not generating thought and consciousness. Shaking the patient, pinching his fingers, shouting at him, or rubbing his sternum may bring him back to thought and consciousness. The all too common alcoholic stupor is representative of this intermittent flicker-fusion-flicker state. (Compare this to the suggested threshold moments of thought and memory in the developing child in stressful situations.) If the metabolic insult continues in duration or increases in magnitude, we may lose the patient to coma and even death.

A significant disturbance in nerve cell processes leads to a disturbance in sensory information (at either the transduction, transformation, encoding, or transmission phase). The disturbance in sensory information flow leads to a disturbance in thought, which may cause a disturbance in memory of the sensory events. Disorders of thought generate a disturbance of consciousness. This sequence may occur at either of the extremes of too high or too low metabolic conditions. This is a simple biophysical relationship that cannot be altered in principle, no matter how hard we may try to out-think it. The metabolic effects on thought and consciousness may be more subtle than the loss of an entire sensory modality or damage to the structural integrity of the prefrontal region, but they no less dramatically determine the content, the quality, and even the presence of the computational product.

In many cases in which metabolic insult has altered thought and consciousness, we may find that not only is the afferent sensory information distorted in its content, but the internally derived temporal dimension is likewise disrupted. Even as the external sensory context and its inherent temporal dimension of background time is degraded into sporadically transduced moments of sensory information, the prefrontal disparity computations between two moments of disrupted sensory representations will still derive an internal temporal dimension. It is the default operation of the module. However, the 4D thought product and its propagation will now contain an erroneous temporal component relative to the actual flow of information in the external world. Illusions, delusions, and hallucinations typically contain components of temporal distortion.

Our model proposes that the most complex operation the nervous system can perform is the internal computation of a unique temporal dimension from two moments of spatial information. It is not unreasonable to propose also that this dimension will be the first to be disrupted in metabolic disturbances that do not fully degrade the operational parameters of the prefrontal modules to below the flicker-fusion threshold of thought production, as in the extreme conditions of stupor or coma. In impaired states such as confusion, delirium, or psychosis, thoughts with disrupted sensory components will still enter the forebrain memory system and form *a structural reality of illusional time*. These disordered memories must be reconciled (or *recontextualized* by transformations) in additional cycles of disparity computations following the recovery of normal function, when and if that occurs. Persistent states of dimensional distortion such as those that may be found in certain dementias or psychoses reflect the biological horror of our constrained existence, tied ultimately to sensory representation.

Dreams

The internal world of dreams reveals the independent referent system of consciousness as a 4D construct. All dimensions, including time, are exposed as biocomputational manifestations of the nervous system during this state, and the threshold from pre-thought to thought may be traversed many times during sleep to initiate the altered generation of thought and thought-memory.

Dreams reveal the sensitivity of our internally derived temporal dimension. The entry into sleep represents a complex genetic modulation of basic metabolic parameters, the exact purpose of which remains uncertain. During sleep, the external sensory environment is prevented from stimulating the brain to a degree that produces thought and consciousness, and output effector systems are blocked from initiating motor behaviors. We can view this process as a metabolic reduction in the operational parameters of the prefrontal modules to a level below the flicker-fusion threshold. The afferent input from the monoaminergic nuclei of the basal forebrain and brainstem and the thalamic projections probably functions to induce and maintain much of this functional comalike state of relative paralysis.

The sleep cycle has distinct stages of neocortical activity that may be monitored and grossly quantified by electroencephalographic analysis. The time spent in each sleep stage changes with development and in various disease states and metabolic disturbances. Dreaming mostly occurs in the phase of sleep that corresponds to rapid eye movements (REM sleep, a period of highly active cortical function). Because we can form memories of dream sequences and experience this state as one of an altered consciousness, we propose that the prefrontal integration modules become activated during these periods and generate thoughts, which may enter the memory system but are usually prevented from influencing motor behavior.

In this time of thought production, we have an altered afferent flow of sensory information entering the computational modules at each moment of processing time. To limited degrees that vary across the REM period and from night to night, stimulus energy from the external and internal sensory worlds may reach the dominant PIM, generating a thought; but in general these stimulus sources are effectively prevented from contributing significant sensory information during these periods. This leaves the forebrain memory system ($R''_a t_{n-x}$), the thalamic input, and the monoaminergic projections contributing the majority of sensory and other stimuli. Relevant to our previous discussion of the minimum amount of sensory information that is required to generate thought, the dream state indicates that in the normal brain under these specific conditions, novel thoughts may be generated with significant inhibition of all real-time sensory modalities.

Thus it appears that the 4D multimodal sensory representations from the memory system may be sufficient to drive the biomathematical computations of the prefrontal modules in the unique metabolic conditions that are present during the REM phase of sleep. Under the modulatory influences of the thalamic nuclei and monoaminergic afferents, memory sequences may enter the prefrontal modules and become propagated across neural processing time. The integrated products, novel thoughts from memory moments, may reenter the memory system and become part of the structural long-term information space. They may also elicit additional memory representations that can enter the prefrontal system and undergo real-time integration with other memory products. This closed loop of private sensory activity would thus generate the dream experience and memory in consciousness.

During this period, the temporal dimension of the external sensory environment would not be a significant influence in pacing and linking the moments of sensory experience. The dominant temporal dimension would be the internally created one within the 4D information flow of thought and memory. The insight that we can gain from our experience of these periods, and from the reports of others, is that the temporal dimension derived in moments of disparity computation by prefrontal modules is indeed unique to the integrated sensory information and not just a reflection of the real-time background temporal dimension.

It is intriguing to speculate that dreams also reveal that the neural processes underlying the conversion of thought sequences into long-term memories do not maintain a highly accurate representation of this relatively new internal dimension. From our evolutionary perspective, this would not be surprising, in that the genetic modifications that resulted in thought and consciousness would not necessarily have modified the entire memory system to provide an absolute structural trace of the temporal dimension in the sensory information entering its computational and conversion pathways. Many realities may occur in dreams, and time may be warped, compressed, expanded, reversed, and replayed. As we noted for illusions, delirium, and hallucinations, *structural realities of illusional time* describe the dream experience.

Biological relativity brings a very interesting perspective to the dream process by imposing a biophysical framework of constraints, bounded by the four dimensions of our existence. We could discuss the ramifications of dreams and illness as they relate to the 4D referent system of consciousness at great length. However, the primary purpose of this discussion has been to show the degree of manipulation of the internal temporal dimension by altered metabolic parameters. Moreover, we found that in dreams the prefrontal computational presence of the internal 4D world of memories achieves dominance as the influence of external sensory stimuli lessens (this relative influence can also be mapped onto our sigmoid-curve function). This relative shift from an external-dominated to an internal-dominated temporal dimension of personal reality may be of great creative benefit in moments of quiet contemplative reflection or daydreaming (when the demands of the environment are at a minimum), but may be horrifically detrimental when it takes the form of illusions, delusions, and hallucinations. Thus, our internally derived time, our integrated time, our personal or subjective time, our sense of individual or *I-time*, is indeed a relative dimension and is created and constrained by the structure and function of the nervous system.

11

Reference Systems of Consciousness II: Interpreting the World

Time, Relativity, and Consciousness

Albert Einstein demonstrated an acute awareness that all the theories, insights, measurements, and realities of which humankind could conceive were ultimately products of thought and consciousness. He wrote and spoke passionately about science as a deeply personal endeavor that colored and influenced all experience. It was common for him to relate complex problems in math and physics in terms of very human situations, perhaps in an effort to reinforce the personal, subjective nature of the all-too-often dispassionate subject matter. It was reported that he would describe relativity theory to audiences of serious-minded students and faculty members in a single sentence that went something like: A minute seems like an hour if you place your hand on a hot stove, but an hour seems like a minute when you have a pretty girl on your lap.

Einstein was, in essence, expressing the fundamental importance of understanding the frame of reference and its personal, human interpretation. His statement evokes the *I-time*, noting how our sense of time is unique to the individual, not absolute, and may be altered by the sensory context. Einstein referred to this subjective time in his formulation of the special theory of relativity as the time within each four-dimensional (4D) referent frame. In our biological model of referent systems, it relates to the function of the prefrontal cortex in that any independent 4D system creates its own temporal dimension. There is no absolute time for 4D systems relative to one another, whether in matter particles, planets, cells, animals, or propagated 4D sensory representations. And, as we have noted, for the human nervous system, changes in metabolic parameters may affect the rate at which thought is produced and/or propagated. Thus, from our emergent perspective, from our frame of reference in organic evolution, external time (a different referent system) feels as if it is passing more quickly or more slowly, depending upon neural metabolic activity. This sense of a change in the background temporal flow rate is the result of a disparity computation of the current passage of external events with the thought-memory of similar past events. This comparison is performed in the prefrontal modules and is therefore unique to the individual, her or his current state of metabolic function, and her or his personal memory of past sequences of events along with their indivisible temporal rates.

The computed relationship between any two independent temporal dimensions is not only relative, but also inverse. Background time, as measured by the clock on the wall, the motion of an object, or any living process, may appear to be proceeding more rapidly if metabolic activity has slowed from its prior (that is, remembered and thus comparative) level of function, and it may appear to proceed more slowly if the rate of metabolic activity has significantly increased. This relationship is an expression of relativity in the biological referent system of consciousness.

In Einstein's statement, the two sensory contexts, hot stove (external) and emotional excitement (internal), may both produce intense, charged memories. But it is the reflection on the temporal dimension as the memories of the events reenter the real-time prefrontal modular processes that creates the perception of a time expansion or compression for each experience. In other words, one would report in the past tense that, "holding my hand on the hot surface felt like an eternity" or "when you were on my lap, time seemed to fly." The relative nature of the temporal dimension comes with the memory of the recent past event compared to the current external time flow. This may not be a perfect example of the relative nature of internal time, but for Einstein it was a wonderful way to bring his magnificent insights into the true nature of the relative universe to anyone who would listen, and think.

With respect to our internal sensation, perception, or feeling of the flow of time in the present relative to some past event, we may pose the following questions: How fast or slowly may one think, learn, remember, write, paint, play music, run, dance, jump, create, discover, or metabolize? We may also ask, How fast or slowly may one see, hear, feel, taste, smell, or fear, hope, love, or be amused? For some of these, such as writing, playing music, and running, we may be able to provide an external measuring stick, a clock by which to make judgments. But, for others, such as creating, smelling, fearing, or wondering, the internal comparison of one temporal dimension with another derived at a separate time is the only metric that can be applied to determine a rate change or *differentiated* experience. We might say, "I used to feel fear more quickly in that situation" or "My sense of wonder when I think about this problem once was more enduring." Each of these statements refers to a comparison of one internal time to another internal time, the metric of which, the clock, was created in biomathematical computations in the prefrontal modules.

Each of us has an internally generated temporal dimension of our personal thought function and experience in consciousness. Subjectively, we can comment on this dimension, but only by comparing two thought sequences from past experience and determining if any relative difference exists. Objectively, we may also correlate, post hoc, one or more biological factors that relate to these experiences with the external background time dimension by measuring heart rate, blood pressure, hormonal release, or brain electrical activity changes. We can then compare the changes in biological parameters with the reported changes in internal time perception. Ultimately, these derivative, comparative constructs will be found to correlate perfectly because internal temporal dimensions are biophysical constructions of neural activity. However, there is no absolute or singular time dimension in our derived thoughts that is wholly a reflection of the current background time flow, as each thought has its own 4D structure that includes a temporal flow of information from the past moment and from the memory afferent component. The combined integration of all these 4D products results in a novel fourth dimension that is of its own metric, unique to the person, the background context of the world, and the universe at large.

Einstein understood the human biology of his relativity very well: "The experiences of an individual appear to us arranged in a series of events; in this series the single events which we remember appear to be ordered according to the criterion of *earlier* and *later*. There exists, therefore, for the individual, an I-time, or subjective time. This in itself is not measurable. I can, indeed, associate numbers with the events, in such a way that a greater number is associated with the later event than with an earlier one. This association I can define by means of a clock by comparing the order of events furnished by the clock with the order of the given series of events. We understand by a clock something which provides a series of events which can be counted."[1]

We are, however, limited to a certain range of normal derivation of our I-time production in thought by our human biophysical system, as Einstein's individual time now becomes the integrated time in the language of biomathematical computations in human prefrontal modules. Even the range of abnormal computational states is limited by the parameters of genetics and context. But either in the normal range or in the abnormal portions of the continuum, each of us is producing a unique 4D information space of thought that is unlike anyone else's. And we may compare aspects of any dimension, including time, from one event moment or sequence with another, similar one produced at a different moment in background sensory world time. The ongoing comparison of the 4D thought experiences of our past and present defines our self and thus our reality in consciousness.

The Emergent Property of Consciousness

We are now embarking on the most difficult of tasks, but we have a strong and detailed framework of information from which to make our observations. We have, to this point, explicitly examined only the computational effect of thought on the function of the brain and of behavior. The emergent property of consciousness must now be fully addressed and conceptualized within the parameters of this model.

We have proposed that life and consciousness are the two organic systems whose structure and function create independent 4D existences, relative to the supporting background systems. The propagating system of the cell physically creates the new time dimension, and life is its emergent property. This cellular-based system has quantifiable effects on other cells and the background environment through unique products created by the 4D processes of life. However, as stated in Chapter 3, the emergent property of life is a propagated organization, the order of matter and energy and its behavior in time. Life as a property has no inherent units of measure, no quantity, and absolutely no force of action back on the generating system or background environment. We cannot measure life; we can only describe its organization in time as processes (e.g., metabolism, transduction, or procreation) or cellular arrangements (e.g., bacteria, carrots, or birds). There is no equation for life as a force; there is no *élan vital*.

The emergent referent system of consciousness has the same general properties and constraints as those for life. The prefrontal integration module- (PIM-) based system and the integrated moments of 4D sensory experience, thoughts, indeed have quantifiable effects on the brain and the external environment through behavior. Thought is computed on a millisecond time scale (≈ 200 ms per product) and propagates within synaptic field activity. These modules of charged organic tissue indeed possess biophysical force and produce an action upon the generating structure (consistent with the basic physics of electromagnetic field phenomena). The processes of consciousness, like the metabolic processes of life, are thus described most generally as thinking and mind, and the quantifiable biophysical products are thoughts, in all their astronomical variations, sequences, and transformations in memory. Consciousness, as the irreducible property emerging from the propagation of the 4D systems of thoughts in time, however, has no inherent units of measure, no quantity, and absolutely no force of action back on the generating system or background environment. No additional new force is necessary to describe the processes and products of this local system in mature human brains. There is no equation for consciousness as a force; there is no *élan conscience* or *élan mental.*

We must keep in mind that all observations, including the present model, are made within this frame of reference called consciousness. The constraints of this reality create many insurmountable difficulties in our attempts to formalize a complete definition of consciousness, as we do not have another referent system from which to view it. We are indeed limited within our own computational minds and constrained by our minds' biophysical walls. We can, however, view the frame of reference of life, as it is a temporally independent 4D system whose moments *we* fuse in sensory representations. In observing life, we can accept that it has processes that we can describe only as 4D rates, products that we may quantify as 3D scalar amounts, and the property of being alive that describes only interactions or behavior in time. Life is unimaginably complex in its order and behavior, but it is not a force.

Consciousness is as *real* as life. We may observe other living humans with consciousness, as they are participants in the life field. We can accept that each person possesses a unique computational process that can only be described as a 4D rate, the rate of thought. We can accept that each person may express the quantifiable products of thoughts in 3D scalar quantities such as language, art, or technology, or in any behavior. We may also accept that we thus observe the process of consciousness in one another and for ourselves as we reflect, in time. Can we accept that consciousness fits the same general model of emergent evolution as does life? Can we accept that the two emergent properties of 4D organic systems, life and consciousness, do not have influence or force? Does a frame of reference approach apply to both systems? Let us examine the processes and products of consciousness further and answer some critical inherent questions that now arise regarding who we are and what we can do in our constrained frame of reference.

Sensation, Perception, Emotion, and Self in Consciousness

In the model of biological relativity, all dimensions of life and consciousness (in addition to time) must be relative to the local system. There cannot be an absolute standard or metric for any process within each referent frame.

It should be as relative in biology as in the continuum of nonliving matter and energy.

We call the most general process of the living cell *metabolism*. We identify other general processes of cellular systems as respiration, circulation, nervous activity, or motion (and collectively we call these systems organisms, fungi, ferns, or ferrets). Each process is a 4D propagation of biochemical and bioelectrical reactions and pathways. From the exclusively human point of view in consciousness, we observe this temporal flow of biophysical events because we have the capacity to fuse these moments of time within our propagated 4D sensory information space. We view the world as a serial path of moments in time, because we generate a serial, internal temporal dimension—a linear fusion of sensory flickers.

Thus, we may talk about metabolic rates, write about blooming flowers, and think about flying eagles. But, as delineated in Chapters 2 and 3 and reiterated many times thereafter, it is most important to remember that in order to apply any standard, any metric, any clock devised in the larger background biosphere referent system to the processes of any living system, the temporal dimension of that process must be collapsed to zero. Only products (static entities devoid of the time dimension) may be measured against a reference coordinate system. Only then can we examine and measure individual biological reactions or discrete steps in a complex pathway of metabolism or any other behavior in terms of scalar products. (Remember that the operational definition of behavior describes actions and processes at any level of matter-energy organization.) We may compare any timeless product to a background standard and report or measure moles of molecular oxygen, micrograms of dopamine, numbers of new petals, or the number of meters that an eagle can fly per minute (in that the time measure of a minute is now converted to a ratio entity relative to a defined spatial dimension). All dimensions of measure are relative to the background referent system's time dimension, biophysical parameters, products, and any ratios or rates derived from them. Each and every 4D process is unique to the individual, internal world of each cell, multicellular organism, and person, and through our sensory transduction of space and time we may observe each such local system within its emergent frames of reference of life and consciousness, behaving, interacting, living, and dying.

Our emergent human processes, contained within the 4D information space, are propagated in our individual, I-time dimension. Yet one person may report these subjective processes to another in terms that capture the entire 4D referent system, since both individuals are local systems within the consciousness field. For example, one person may say to another, "I'm thinking about the mathematical formula for integrating the area inside of that donut." And the other person will understand what is meant, because both individuals are simultaneously moving through the same 4D time line that is being verbally described. They both are embedded, if you will, in the consciousness field of space-time and therefore may communicate their ongoing experience to each other.

We must note at this point that any observation or thought that one person may experience privately or report to another individual was formed in the past. All descriptions of processes transduced through the nervous system are, in effect, after-the-biophysical-fact computations and reflect a memory-dependent process. Everything we experience—that is, everything that we can comment on, make judgments on, compare, or relate—has already taken place.

The general categories of processes in consciousness have many names, but we will select a set of commonly used descriptive terms that encompass our human sensory experience: *sensation*, *perception*, and *emotion*. These complex sensory processes, as 4D propagated sequences of information, are converted into long-term structures in the forebrain memory system as sequences of computed thoughts produced within the field of PIMs. They may then reenter the prefrontal modules for future comparative computations. That is, past sensations, perceptions, and emotions may be compared with a recent experience thought by thought, linked by the derived internal temporal dimension of I-time.

If we attempt to compare our internally derived and experienced sensations, perceptions, or emotions with another person's experiences or with any type of background standard or metric, we must collapse the temporal dimension (the I-time) to zero before doing so. Only then may we measure the scalar products of an informational component of the 4D sequence of sensory experience. Examples of a sensory information component (a measurable scalar entity) of a 4D internal perceptual experience include measures of blood pressure, heart rate, pupil dilation, and skin conductance. All readings, measures, and even verbal statements that estimate magnitude (e.g., "it was heavier than the other weight" or "it seemed to take longer this time") are *always* relative to the background field referent metric of space and time. These internal 4D processes do not create an absolute referent for the 4D local system of consciousness any more than they do for the 4D processes of the local system of life. We can better comprehend this when we apply our frame of reference model to individuals as independent biological referent systems, relative to one another and the background field.

As we will discover, now at a deeper level of existence, context is indeed everything.

In the most general (dictionary) definitions, a *sensation* is described as a mental process such as seeing or hearing. It is further differentiated as an immediate response to physical stimuli that may precede an awareness, perception, or emotion. Synonyms include terms like *sense* and *feeling*. A *perception* is regarded as awareness in consciousness of the physical elements of a sensation. It is a cognition, mental image, or interpretation that comes through an experience of sensations. *Emotion* is commonly defined as the "affective aspect of consciousness," or a feeling. It is considered as a *psychic* and physical reaction (as anger or fear) experienced as feeling and involving changes that prepare the body for immediate action.

The historical debate on the differences among sensations, perceptions, and emotions has alternately led and followed the debate on thought, mind, and consciousness. They have been inseparable. Now, in our model, we propose that they are not only semantically inseparable from the perspective of intellectual discourse, but also physically indivisible as 4D constructs, and that as such, they are exclusively produced in the thought and memory processes of the human mind. (There is a final constraint that we will discuss in the last section of this chapter.) To be explicit, sensation, perception, and emotion apply only to thought and consciousness; therefore, they cannot have application to the 4D processes of the pre-thought, preconsciousness life field.

To place these three general processes of consciousness in the context of our model, they must fit within the fundamental 4D information space that is generated and propagated in prefrontal modules and entered into the dynamic structure of the memory system. For the purposes of our biophysical model of thought and consciousness, sensation, perception, and emotion are operationalized as very similar sensory processing operations that vary only in the differential weighting of their unique combinations of sensory information or in the time at which each process is initiated relative to the reference stimuli. This classification scheme would thus define a sensation process as one that produces a thought sequence based on immediate, realtime sensory experience. Perceptions are generated later in time, following a reference stimulus event, and thus contain a strongly weighted memory component of sensory experience. Emotional thoughts are primarily produced from internal stimulus energy sources (visceral-autonomic) in reaction to the external context, and they may also be influenced by the memory system.

We have constructed a physical model in order to better understand how and why we operationalize these terms, and how they may be appropriate tools to describe the majority of our 4D thought processes in the consciousness field. The 3D cubic space represented in Figure 11-1*a* is created by connecting three orthogonal axes or dimensions: stimulus modality, stimulus location, and time. Thus, for the modality dimension, the axis runs from unimodal to multimodal; for location, the axis runs from external to internal; and for time, the axis runs from present to past. Now, if we freeze-frame a PIM in its thought-generating operational cycle, we can take the complex afferent sensory information contained within its boundaries and analyze it along the three dimensions of our cubic space. We can now project (map) the sensory information of a PIM onto the 3D space by marking the region that most closely relates the hypothetical thought content to the axis dimensions. This model of thought mapping may be used to visualize the concepts of sensation, perception, and emotion, and how they are related, but also differ, by the operational definitions applied.

The 4D process of a particular sensation, perception, or emotion must, by definition, include the propagation of a thought sequence if the individual experience extends in time beyond the ≈ 200-ms integration of a single PIM computational cycle. Region A (Figure 11-1*a*) represents sensory information that is unimodal in content, was initially transduced from internal sensory receptors, and has arrived in the relative present. The represented process might be imagined as a sensation of acute (present time) abdominal (internal location) distention (unimodal mechanical energy). Region B represents unimodal, external sensory afferent information transduced in the present time, and may be reported as the sensation of a rapid shift in the color (photon energy) of a traffic light. Location C represents multimodal sensory information from the external world that was originally transduced in the relative past, but has now been reentered into a PIM from the memory system, in real-time comparison with the current context. This might be considered as a perception process, where a room and all its integrated sensory information is reported as unchanged or changed from a prior exposure to it. In region D, multimodal sensory information from the internal world from the past is brought into the current modular computational activity. Here we may report the emotion of joy as a name given to a complex, visceral-autonomic state experienced many times in the past and now reentered from memory because of a real-time event, such as the question, "Do you remember how you felt when that happened?" The memory component is the dominant source of the 4D pattern of sensory stimuli that brings a physical representation of a complex internal stimulus environment. The result of evoking a past experience and entering it into the current prefrontal computations may,

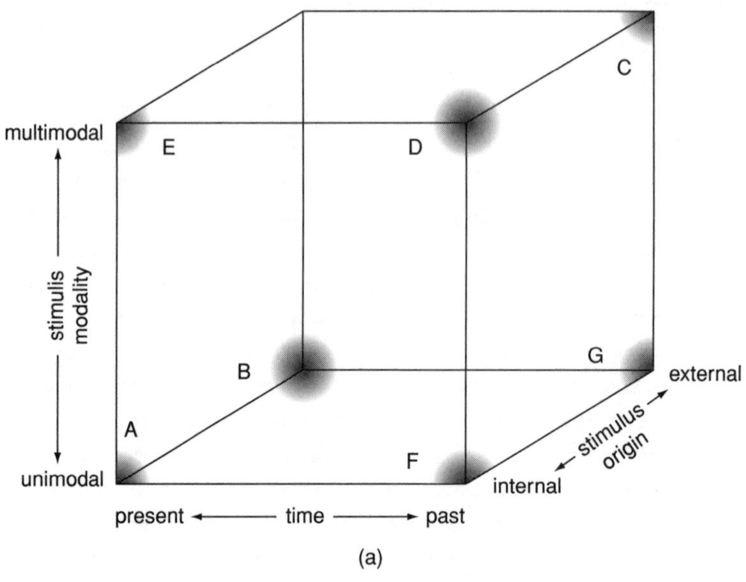

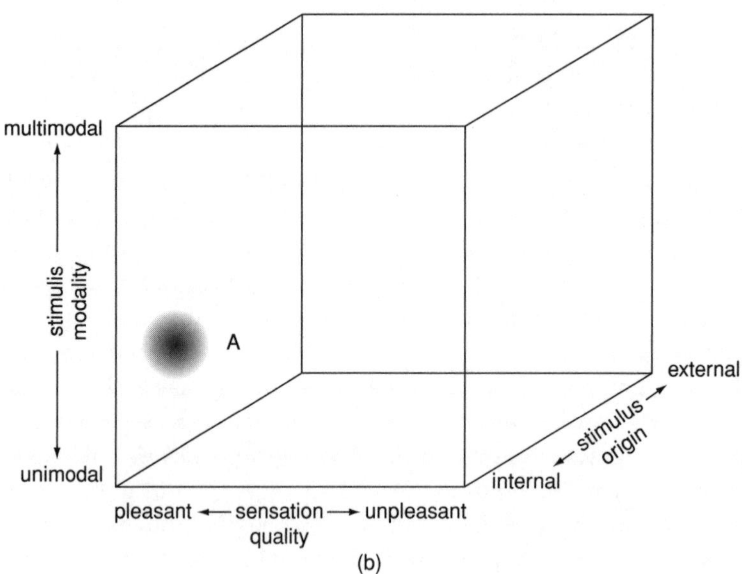

Figure 11-1 (*a*) The components of thought as represented within a prefrontal integration module (PIM). This operationalized representation of the sensory information that each thought may contain helps to define concepts of sensation, perception, and emotion. The axes depict the time of the information (past or present), the sensory type (unimodal or multimodal), and the origin of the stimuli (internal world or external world). Locations A through G are discussed in the text. (*b*) By replacing the temporal axis with an axis for an arbitrary quality such as pleasantness, emotions like affection (A) may be mapped onto this space.

in a feedforward manner, partially recreate the internal conditions that originally produced the sensory wavefront.

If we move along the time axis toward the present, we have region E, which, like D, brings multimodal, internal sensory information, but now the complex stimuli transduced from the internal world are the dominant source of information to the PIMs. In this example, one may report the onset of the emotion of satisfaction following the ingestion of a large meal. In region F, we find unimodal transduction of internal sensory stimuli that were previously experienced, either in the distant past or in the past of a few moments gone by. Watching a television show about coronary artery disease may evoke a memory of chest pain from a prior heart attack or heartburn. Finally, location G represents sensory information related to a unimodal, external stimulus from the past. This perceptual process may involve the tuning of a guitar string. We may perceive that the current sound of a vibrating string is out of tune through the process of disparity computation of a recent (working) or distant memory of a different tone.

In summary, we reiterate that the stated focus of our model is the principles of thought generation and the process of thought propagation to create the emergent referent frame of consciousness. Thus, the fundamental processes of the PIM operate on all sensory representations that reach a threshold order, regardless of the relative weighting of the afferent information contained in $R_a t_n$, $R'_a t_{n-1}$, and $R''_a t_{n-x}$. The examples described above are but an infinitesimal sample of the sensory process moments that can be projected into the thought-mapping space during a lifetime in consciousness. The ≈ 200-ms process of 4D thought generation produces all the subtleties and refinements in each sensation, perception, and emotion we experience, learn, and reexperience throughout our life. Our internal experiences of sensation, perception, and emotion are private, subjective, individual, and relative. They are collectively the *I-experience,* which is indivisible from the internally derived temporal dimension, or *I-time.* Together, in the 4D information space, they embody all the propagated and recombined thoughts of sensory representations, from the most crude to the splendidly sublime.

The personal process of thought and thought-memory is a relative process, derived from sensory stimulus energy of the external and internal worlds that reaches the prefrontal neocortex in a multitude of patterns of order or information. And, as with our internal temporal dimension, there is no absolute coordinate system for sensations, perceptions, or emotions. We construct our unique subjective sensations, perceptions, and emotions within our own referent frame. They are indeed a function of the sensory stimuli of the external and internal environments that the brain binds in time, but they are not an absolute and unaltered projection of the sensory moment into a thought product.

In the thought process that interacts with the memory structure to derive sensations, perceptions, and emotions over time and ongoing experience, we see the true relative nature of the individual reality that cannot fully be measured or scaled. For example, one may say that she did or did not sense or perceive a change in a particular stimulus or setting. Or, one may report that he did or did not feel a touch or pinprick. Any attempt to describe, measure, or express these processes in any way must reduce the 4D experience to a freeze-frame comparison of a single component or global gestalt in background time and structure. A comparison in magnitude or quantity, a scalar product, is all that may be expressed for the internal 4D process. We can collect statements or thoughts, such as, "I felt more/less"; "I sensed the same/differently"; "I am happy/sad"; "It is louder/quieter"; "It is unpleasant/less unpleasant"; "I perceive it to be wetter/dryer"; "bright/dim"; "salty/sweet"; "acrid/pungent"; "there/not there"; "all/nothing"; and so on, *ad infinitum*. These simple statements do not, however, impart the individual's experience in 4D thought and consciousness; they impart only the collapsed dimensions of propagated order expressed in relative 2D scales of quantity, quality, or magnitude.

But within each person, the refinement of thoughts that may be classified as sensations, perceptions, and emotions is an ongoing recombinant process that takes time and has quantifiable limiting and constraining parameters. If we were to replace the present-past axis in Figure 11-1*a* with one that had pleasant at one end and unpleasant at the other, then every region in the space would denote a sensation, perception, or emotion that was a combination of unimodal or multimodal sensory energy from the internal or external environments, and each would have a relative positive or negative quality attributed to it that lay within a range of relative pleasantness values (Figure 11-1*b*). If we were to select one region in that space (A) that was somewhere toward the multimodal end of the *y* axis, nearer to the internal end of the *z* axis, and more toward the pleasant part of the *x* axis, we could hypothetically name this the emotion of *affection*. Affection is something personal and unique, a dynamic, complex construct created within a single person over time and experience. To demonstrate the relative nature of any 4D process in thought and consciousness, whether in the sensory information content of the I-experience or in the temporal flow of the I-time, we will take this one single region, affection, out of the larger sensory space, which will be densely filled over a lifetime of experience, and look at it closely.

Now, we could average or integrate a number of operant definitions gathered from many people to create a consensus or group opinion of just what affection is or is not. But any definition that takes the form of a set of words or graphs must still represent the collapse of the temporal dimension of the process to zero, no matter how complex and inclusive of all known facts about anatomy, physiology, biochemistry, and mathematics the definition may be. Within a single individual's thoughtful mind, through experience, learning, and memory, affection may be subdivided, partitioned, or differentiated along personal continuums or dimensions of component informational structures (attributes of the global sensation or emotion).

We will now make a one-dimensional map (a line) for the singe emotion of affection (Figure 11-2). The range of this single dimension is defined as from −1 to 1, and we see that it follows the same S-curve as the prefrontal output effect on behavior. It reflects the same type of integrative function, but it is now focused on just one complex 4D entity, affection. The extreme of −1 marks the antithesis of affection (whatever descriptive word or set of biomathematical equations we want to place here would be a relative selection). The other extreme on the y axis, +1, denotes the maximum amount of affection (again, we could agree upon some words here or just leave it as an unnamed emotion, unique to each person). The midrange of the sigmoid curve represents the extended region of intermediate sensations or emotions that would express the feeling of affection between the theoretically difficult-to-reach extremes. The crossing of the zero point would correlate with the state of relative ambivalence, a negation of all the positive and negative aspects of affection that a certain situation, object, animal, or person evoked at a particular moment in time.

We must note that affection, as the internal derivation of a multitude of sensory information in real time and from memory, can also be mapped in a mathematical multidimensional space. This type of space would be defined by several orthogonal axes that would represent continuums of the component parts, such as the particular settings in which some degree of affection is felt, the particular objects or people that evoke an emotion of positive or negative affection, the external qualities of affection (visual, auditory, tactile, olfactory, or gustatory), and the internal qualities related to affection (visceral-autonomic sensations, such as changes in heart rate, blood pressure, pupil dilation, hormonal secretions, sweat secretion, gastric acid secretion, etc.). Now collapse all of these variables and dimensions of affection onto the one-dimensional S-curve that represents the entire potential individual range of the single emotion. Next, mark any two points adjacent to each other on this curve, say between a little positive affection

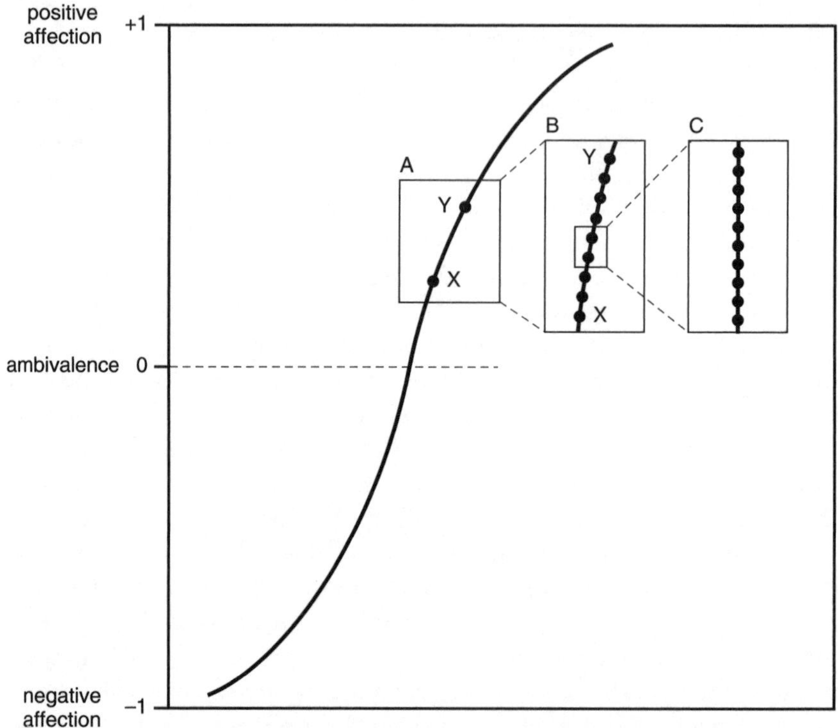

Figure 11-2 Relative and individual nature of thought as demonstrated for the emotion of affection. (*a*) Between the extremes of negative and positive affection (*y* axis), two points may indicate a small difference in the quality of experienced affection. (*b*) A change in external or internal sensory conditions or a change resulting from learning may create new discriminative points of emotion between the previous ones. (*c*) Over a lifetime, the degree to which one may express the emotion of affection may become increasingly refined.

(*X*) and a little more positive affection (*Y*) (area A in Figure 11-2). We can see that the distance between these two points could theoretically be subdivided again by a shift in one or more of the components that make up the emotion (area B). To the extent that a given person can transduce and integrate sensory information and transform it in memory, the points along the curve may grow in number, thus representing an acuity, subtlety, or differentiation among emotional degrees, states, or feelings (area C). Theoretically, any two points may again be divided by a new, learned microshift in any one of the contributing parameters from any one of the many dimensions projected in multidimensional space!

Any process in consciousness, whether it falls into the general category of sensation, perception, or emotion, may be seen as a potential infinite regression function relative to background metrics. From absolute negative affection to absolute positive affection, each individual would have his or her own dynamic continuum that would change in time as a result of changing experience, memory, and metabolic conditions. This internal process, which proceeds along a long-term progression embodied in Piagetian concepts, may lead to a refinement of the way one expresses affection or any emotion in various situations and in association with objects or people. This internal process of consciousness is personal and subjective, and it cannot be fully understood once the 4D process is decomposed into 3D attributes or scalar quantities.

Emotions and the Sensory World Inside

In most working definitions of sensation and perception, we note a tendency to refer to sensory representations that are transduced only from external stimulus energy sources. We report sensations of brief visual or acoustic stimuli, or the delayed awareness of a perception of the entire visual scene. And, while this is not exclusively true for all possible uses of these general terms, it separates sensations and perceptions from the typical definition of emotions. The model of biological relativity defines emotions in terms of the complex patterns of sensory stimuli produced within the internal structure of each individual's body and transduced by the sensory receptors primarily of the peripheral nervous system.

Affect or emotion is nearly always defined in terms of feelings, internal states, and visceral or autonomic processes. The classic investigations and theoretical constructs regarding what emotions are and how they are created may be dichotomized as the James-Lange and Cannon-Bard debate.[2] While this has never been truly settled, it may be summarized thus: Either emotion begins in the internal world and drives the brain's perceptual process, or it begins when higher-brain functions sense external-world stimuli and then cause changes to the internal state. The current investigations into the neurophysiological and neurobiochemical basis of our emotional experience are wide-ranging in approach and theoretical basis, and are producing a wealth of scientific and clinical information (McEwen, LeDoux, Rolls, and Damasio, to name a few).[3]

For the purpose of the presentation of our model, we want to focus on emotions as a component of the 4D information space. For the general function of the human nervous system, we hold that the transduced internal world of sensory energies that reach the prefrontal modules as a component of $R_a t_n$ and the propagation of these energies through $R'_a t_{n-1}$ and $R''_a t_{n-x}$ typically dominate the processes of thought in consciousness. We consider all affect and emotion to be operationally defined as functions of the internal world of sensory energies, integrated in prefrontal disparity computations and entered into the dynamic structure of the forebrain memory system. As we will see, consciousness is indeed not a *disembodied* phenomenon!

From an uncomplicated evolutionary perspective, we note that all animals with nervous systems approach stimuli that augment internal order and avoid stimuli that decrease internal integrity. To some degree, more complex animals whose genetic expression resulted in behavior that led to the avoidance of internal damage were able to maintain their existence and thereby increased their statistical probability of reproducing. Internal homeostatic functions and their neural representation in the brain (as the feedback system) continued to advance in complexity and influence under the evolutionary process.

Two other obvious, but fundamentally important, points must be made. First, from the original living cell forward, the intracellular environment has remained the most stable part of the entire sensory context. The sensory energies of the external environment change along various time courses, but the internal representation of that world remains far more constant. This is the basis of the internal order that brought life into existence. From that first cell to the human body, the internal milieu remains the most stable 4D sensory context. There may be rapid sensory energy fluctuations in the external world, but the internal world tends to change along a slower time course, and it does not ever leave. It is always with us, regardless of the wide range of external environments through which we may roam. Second, in evolutionary time, as single cells and then multicellular animals developed response pathways that resulted in motion, life moved toward gradients of organic and inorganic energy sources that enhanced and maintained internal order. It was either that or die. Those that happened to move in this manner lived. Thus, a statistically nonrandom shift in the distribution of living systems occurred along long time scales; this is evolution.

As genetic complexity increased and motion behavior became more prevalent, feedback mechanisms evolved that in some way promoted or rewarded the behaviors that gave more energy or order to the system. All this occurred in evolutionary time, prior to the first nerve cell or nervous system. We hold that these basic operating parameters of organic evolution on Earth have not changed. The forces of nature and stimulus context that were at work on the first nervous system and that are now at work on the human thinking nervous system are exactly the same. We have reward pathways in our internal milieu that have always been with us, through evolution and development. Neural networks, neurotransmitters, neuropeptides, hormones, glands, and the circulatory system all coordinate to produce these reward systems. The evolutionary modifications that focused on the prefrontal neocortex to bring about thought and consciousness may not have altered the internal systems to a great degree. (The fact that we cannot think our way out of addictions and other disorders of internal reward systems may relate to this all too human condition.) They are systems like any others we possess that conduct biological processes (e.g., the cardiovascular, lymphatic, or digestive system).

The influence of the internal milieu and the multisystem reward pathways upon thought and consciousness is profound. The drive states, no matter how one may wish to define them—or even if one tries to ignore them—are the difference between life and death, even for mindful humankind. It is not an insignificant nuisance that each thought, and thus our experience in consciousness, contains an afferent component from the internal sensory world. The disparity computations of one sensory moment with the next involve the weighting of an internal world whose operating parameters are largely set by neural mechanisms below the neocortex.

The degree of influence that this ongoing drive or reward system has on our thoughts and behaviors, and thus our experience in consciousness, remains to be determined. Lesions in certain regions and combinations of the amygdala, septal nuclei, or thalamic nuclei can result in impaired spatial working memory. Even with a working hippocampus and temporal lobe, the animal cannot recall important locations or places. Perhaps this impaired memory function is the result of a decrement in the internal reward system (in its most general definition) that provides the relative importance to places in external space.

From a neurophysiological and neuroanatomical perspective, it also appears that the visceral-autonomic sensory system functions along a unique time course with respect to other sensory modalities. And, unlike the other major sensory pathways, the orbitomedial regions of the prefrontal neocortex receive a significant amount of these sensory projections. Within the prefrontal integration modules, afferent sensory representations from all modalities may converge. The time that a sensory representation may remain as an ongoing, incoming pattern over prefrontal computational cycles may be very different for each sensory modality.

These basic relationships are related in Figure 11-3. The three curves (A, B, and C) represent different sensory modalities. The *y* axis represents the decay of a sensory representation from 0 percent to 100 percent loss of the information. The *x* axis is a relative time line for prefrontal modular processing. Our analysis here does not place an exact time scale on this axis. The curves then represent the decay of a real-time sensory representation in the prefrontal modules over processing time. Curve A, the steepest, drops from 0 percent to 100 percent loss between the two time points (t_0 and t_x). This curve reflects the quick shift in sensory information that can occur for visual, auditory, or light touch stimuli, or even for the vestibular system. The nature of the sensory energy source (photons, sounds waves,

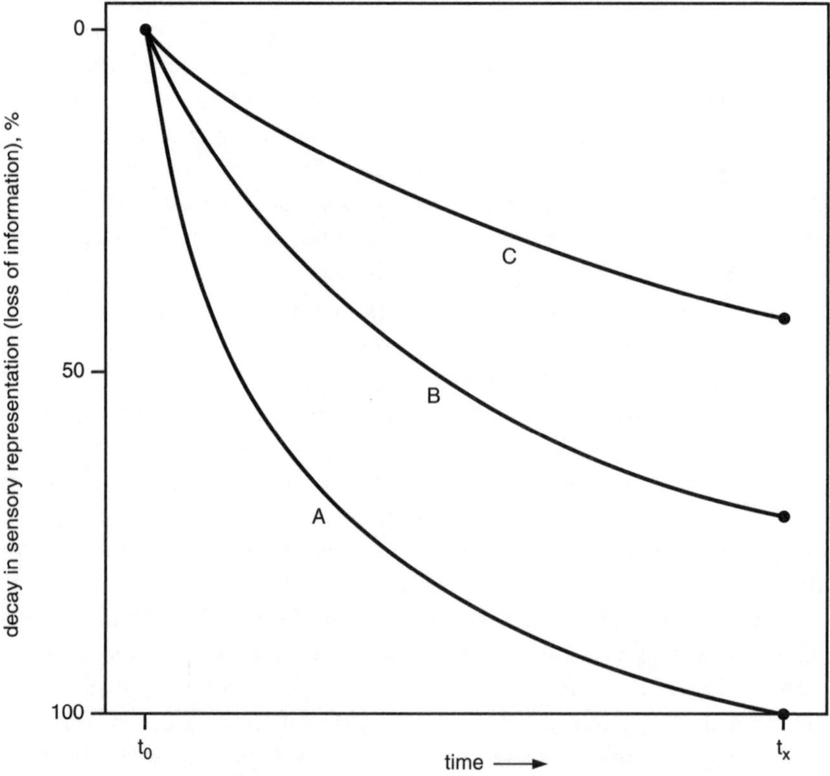

Figure 11-3 Relative decay curves for sensory modality information as processed with PIMs. It is hypothesized that certain sensory representations (e.g., visual, auditory, or touch) change rapidly within the prefrontal cortex (curve A), while olfactory and gustatory stimuli appear to last longer (curve B). The internal sensory world of visceral-autonomic stimuli may generate the longest-lasting representations in thought processing (curve C). Thus, emotional states may persist even while external sensory information changes.

pressure waves, or mechanical stimulation by acceleration change), the receptor transduction physiology, the neurons and neuroactive compounds involved, and the brain nuclei in the pathways to the neocortex all contribute to the shape of this curve.

Curve B, the middle line, represents the temporal change in sensory representation by the two primary external receptor systems for chemical energy, the olfactory and gustatory systems. Relative to those that produce curve A, the parameters that combine to generate curve B result in a slower decay of one sensory pattern to the next. Thus, smell and taste sensations are experienced relatively longer than are visual stimuli, even after the initiating event is gone (the source of the odor or taste is removed, or the light is turned off). We could just say that the molecules that generate a taste or smell remain in the local region of the receptors longer than does a photon or a sound wave.

Finally, curve C is a very shallow decay curve relative to curve A or curve B. This curve represents the internal milieu as transduced by the visceral-autonomic nervous systems. The stimulus energy-receptor interactions that generate this curve would include chemical, thermal, and mechanical energies. The free nerve endings, chemoreceptors, thermoreceptors, and a variety of mechanoreceptors are present in these systems. The body structures and processes that generate the afferent sensory wavefronts include the smooth muscle of all internal structures that may undergo contraction, dilation, and distention; the internal temperature gradients; glandular secretions and the chemical milieu; blood pressure; heart rate; and basic muscular tension. These sensory patterns are generated within a relatively stable 4D internal world and tend to remain stable across prefrontal modular activity. Thus, the recurrent wavefronts of real-time afferent activity tend to bring a slowly undulating sensory representation to the prefrontal regions. This is very different from the typical shifting patterns of sensory information transduced from the external environment, and it may have a very profound influence on our experience in consciousness.

We are proposing that the internal sensory flow creates the *waves of emotions* upon which thought rides. The patterns of sensory representation that reach the prefrontal modules (initially in the orbitomedial portions) are integrated as the emotional state and determine the feelings for the duration of their computational existence. This provides a powerful constraint on our experience of reality. For, even if the external context of visual and auditory stimuli dramatically changes, our emotions *cannot* change (especially after a sudden rise in the transduced sensory energies) until a particular point in the decay function of the internal state representation curve (Figure 11-3) is reached. Only then, at a critical competitive threshold, can another sensory pattern become the statistically dominant afferent influence and shift the prevailing emotional sensation, perceived as a change from the remembered recent past.

Let's explore an example of this significant constraining parameter of thought and consciousness. A relatively well-adjusted and healthy man living in a large city has just narrowly escaped being hit by a car as he crossed the street. We could say that he has just experienced an acute, *emotionally charged* (note the vernacular) event. We note that the change in his internal state will persist well beyond the external visual-auditory and nearly tactile event. The gentleman, shaken by his near-death experience, returns home and enters his living room, a place that typically induces a feeling of calm, security, and comfort. However, we find that he is experiencing completely different emotions, even after spending some time in his beloved home. He is still feeling agitated, insecure, and very angry. These emotions will eventually fade, but the time required for the fading of the emotional state is orders of magnitude longer than that required for the fading of the visual-auditory stimulus that initiated it.

The car is gone and the warm, cozy living room is in view, but we may still hear the man say something like, "I've got to calm down. I've got to get control of myself!" The external sensory context cannot override the internal sensory context—not for a while. It is not a reverberating afterimage of the car that is continuing to set and maintain the internal sensory state; conversely, it is the internal sensory conditions that continue to elicit the remembered image of the car. This is important; it has many ramifications in our daily existence, in illness, and in chronic disease.

The emotional state persists and permeates our thought processes in consciousness. It colors and tones our 4D information space as this space is generated in prefrontal modules and revisited in memory. When the emotional state has a statistically dominant influence, it determines paths of thought and constrains their operating scope for a considerable duration of time. Important parameters that determine each individual's emotional capacity with respect to intensity, duration, and even emotional complexity include metabolic conditions, the genetic patterns of nervous system development, and alterations to these patterns during maturational experience, trauma, and illness. In our constraint analysis of structural and functional parameters that affect the thought processes, we noted that metabolic changes induced by toxicity, infections, medications, other drugs, and alcohol may alter the internal sensory world to a degree that significantly changes the emotional component of thought. However, metabolic influences may affect many cells in the body, and it is at times difficult to assess the location of maximal change in nervous system activity. Finally, many reports of patients with spinal cord injuries (e.g., Hohmann, 1966) indicate that as visceral-autonomic sensory information is prevented from reaching the brain, the experience of emotions in consciousness is diminished. In emotion, too, we are bound to a biophysical reality and its many constraints.[4]

The Self in Consciousness

The self in consciousness is a combination of sensations, perceptions, and emotions related to our body, all its motor expressions, and its interactions with the world, other animals, other people, and its own structure. We may observe and transduce the visual sensory representations of our own body in motion, and the auditory sensory representations of our own voice as it makes noises, words, and sentences. We can see our hand reach out or our image in a pool of water or in a mirror; we can perceive our sights, sounds, tactile sensations, joint positions, smells, and tastes in a growing multitude of thought moments. The self develops and matures with the person. It is the I-experience in the I-time, and like all processes in consciousness it is human, private, subjective, and individual. The self is the 4D *I*.

The 4D information space develops and matures along the general path defined by Piaget, and the internally constructed image of a self as an *I* that may perceive its own actions slowly emerges. As each disparity computation is performed, the sensory representation of the self, or a part of it, from the memory system may be compared to a present representation. The outflow of novel thought products contains the updated self, or information about the differences derived. This novel information may then be reentered into the dynamic memory structure to further update the self construct.

In essence, the development of the self is the construction of an internal, context-independent 4D mirror. It is a reflection of the individual in all sensory modalities and combinations constructed from sensory information from the past brought into the present computational cycles. The mirror of the self grows in its scope, detail, and multimodal attributes (words, sounds, rotations, feelings, and perspectives of the self in a variety of external contexts in memory) across decades of experience. The context-independent nature of this 4D construct allows this mirror image to travel in time and place. As portions of the remembered self-image enter into a dominant prefrontal module producing real-time thought, they are compared with new sensory information. An ongoing internal reflective disparity computation updates the image of the self with new information and enters this into the memory system to modify the long-term image with which all associated information is linked. The self-to-self disparity computation is propagated across the prefrontal modules in computational moments, creating a fused ongoing reflection after reflection in personal time.

The self is thus perceiving the self, in a self-*awareness* (as we like to call this 4D process in consciousness). This reflective disparity computation and the reflective response (as the efferent output to effector systems) permit the individual to collapse the temporal dimension and write, speak, draw, paint, or even dance in a way that represents how he or she thinks, feels, and senses the world. The expressions of thought through effector systems are about past moments of information processing, including past representations of the self.

If we stand in front of a mirror and have another mirror held behind us, we see a repeated self-image in real time propagated across reflected space. In the 4D information space generated by disparity computations, the self is reiteratively compared with another past self and propagated into future time. Thus, as we can create thoughts about the reflected image in the external mirror and comment or report on these relative to background time and background metrics, so in exactly the same manner we can create thoughts about the reflected self in our internal 4D propagated mirror of the past and express them relative to background standards. This flow of information is not the subjective experience of self in the 4D process of consciousness. It is a collapsed product that describes only a component of the process. Over time, we learn to describe what we feel, what makes us sad or happy, what we like, and what we believe by comparing the actions and reactions of the past self in real-time disparity computational sequences and associating this information with background standards like words.

We learn about our self. We do it in 4D information space that creates a reflection for future comparisons and changes. We thus describe the learned and remembered past when we express something about our self, relative to a background metric. This indicates how we can see and listen and feel our self behave. It also indicates how we can hear our self think. As one speaks, his or her own auditory receptors may immediately return this external sensory representation back to the neocortex as a new afferent wavefront. This information enters the memory system and may become part of the reflected self as sequences of thoughts that contain the sensory representation patterns of our own speech, as the thoughts are propagated in time. Finally, we note that as we learn to associate emotions with external objects, people, and situations, so may we associate emotions with the reflected self. These associations of self-feeling are dynamic and may change in developmental time.

Reiterative, Recombinant Refinement in Consciousness

We may now ask, what is the fundamental process in consciousness that creates our rich experience of life and mind? How do early pre-thought learning and thought function to produce individuals who perform math, paint murals, write books, build cars, cook meals, and explore the universe with all manner of microscopes, telescopes, and robotic sensory devices? The learning and memory systems that developed in evolutionary time added plasticity, specificity, and thus flexibility to the basic behavioral reactions of approach-avoidance in the natural setting. As animals, then mammals, then primates, then *Homo sapiens* evolved onto the scene, we may ask, when did the basic bias toward behavior, however modified by learning and memory, get replaced by a better system of learning and memory?

For all our behavioral flexibility and the variety of contexts in which we may exist, most of our behavioral sequences may be understood, to a reasonable degree, if we have an accurate accounting of both the history of the contingencies of reinforcement and the information contained in the present context (as we demonstrated in Chapter 7). The basic homeostatic drives for nourishment, water, temperature control, and reproduction, and the reward systems that developed to promote them, thus produce a tremendous amount of ongoing behavior, and the prefrontal outputs provide influence in the form of the inhibition-reinforcement S-curve that we have discussed.

As a young child crosses into the emergent referent system of thought and consciousness, all the learned pre-thought associations and the basic functions of learning and memory, homeostasis, and reward systems remain unchanged. The newly developing 4D information space (within which sensations, perceptions, and emotions grow into an internal, reflected self) produces associations that continue to be reentered into the dynamic memory structure, transformed, and recombined at the limiting pace of neural modular activity. This refinement process proceeds along the general conceptual lines observed by Piaget. Thus, we say that the fundamental processes of knowledge and emotional development in the 4D information space consist of the generation of novel thought products, their propagation across the prefrontal modules, and their entry into the dynamic forebrain memory system. From the memory structure, thought sequences (and pre-thought association sequences) reenter or reiterate through the prefrontal cortex-to-memory system connections as they are elicited by internal and external contextual stimuli.

By definition, a reiterative process is not symmetrical, linear, or without change. Any information integrated in the prefrontal modules that produces a thought creates new information and its derived temporal dimension. The recombination of sensory representations occurs in the prefrontal modules, and perhaps within the dynamic activity of the forebrain memory system. Over time, a refinement process based on these reiterative, recombinant cycles creates nonrandom groupings, comparisons, and information differentiation by disparity computations. The accumulation of a 4D information or knowledge space is thus a process that increases order in a local negative entropy region of long-lasting structural information codes. It is a process that requires a large amount of metabolic energy to support. This fundamental process operates on any information that enters the prefrontal integration modules and derives novel solutions concerning comparative differences.

With the refinement processes described, 1 and 1 may easily become 2 in the 4D informational space. And, reiteratively, if the distance between 1 and 2 is cut in half (as one can do in many physical settings), and that ½ is cut again to make ¼, the 4D information space and the prefrontal disparity computations combine to create the basis for an infinite regression—an infinite refinement of our concept of the physical dimension of space and its relationship to numbers, or any area of human knowledge that is the focus of extended study. The natural, irresistible process of brain activity reduces any general set of sensory information to finer degrees of specificity.

Natural reductionism is the neural process that penetrates, refines, and unveils the beauty and richness of life, producing the emotions of awe and wonder as our reward for new discovery. At a fundamental level, these processes define who we are and what we do at every moment of consciousness. We indirectly introduced this process for the emotion of affection, and we mapped the refinement points along the S-curve between absolute manifestations of positive and negative (Figure 11-2).

However, we must again reinforce the fact that the disparity function doesn't care about the afferent information that undergoes biomathematical transformation. Thus, many novel solutions derived in modular computational moments are inaccurate or erroneous when compared to external standards. From the onset of thought production, these computations may contain mistakes, misinterpretations, mismatches of external and internal representations, illusions, unique perspectives, creative insights, or profound revelations; in the context of dreams, metabolic abnormalities, or illness, they may be filled with bizarre disconnections from even the broadest of realities experienced by most others.

At the extremes, through both great moments of insight and tragic moments of illusion, the thought processes of information comparison and refinement have changed the world. Across a spectrum of near-infinite potential, we produce an internal library of moments, short stories, poems, and novels in all sensory modalities that grows and expands in our lifetime; and it is private, subjective, individual, and absolutely relative in all four dimensions.

As a child, a young girl hears the sounds of music at home, in the car, at the store, and in many other settings. She is attracted to these complex melodic sounds by the positive internal sensations they arouse. In time, she learns that these types of sound patterns are called music. She is attracted to music. She learns to say, "I like music." This is important: The child is learning about the interface of her internal emotional sensory world with the external environment. If we recall Chapter 8, we know that she is most likely well into her emergent twos.

At the same time, she is making distinctions and refinements in the general sensory representations from both the internal and external worlds. Their points of intersection are creating more subtle and varied feelings and emotions concerning things, life, people, and self. In our example for the emotion of affection (Figure 11-2), we noted that our natural reduction process leads to finer and finer resolution of our experience of visceral-autonomic variables and the names and relative positions on a scale that we assign them. In the same manner, the child is learning about her inner world, unveiling the nuances of her shifting waves of emotional representation. The emotion that is associated with the word *like* may in fact fit on the affection curve. This, of course, is a personal experience for our child, as it is for each of us. (She would have to agree that what we want to express in the affection spectrum includes what she feels it is—hence, the insurmountable difficulties in this type of research.)

Let's assume that the S-curve we constructed for affection in fact does encompass the little girl's experience of emotion using words such as *like, dislike, love,* and *hate*. In the figure, if we place *love* at the +1 extreme and *hate* at the −1 position, we could locate *like* somewhere between the *X* and *Y* points plotted. Thus, in time and experience, the child begins to put more points on this curve reflecting her basic feelings.

Simultaneously, she is learning about music. She is learning to note disparities between different patterns of this peculiar form of 4D sound. She is building an internal library of sound types. In time, she learns names that classify some musical forms. Classical, orchestral, contemporary, popular, folk, opera, jazz, and many other terms begin to populate her vocabulary as she grows and matures. The fundamental refinement process applies to music as well. Within each general category, we can discriminate among an ever-increasing number of particular characteristics, each of which may be assigned its own identifying term. For the young child, the difference between classical and popular is now known. She is also learning to report differences in her emotional experience, and so she uses the terms *love, like, dislike,* and *hate* with increasing regularity. We hear her say that she likes both classical and popular music, but she likes popular music more—a subtle distinction in her growing information space. The young girl's parents have different tastes in music, however, and they feel that she should have a solid grounding in the classical arts, including classical music. As her knowledge of composers and their works increases, she continues to make ever more refined distinctions concerning music, composers, and emotion—she is attracted to some music and composers and repelled by others. On her personal continuum of attraction-repulsion, or love-hate, she is now mapping objects and people onto each point between the two extremes.

Over several years of listening, studying, learning, and feeling, we may hear her say, "I love Beethoven, and I like Bach, but I really dislike Brahms." These associations that reflect her development of points of relative attraction for composers also represent her development of the same distinctions in her emotional patterns. She is integrating the two worlds in her mind. It is a fundamental process that continues moment to moment, day to day, and year to year. It cannot be stopped. The girl, now about 9 or 10 years of age, may continue to refine her associations and express distinct emotions about each work that Beethoven produced. She may even be able to say which movements within a single work she enjoys most, and which she enjoys least. This example of the child's changing sensitivity to music and her internal sensory patterns shows the process of infinite regression for any experience in consciousness, over time. Sensations, perceptions, emotions, and self all become more distinct in time through the basic thought and thought-memory processes of reiteration, recombination, and refinement.

Piaget's observations indicate to us that as each child crosses into thought at the beginning of the preoperational stage, the basic processes of transformation begin to operate on the new order of information, the 4D order. Of course, for each human infant and all other animals, these brain processes function at the pre-thought level of associative learning. The difference in thought is that now the disparity computation derives a unique temporal dimension that links together each moment of sensory representation in the internal 4D information space. 4D products in propagated sequences provide a context-independent knowledge source that develops all the sensation, perceptions, and emotions of the self. A relative internal world travels with each of us, regardless of where we wander.

Each child in thought and mind begins to rediscover the world and reinvent all its laws, rules, and inventions. Piaget observed that every child proceeds along a similar developmental path (the development of the 4D information space, from our perspective), creating a world that is at once unique to the child and common to the history of human discovery and understanding. At some point in development, a child demonstrates the belief that inanimate objects are as alive as an animal or a person. This *animism* is no different from many religious constructs of ancient history and some current belief systems. Most children learn that there are disparities between rocks and dogs, and they incorporate these distinctions into categories of nonliving and living, but this takes time and experience. There is no shortcut for the basic process of refining the internal continuum for any aspect of learning. It is personal and relative, and it develops in each child along a time line that follows Piaget's general guidelines.

Children also pass through the discovery, and ultimate rejection, of the principle of *centrism*. At first, the child sees himself or herself as the center of the universe; later he or she feels that the center is the Earth, then the Sun, then the galaxy, and finally, in his or her teens, the child may understand concepts such as the origins of the universe and cosmic expansion. Of course, these concepts, like animism, have undergone a similar progression across time in the social process of reiteration, recombination, and refinement of shared information. It was not long ago that most people thought that the Earth was at the center of the universe and that the universe was static, not expanding, and eternal. The child continues to reinvent the foundations of nature, such as gravity, inertia, mass, force, dimension, and time. Children obviously do not know these things at birth, and it takes time for them to process enough experience to be able to express an understanding of them.

Piaget's great observation skills provide us with insight into the limits and constraints of brain function. First, it takes time for the 4D information space to grow and mature. At a fundamental level, this process cannot be pushed or rushed by any amount of training or experience. From our perspective, this reflects the reiterative, recombinant refinement process in thought whose rate is set by the computational activity of the brain. We cannot know certain mathematical or physical properties of nature until we have experienced, recombined, and refined a threshold amount of basic information. This is the limit of time and information processing.

Second, we propose that Piaget observed and described a fundamental constraint on the biomathematical transformations performed by the brain, as manifested in patterns of thinking. The commonalities in the patterns of thought that all children express as they each reinvent and rediscover the basic rules and operating procedures of nature, life, and humanity are the products of the same few and identical processes of information transformation in thought and thought-memory that exist in all human brains. This is why we have used the singular term *disparity computation* for prefrontal module activity and the terms *reiterative, recombinant,* and *refinement* for the ongoing, most fundamental processes that produce and develop the 4D knowledge space. People think like other people. Logic, conservation, deduction, inference, syntax, metaphor, allusion, perspective, empathy, reflection, space, time, past, future, imagination, and other classifications of basic patterns of thought that do not necessarily refer to any single type of information or sensory modality define important constraints on human consciousness. The information may change, but across the developmental changes observed by Piaget, the fundamental operations that the brain can perform are expressed in common patterns throughout humanity. The lyrics, instruments, players, and settings may change, but *the song remains the same*. Variations in genetic endowment, developmental experience, information exposure, illness, and many other factors will and do provide the unimaginable diversity in individuals' thoughts, but the biophysical manner in which they were constructed, remembered, recombined, and remembered again is virtually identical in each of us.

In each general area of human experience, from language to science, art, and music, many theories about how and why each person develops certain common abilities and unique variations have been proposed that express positions similar to this one. In our model, it does not matter which aspect of human experience we choose to focus on, because the principles of thought generation, propagation, and transformation along the time scales of development and in real time operate on any source of afferent sensory representation (the brain doesn't care if it is processing words, sights, sounds, or temperatures). While Piaget and others since have watched this process in the young as they discover the universe through a common pattern of relationships in space, time, and emotion, another prominent individual in history made similar remarks about the commonality of fundamental thought in adults from diverse cultural backgrounds. Albert Schweitzer, in his book *Reverence for Life*, wrote about his deep feelings of a fundamental human connection with the members of the African communities with whom he worked and lived.[5] The doctor and the tribes' people were very different in terms of the types of information they had been exposed to, the training they had received, the social customs they had learned, the language they used, and almost any other aspect of learning and experience. A well-educated physician, musician, organ maker, and philosopher, Schweitzer reflected on his experience while sitting around the nightly fire with people whose primary education had involved the struggle to stay alive. He noted that while there was a great divide between himself and the tribespeople in many areas of knowledge and experience, when it came to the understanding of living nature, human thoughts and feelings, and humanity's place in the cosmos, they were of one mind.

This struck Schweitzer as profound and meaningful, and indeed it is. The important things—the basic, fundamental perspectives of life, love, and the mystery of existence—do not depend upon a specific type of information or training. While the individual opinions of the various people sitting around the fire may differ widely (a reflection of the refinement process and differential experience), there are common patterns of thought in consciousness. (Jung and many others have described related concepts with such terms as *archetypes* or *synchronicity.*)[6] These commonalities not only bind us together as a single species, with similar genetics, similar nervous systems, and similar patterns of thought but they also define our significant constraints. We think in similar patterns that develop in brains that are constrained to process information according to a basic set of operations. This further begins to define the boundaries of our humanity.

Sensation, perception, emotion, and thus self are developed by the process of reiterative, recombinant refinement of the 4D information space. In each individual, this internal multidimensional space contains personal and dynamic axes or continuums for every possible combination of sensory experience—S-curve intersecting with S-curve, layers upon layers of emotion and feeling in association with facts, objects, and people. Our examples for affection, basic math, and music demonstrate how any two points of relative difference may expand to a nearly infinite set of distinctions. This fundamental refinement and natural reductionism, which begins with our inherited set of evolutionary biases and rewards to maintain homeostatic tolerances, leads to our uniquely individual qualities of predisposition, tastes, preferences, discrimination, knowledge, judgment, maturity, compassion, and wisdom. This is our genetic personality refined in consciousness.

Our most complex human experience in consciousness is driven by the same basic push-pull, approach-avoidance dynamic that characterizes all biological systems. Contemporary research with infants and children often acknowledges this fundamental dichotomy and its refinement. As Fischer and Rose (1994) reported, "[C]hildren from an early age organize their social understanding in terms of [a] positive-negative split. For example, 3-year-olds categorize people and their actions as either nice or mean, and they see nice and mean as incompatible, even when the actions they witness were not split in this manner. With development of more complex control systems, children eventually become able to bridge this split, understanding how 'nice' and 'mean' (or other positive-negative splits) can be combined in people's actions."[7] They finish this line of thought with, "Still, the split into positive and negative or approach and avoidance remains a basic dimension of the organization of behavior throughout life. Even adults who can bridge the split still use concepts of good and evil, for example." Fox (1991) proposed a similar model for the development of complex emotions from a basic, initial dichotomy.[8] As the self develops, this bridging of the basic positive-negative split is achieved by the refinement of sensory representation patterns as they are associated with genetic-homeostatic dichotomies, through moments of disparity computation whose solutions produce ever more distinct places along internal continuums of remembered sensations, perceptions, and emotions.

Considerations of Free Will and Thought

At what point in the flow of neural information encoded in 3D axon arrays that begins at the moments of sensory energy transduction and courses through transformational networks of brain tissues to enter the prefrontal modules do we get to exercise our will? At what moment or moments in the progression of thought generation, thought propagation, entry into memory, and reentry into the thought process do we have control? Equally important is the question of where. Do we exert our will on the biomathematical processes of brain tissue? Can we decide what information we wish to compare and then command the brain to perform a certain transformation? Or can we direct the efferent solutions to specific motor outputs and not others? May we rearrange memory to suit our needs? What abilities do we have in consciousness, where do they exert their influence, and what are their limitations? Do we have a choice about reading the rest of this sentence? Or perhaps this one?

Our model of thought generation utilizes a temporal sequence for sensory representations that enter a thermodynamically dominant region of prefrontal neocortex. The focal PIM receives the afferent sensory information of a *now* moment ($R_a t_n$, $R'_a t_{n-1}$, and $R''_a t_{n-x}$) and performs a biomathematical disparity computation as the wavefront of ordered energies flows through the modular tissue of the brain. The solutions to this process derive the embedded temporal dimension between past and present, as encoded in axon arrays that project to the next dominant PIM, the forebrain memory system, and other brain regions. We proposed that the time of each thought generation, as a single product of modular activity, was on the order of ≈ 200 ms. We may follow the flow of thought across prefrontal modules (in ≈ 200-ms moments) and into the memory system, and the modules' reiteration back into a dominant PIM for recombination and thus refinement. The sensory wavefronts in afferent projections enter the synaptic zones of the PIM, the biophysical transformation is conducted, and the code for the 4D product is transmitted as patterns of nerve impulses in structured axon projections. Where, when, and how does our free will manipulate the process?

We selected an ≈ 200-ms window of time for the production of a single thought product for many reasons. The time from stimulus energy transduction by a peripheral receptor organ to the arrival of this stimulus energy in the prefrontal cortex, and the unknown biomathematical processes that occur in each prefrontal module (as the afferent fibers bring the highest order of sensory representation, what we called the point or gestalt representation of the moment, and transduce nerve impulse patterns into the release of neuroactive compounds that initiate a flux of biochemical and bioelectrical energies though the most complex arrangement of brain tissue and synapses known) may reasonably take place within this time frame. The long productive history of behavioral research into sensory awareness, stimulus processing, and reaction times also indicates that this time frame for our theoretical construct of a thought as product is not far-fetched. Finally, the conceptually alluring phenomenon of neocortical brain-wave or electroencephalographic (EEG) activity following various sensory stimulus events provides additional support for the temporal sequences in our model. An average evoked potential, now commonly referred to simply as an evoked potential (EP), is a wave of negative and positive fluctuations in brain electrical activity as recorded by electrodes placed on the scalp. In healthy adults, there is a general pattern to this activity following a wide range of stimuli presented in various modalities, settings, and sequences. For our purposes in this section, it is noted that on average, a peak (P) in the amplitude of a wave of brain electrical activity can be recorded at around 300 ms (P300) following stimulus onset.[9] Many practical and theoretical issues surround these observations and their interpretations, but in general we may state that an early phase of the brain activity that will lead to this peak may be detected in the prefrontal regions of the brain at about

250 ms after the stimulus onset. Thus, the molecular-scale biochemical processes of the prefrontal integration modules that generate a thought product may correlate with these large-scale electrical measures. We speculate that the critical biomathematical computation whose solution is a thought may slightly precede the electrical changes detected in the scalp electrodes, placing thought generation in the 200-ms range. Functional interpretations of the P300 wave vary in terms of the central issues of awareness, attention, update of working memory, and matching of real-time sensory stimuli with memory representations. All are aspects of human thought production, from our perspective. Interestingly, this phenomenon is not found in other nonhuman primates, and infants under 2 years of age may not be able to generate the adult pattern of the wave.[10] Perhaps it reflects thought generation and propagation in consciousness.

Let's revisit two individuals we already know and walk with them through their experience of the temporal flow of sensory information and thought in consciousness. Helen Keller lost her ability to see and hear near her second year of life. From our perspective, her development of thought in consciousness appeared to proceed rather normally, and she reported a full experience of life and mind. If this implies a free will and control of behavior, it appeared that she was in full possession of it. She just could not see or hear. She could not *will* herself to see or hear (no matter how many hours, day, and years she most likely tried in silent, dark, frustrated agony). It may be inferred, then, that the power of will cannot work on something that the brain does not provide. She could not choose to see or hear because the brain did not bring the necessary information into her thought processes. It would have been a profoundly abusive assault upon Helen if someone who claimed to have professional knowledge had told her that she just *lacked the will* to see and hear or that she was just suffering from a hysterical reaction to repressed memories of sexual abuse and would be able to see and hear again if she would only get in touch with her emotions and try really hard. In our enlightened times, if a thorough examination of Helen's eyes, ears, and brain scan did not reveal obvious damage, how many would begin to think of these other explanations? Compassion, in ignorance, is nonetheless cruel.

We might then say that free will depends upon information from sensory receptors. The brain needs to be working, and free will may act only on the information the brain can produce. In Helen's case, she lacked the spatial information concerning the visual and auditory worlds, and so she could not command it to appear or make decisions based upon a disembodied perspective that would have allowed her to view the world without vision or to listen to the world without hearing. This may seem to be obvious. However, if we agree with the assessment of Helen's private experience in consciousness, then we must accept that free will, control, and command act only on sensory information provided to and processed by the brain.

The gentleman known as H.M. also appears to be thinking in consciousness, because he is aware of the real-time world and all its sensory stimuli and because he has no known damage to his prefrontal neocortex. In addition, prior to his surgery, he had functioned as an adult with relatively normal thoughts and memories, although critically impaired by recurrent seizures. Thus, we observe H.M. generating a real-time thought function that is propagated across his prefrontal cortex, providing him with an internal temporal dimension, but of limited duration. If we were to sit and talk about politics with him and we asked him to tell us whom he would *choose* to vote for in the next election, he might say that he will vote for Ike. He might even let us know that he has the free choice to decide if he wants to join the Workers' Party or not.

The damage to H.M.'s hippocampus and temporal cortex has restricted his sense of free will or control to fleeting moments of real-time thought propagation in the prefrontal region, and any reports by him about how he is going to control his future are based on a 4D knowledge space that was entered into structural memory more than 40 years ago. For H.M., in the memory afferent source of $R''_a t_{n-x}$, the x is at a minimum equal to the number of years since his surgery, and it has even larger values for revived memories of earlier experience. The pathway from the prefrontal modules to the memory system is essentially nonfunctional. If he tells us, in real-time thought, "I choose to have a T-bone steak for dinner tomorrow night," we think about our recent memory of what a T-bone steak is, and we sense the potential future of tomorrow night as an agreed-upon duration on an external clock and as a sensation of duration within our own individual referent frame. But H.M. is freely choosing a steak from the 1940s, and tomorrow night is a tomorrow that occurred long, long ago. For him, the tomorrow that is measured by the clock on the wall or the rotation of the Earth will never come. It is always *now*, as the fading of thought in computational dilution untethers him from background time, and the inability to form new memories chains him to an internal distant past. H.M. cannot *will* himself to be aware of the past moments that fade from his mind. The power of his potential control is limited to seconds in real time and to the far distant past.

From H.M.'s perspective, it appears that his free will, intent, volition, and choice are very much intact and exerting their influence. From our perspective, his internal force of will may be working just fine, but it is trapped in a cell of past 4D experience. Again, the will needs a healthy brain to exert command and guide one into the future. But, strangely, as we think about H.M.'s world, it appears that his will still chooses to exert its effect on past information. Doesn't it know that this is foolish and illusional? Can the will stop itself from saying and doing things that are in error in the present context? Or would this type of control also require the will to have a disembodied perspective that would enable it to understand and know that the thought memories of the 1930s or 1940s are out of date? Let's imagine that H.M. had drifted to another city after his operation and lived there for many years. In time, as he continued to be forgetful and to talk only about the receding past, perhaps complaining about things that appeared bizarre in the current context, he might have been sent for help. Without knowledge of his surgical past, how many would have tried to get at the *emotional* roots of his *amnesic* reaction? How many would have tried to tell H.M. that he had to think *real hard* about what is happening right now, to *command his will* to focus and stop drifting every few minutes? And to stop living in the sentimental past!

Even in an intact individual, is the force of will that is generated by the brain and dependent upon the information provided by the brain acting on *past* information? Remember that the frame of reference of consciousness, like that of life, is not producing a new force controlling all behavior. There is no *élan vital* or *élan conscience*. Could it be, then, that the sensations, perceptions, or feelings of free will, intent, and control are generated in the same manner as *all other* sensations, perceptions, and emotions? Does the process of reiterative, recombinant refinement of all sensory information that slowly constructs a self in memory (and that we further refine in real-time moments of disparity computation) also generate a sensation of free choice and command as we reflect on our self as we interact with the world? As we experience the internal and external sensory worlds in our private 4D referent frame of consciousness, across moments of I-time, does the flow of background 4D sensory information precede or lead the internal generation of our subjective existence? Are we reflecting on information that has already occurred in one frame of reference and experiencing it as a personal real-time event within our unique local system of I-time? Could our sensation, perception, or feeling of will and control be a private experience, contained within the thermodynamic boundaries of our individual reference system and experienced as our reflected self behaving in, yet wholly disconnected from, the background clock of real-time stimulus energy or sensory information? Is the information that controls our behavior and our thoughts already present in the background context, *one tick ahead* of our internal 4D sensation or perception of time, decision, choice, and will? Is our sense of the temporal flow of information in the background referent frame *mismatched* with our internal 4D experience of that information as it enters into thought? Are we producing an *internal illusion of information in time*, relative to the information in the background system? Do principles of relativity apply to biological systems in four dimensions?

Illusions in Consciousness: Of Time, Information, and Motion

Animism, centrism, anthropomorphism, and cause-effect relationships are general categories that define the illusions of our existence in thought and consciousness. Each child discovers the world and invents the laws of nature during development. Illusions, *as mismatch errors of information in time*, are a normal part of this progression and undergo refinement as each child passes through adolescence and adulthood. In a parallel process, the history of humanity has moved along a course of collective illusions that have also undergone refinement over time. For every child, as for humankind, the Sun, wind, trees, and fire were once alive and willful. The Earth was at the center of the universe, and the horizon marked the edge of existence. Yet, while a growing child and a maturing humanity learn to make distinctions among insects, fish, birds, and mammals, no clear understanding of intellect, awareness, thought, or consciousness seems to emerge. These appear to be very relative ideas; one individual's truth is another's illusion.

History and development are filled with illusions of cause and effect. The basic phrase that we use to describe this type of illusion process is *contiguity implies causality*. When two events happen together in time, we perceive a cause-effect relationship. Applying our model of thought production, we can understand how this happens. What we sometimes fail to appreciate is that this happens all the time, throughout life and throughout human history. Historical examples of great magnitude would include the belief that someone's personal actions would cause the Sun to be blotted out (in an eclipse) or that a human or animal sacrifice would cause a better crop or better weather. More mundane daily events that produce exactly the same perception in our minds would include receiving a phone call from someone whom we were just thinking about or receiving a phone call as we were reaching for the phone. Another common occurrence in which contiguity implies causality is when we make a movement, such as standing up, and at the same time we hear a strange noise. If the noise is not a very familiar one and the two events occur close together, we pause and wonder if our motion caused the noise. A person may even sit back down and repeat the motion to investigate the cause-effect relationship he or she had perceived. Our lives are filled with these moments, and the story of human history is significantly based upon them.

The fundamental brain process of disparity computation in the prefrontal integration modules provides the basis for this type of illusion. The brain doesn't care about the information it is processing. It cannot predetermine the sensory representations before they undergo biomathematical transformation in the prefrontal modules. Any sensory information that is present as a 4D thought is produced will be incorporated into the structure of that thought. Thus, two closely occurring events are linked in our brains by the temporal dimension that we derive in thought. We create information as a temporal link that constructs the cause-effect relationship. The contiguity is the time factor that implies causality, the illusion. Now, of course, this system of event-linking in computational moments also makes correct associations that form the basis of all animal learning. But there is no *a priori* manner in which we can distinguish the illusions from reality. In our development, we learn to ignore a tremendous number of contiguous events, but many still enter our memory and affect our behavior in a subtle or significant fashion.

The creation of a formal approach of asking questions, gathering information, checking the information with others, and then repeating the process became a method—the scientific method—of determining whether contiguity does imply causality for any two events. This is the only method of illusion reduction that our computational systems can utilize to refine our internal information space through our reiterative, recombinant processes. It is an *interpersonal* refinement process that helps to refine our *intrapersonal* knowledge base. But it is a human method, and thus it also is filled with illusions and misinterpretations of events linked in external or internal time.

The information that is present and the order in which events occur relative to a particular information source define the core relationship that generates illusions in our thoughts and memories. In pre-thought association learning, this problem is reduced to a single temporal dimension of background time. All contiguous events are learned as associations without further refinement, unless the events are paired again at a future time. In thought and thought-memory, associations made between contiguous events in background time may be further compared to external stimuli in very different contexts and times. Our unique ability to form our personal

4D information space and have it available in other contexts and at other times gives us both great learning power and great potential to make associations that have nothing to do with reality.

The magician takes full advantage of our illusion-generating capabilities. Magic is the manipulation of information in a way that causes the observer to perceive a temporal flow of information that is in error. The *a priori* arrangement of information creates a contiguity that implies a causality that can happen only as a result of supernatural or magical powers. The sequence of behavior that one observes—a rabbit appears from a hat, an assistant is bisected with a saw or impaled with a sword, or a tiger vanishes—is prearranged. Thus, *the behaviors have, in effect, occurred before the observer perceived them happening.* The rabbit is already there, the assistant is already out of the path of the saw or sword, and the tiger has already been removed before the observer thinks it is happening. The observer is provided with only partial information. As we have stressed in earlier chapters, if we could account for all the information that is present before the act even began, there would be no illusion.

A stacked deck of cards contains information placed there by the scam artist. The gambler or mark does not have this information. The hand of poker will play out along a predetermined path, without any choice. The mark (or observer) perceives a semirandom event and thinks that he can control the outcome. In reality, the context is set, and his information account book (and perhaps his bankbook) is unbalanced. He is fooled. He is experiencing an illusion. Without additional information, he cannot know that his behavior was determined. He has no other perspective from which to derive the necessary information.

Our tendency to form illusions by misinterpreting the flow of information in time makes it difficult for us to assess intelligence, awareness, thought, will, and control in all living things. Vitalism and the concept of *élan vital* are illusions of this nature applied to any cell or organism. As we saw with the African termite cities and Clever Hans's calculations, we can easily form illusions of intelligence, thought, free will, and personal choice when we do not take into account the information that is already in the context.

When we do balance the information books, all illusions of these powers and abilities *disappear into the background,* because it is the background—the context—that has the information that elicits and guides each moment of behavior. When we do this, we have figuratively put the horse back in front of the cart. From our referent frame of consciousness, we can integrate moments of background time and thus observe the flow of life. This relative perspective of a different frame of reference, in theory, gives us access to all the information contained in the life field. If we examine the informational content and the history of information flow, we may accurately assess any cause-effect relationships within the context.

When hummingbirds fly between flowers to feed, we may observe the larger scene and fuse its information moments within our thoughts. If we freeze-frame each sensory moment and line them up in discrete snapshots, we note that there is no information about the behavior of the hummingbirds relative to the flowers in a single moment. Only when we fuse the flickering moments of information within our internal 4D information space do we derive the motion of the birds within their context of atmosphere and flowers.

From the hummingbirds' perspective, they are immersed in a dense, stable 4D sensory context that is transduced in disconnected moments of existence. They do not fuse these moments in time, and thus they do not experience the fluid behavior of motion and paths of travel that we compute in consciousness. Each sensory transduction moment (or frame) for the birds is filled with information about gradients of molecules in the air, and perhaps the visual coordinates of the nearest flower and other patterns of stimulus energies. The information about the next moment of behavior for each hummingbird is already present in the background 4D environment and guides the hummingbird across time. The hummingbirds have no way of perceiving the 4D process of flight or foraging because they do not have another frame of reference from which to view the 4D progression of their own behavior.

We derive the internal neural movie of the hummingbirds' behavior from the still frames of sensory representation as we fuse them in the thought process. The illusion that is created, which is inherent in this exclusively human process, is one of the temporal flow of information. We see the hummingbirds choosing a path of travel and deciding which flowers to feed upon. *We do not see the richer context in which each bird is fully embedded as a structure that by its shape of information gradients moves the bird along dynamic, emerging 4D pathways*. We see the birds climbing in the sky as a result of the rapid force generated by their wings. We do not see the thick atmospheric currents lifting the birds aloft. We project our large-scale information onto the small referent system or object in motion.

For a moment, imagine that we do not know the difference between a hummingbird and a flower. Next, picture two hummingbirds hovering in the sky, their wings beating so fast that we cannot perceive them. The hummingbirds appear to be frozen in position. Now, imagine that the entire 3D scene were to move around, but the birds remained in their places in the air. If the flowers, now in motion, moved in a path that took them from bird to bird, we would have a very different perception of the 4D process fused within our minds. We would describe the behavior of the flowers, and attribute to them information regarding the birds and the paths of travel they took to reach the birds. We would say that the flowers planned and executed their food-giving actions—that they knew what they were doing and willed it to happen. We could not help it.

This example of a *figure-ground* relationship reveals the error in thought that comes with our ability to integrate moments of sensory representation and derive the embedded information about time—and thus motion—in a sequence of events. It is an illusion of fluid motion, intent, volition, will, and cause and effect. If we had performed a freeze-frame analysis of each moment in background sensory time and looked at the discrete snapshots of the birds, the flowers, and the 3D environment, we would not have been able to see any information about their relative behavior. The information about who was doing what and to whom came from our internal 4D knowledge space. Nothing in the life field—no flower, no bird—has any ability to process this 4D scene. Each element of the life field exists in moments of background time, discrete, flicker sensory events.

Thus, in reality, the nervous systems of the hummingbirds process moments of a sensory information space that by its structure leads and controls all their actions. The *figurative horse* of the entire sensory context (including the bird's internal homeostatic conditions and any learned associations) pulls the *figurative cart* of the bird. Our tendency to see the bird purposefully moving through its environment is derived from an illusion process that is our inheritance for temporal flow, information, and motion. This illusion process is always with us and has permeated our history, as is evident in our songs, poems, stories, drawings, philosophies, religions, and laws. Moving streams were once alive, and the wind, the Sun, and the moon, as moving objects, were either alive or controlled by individual gods. The motion of such objects against a perceived static or flat background creates for us an illusion of intent, choice, and will. This is an exclusively human process of thought propagation and memory in the frame of reference of consciousness. It may apply to all things in motion, including us.

We do not choose to breathe, maintain a circulatory system, or keep watch on our heart rates and digestive systems. We do not decide when to sweat or salivate. The entire world of bodily functions is not subject to our presumed free will. We cannot control a reflex, a cough, a sneeze, a headache, vertigo, or sleep. We do not have any say in the pathways along which color information proceeds through the cortex, parallel to other visual information. We do not have any choice in the matter of when or where we derive the third dimension, depth, as it is integrated by the disparity computation performed in the cortical modules. We will perceive a floating square above a random dot stereogram, even though it is not really there. We cannot will it away. Through learning and memory, when the letter A is traced by a finger on our palm or back, we will automatically see the letter, think of the written letter, and perhaps hear the sound of it in our thoughts as the information is elicited from the multimodal stimulation of the parietal region. We cannot stop it.

Our map of the local external context and the places within it that have positive or negative (visceral-autonomic) attributes is constructed in the hippocampal system. This neural construct determines how we see ourselves in the world and how we feel about it. We cannot decide to rearrange the neural representation of the physical environment through some *mental feng shui*. We do not determine the flow of multimodal sensory information as it courses into the prefrontal integration modules, or its timing, or its content of real-time information, the information from the past moment, or the information from the memory system. As this gestalt sensory representation is integrated during one modular operation—during ≈ 200 ms of synaptic zone activity and dynamic flux through a charged field of brain tissue that results in an efferent axon output—we cannot decide which information to keep and which to discard. The computation is made and the efferent outflow is transmitted, all within the known properties of the biophysical world. We do not know the biomathematical functions, but we have clues, and these functions will ultimately be discovered. We may then ask, Where does the power of will enter into this process? If it comes after the prefrontal computational moments, then it can change only the past.

Our experience of I-time is a narrow serial flow from one dominant prefrontal integration region to the next. Because of this strict limit, we cannot be aware of, cannot be thinking about, and cannot be attending to many things at once. We process all sensations, perceptions, and emotions—and even the self—in a serial manner, at the level of thought generation. This severe limitation is readily exposed when external demands bring us more than one thing to be done at a time. Essentially, we can do only one thing at a time.

Our memory for past behavior also reflects the serial flow of computational events and solutions. This limitation can be easily tested by having two, three, or more simultaneous stimuli presented, such as one verbal question, one or two visual tasks, and one tactile question traced on the skin. We may shift back and forth among them, especially if we have prior information about the events and what they will entail, but we cannot process all the information on parallel thought streams. As each successive dominant PIM processes the *now*, it is the only information generator that reaches the thought threshold. It is a linear 4D product stream that defines our external and internal worlds and creates the experiences we remember as sensations, perceptions, emotions, and self.

Behavior is ongoing, and the great majority of it does not require a prefrontal contribution. Most behaviors consist of expressed sequences of basic reflexes or learned associations from the memory system directed through subcortical pathways. The influence that thought has on ongoing behavior is focused and restricted, and thus extremely limited. The duration for which PIM-to-PIM sensory information may contain a relatively constant pattern of content (*focused attention*) is also relatively brief and shifts over short time frames. External and internal sensory stimuli dynamically interact to alter the statistical dominance of information content that forms a thought, and our attention shifts. This is why it is possible for us to suddenly recall that within a brief time frame, we have performed several tasks that we were not completely aware of and did not feel in control of.

Other limits on the duration of thought content (focus) may come from the constraints of the prefrontal system in the propagation of thought across its fields. Perhaps at these boundaries of thought propagation, a break in the stream is created at restart or reset moments. Furthermore, at a certain point in decay, *the fade of the now* may create a shift in serial thought. In other words, there is a very limited duration in which a past *now* can maintain a computational presence as it is progressively diluted in information from PIM to PIM as a propagated component of the $R'_a t_{n-1}$ corticocortical afferent source. The reentry of more distant past moments from the forebrain memory system may reinforce the current focus of the thought stream, or it may prompt a shift to another subject or object.

So where in this flow of activity does choice, decision, free will, or control exert its effect? Our nervous system interprets the sensory worlds by transducing stimulus energy (from the external and internal environments) and binding in time the wavefronts of information on a millisecond time scale. A relatively minor genetic modification in evolutionary time produced a structure and function in our brains that achieved the disparity computation of two 3D sensory representations and the internal derivation of the temporal dimension embedded in the informational order. Thoughts are propagated in a serial stream across our prefrontal modules in ≈ 200-ms wavefronts of 4D sensory representation.

In reiterative and recombinant transformations, thoughts enter the forebrain memory system and are converted into a long-term, dynamic 4D information space. With thought upon thought, moment upon moment, the growth and refinement of our personal, internal 4D world of representations begins at the crossing of a thermodynamic boundary line, a developmental milestone into consciousness that occurs at around 16 to 24 months of age. In the real-time thought processing modules, we compare our past with our present. We reflect our maturing self-image onto our past self-image, moment by moment, year by year, decade by decade. Our developing sense of self and all its attributes, feelings, emotions, and actions is an internal reflection that continues to undergo disparity computations until our dying day, or until we suffer a permanent loss of memory function or loss of thought and consciousness.

The illusion of will, choice, and control is the result of an error in the temporal order of information, made in the reflective process of disparity computation. The illusion occurs when the information that is currently present in the external context (which determines the next moment's actions) is not derived as distinct from and preexisting the information currently present in the 4D afferent flow from internal memory, as both types of information are integrated in the prefrontal modules. In other words, when the external stimulus world (the relatively stable flow of the 4D context) elicits a behavioral sequence from memory (a learned pattern of information originally created within similar surrounds), the real-time disparity computations performed by the prefrontal modules mathematically cancel out what is similar in the two representations. If two sets of 3D representations are congruent, then there is no distinct temporal dimension to be derived between them. In such a situation, the remembered representations will eclipse the information coming from the external stimulus world. In each moment of disparity computation under these particular conditions of the temporal flow of information, the flow of the internal (recalled) temporal dimension for a particular behavioral sequence of any content type will be dominant and will involve our reflected perspective of the self in time. Thus, we report that it was *I* who decided, chose, willed, or controlled the behavioral sequences as they unfolded, when actually our behavior was preceded by stimuli in the external context. Although this does not appear to us to be the case, our personal sensations or perceptions are actually created after the fact, in past moments of neural representation (relative to background time)!

When a critical threshold of similarity or congruence exists between the external background 3D spatial context, as it flows along its temporal course, and the remembered 4D context (and associated learned behavior), as it reenters the prefrontal modules from memory, the background temporal dimension becomes biomathematically indistinguishable from the temporal dimension of the memory sequence within the disparity computations. That is, there is no disparity information in the two framing contexts by which to derive a mismatch between the two temporal dimensions. In these moments, even though the surrounding context evoked the behavioral sequence from our memory and continues to lead this behavioral sequence along or change it, the fact that the behavior from memory contains information about our self causes our misperception of self-initiated and self-guided actions or thoughts. We report, from our immediate memory of real-time behavior, that *I* had the idea, *I* decided to do this or that, *I* willed something to take place, or *I* controlled the situation. When subthreshold disparity exists between the surrounding, real-time external world and the simultaneously integrated memory of a similar context, our phenomenally complex—but biomathematically constrained—operations compute the relative temporal dimensions as one and the same. Therefore, all information in each 3D sensory moment that relates to any behavior, whether thought or action, is regarded as belonging to the set within the 4D information space from memory, and the internal temporal dimension provides the link between each moment of remembered thought or action sequence.

This process creates the normal, human illusion of will, choice, and control that guides our behavior. The illusion process misplaces the information that, in reality, determines which behavior will occur and the path it will follow. It appears that a magical, disembodied presence (I) is determining our actions and our thoughts. The process is exactly the same as that in any magical act: An observer feels, perceives, or believes that some force of magic causes a rabbit to appear or a tiger to disappear. The illusion of magical force was produced by a mismatch in the flow of information from the perspective of the observer. The observer did not integrate the background flow of information because it was deliberately hidden.

For the illusion of personal force of will and control, the *now* self (the observer) is comparing a remembered *past* self in action as *now* computed past moments relative to the flow of (determining) information in the background context. The determining background information is hidden, in a computational manner, because the similar information that is reentering thought from memory becomes the mathematically (sensory) dominant 4D referent system. And for every moment after this illusion process begins in each child, it is reinforced by the novel memories of sensation, perception, emotion, and self that are derived during daily activity. Over time, a large knowledge space, our internal library, becomes filled with images, sounds, sensations, emotions, sentences, and stories about the self and the force of will, command, and control. At some point in our development, the illusion becomes virtually all-encompassing.

There are situations, however, in which the illusion is exposed, in which the temporal order of information becomes apparent in our computational moments and we see the context that is determining our behavior. It is like finding out about a magician's tricks or a card shark's manipulation—or that the Sun is not alive, the Earth is not at the center of the universe, and a horse cannot solve mathematical equations. And when the illusion is exposed, our individual reactions vary widely. A significant percentage of people who are shown a magician's tricks remain convinced that the magician commands special powers, and they continue to accept the illusion as real. Others enjoy the moments of deeper insight into the real nature of the act. An individual who has lost money to a card shark may respond with great anger at being the victim of an illusion.

The frame of reference approach to time, information, and illusion, as a model of thought and behavior, evokes a similar range of reactions. Most people feel certain that animals think and have a force of will that enables them to decide which flower to visit, which bone to chew, or which button to push, and they thus reject the notion that this is an illusion. They do not want to hear that the temporal order of information as it exists in each and every frame of reference determines the path that each object, animal, or person will take, moment by moment. Some people enjoy the discovery of deeper information, some get angry at being reduced to a victim of context; and others reject the notion, but aren't sure what the reality is.

A Moment of Recapitulation

In our earlier description of the random dot stereograms, we noted that there was hidden information that was derived by the disparity computations performed in neocortical modules. From the perspective of an observer looking at the two unfused sheets of dots, there is no other dimension, no additional information. When the two sheets are fused by disparity computation, however, the brain perceives the hidden information, and the illusion of a floating square is detected. We didn't will the square to appear; it was already contained within the 3D image, hidden in two regions of 2D space.

Illusions of motion are produced by the same process, as illustrated by the flicker-fusion of a Muybridge image set or any television, computer monitor, or motion picture sequence. Each picture of the Muybridge horse is framed by the background context. As we flip the images, our brain cancels out the similarities in the background part of the images in disparity computation. The result is that the horse appears to be moving across the stable background setting. It is an illusion. Every television monitor or movie projector generates the same illusion in our brains. The similarities are cancelled out, and the disparity information appears to be moving in space and time. Understanding the mathematical expression of this informational flow and the biophysical illusion process of the brain has led to the information compression technology (e.g., MPEG) that is truly revolutionizing our daily lives.

We see the same illusion in our memory of the immediate past, when our brains cancel out the information about the background context of a similar time and place. We perceive ourselves as moving in that fused context of external now and past memory of a similar context. And we perceive the remembered information and its unique temporal dimension as guiding the behavior. The floating square, the running horse, the kissing screen stars, the freely behaving self—all are illusions of time and information computation.

When we have enough information about the background system, the illusion is exposed, but the perception may not change. We know where the information lies in the random dot stereogram, the Muybridge images, and the television projection tube and screen, but our brains cannot choose *not* to fuse the images and derive the new dimension, even if we know it is an illusion. Likewise, even if we learn that the background context holds the information required to evoke each and every moment of our complex behavior, we cannot choose not to experience the internal temporal dimension of our behavioral sequence as it is reentered into thought. And since this temporal dimension came from within, we inevitably perceive it as the cause of our behavior, as our exerted will acting on our own actions.

This is the two-edged sword of our existence in consciousness. We have great flexibility of behavior and thought as a result of the generation of an internal 4D information space that contains all our learned behavioral sequences and their dynamic refinements. This 4D internal existence moves with us in space and time, and these complex behaviors may be elicited in distant futures by context stimuli that need have only a threshold amount of similarity that persists for a critical amount of time. But the evoking context information is mathematically cancelled out by the similar information from the internal memory of the context in which the original behavior sequence was learned, and an illusion of an internal force of will is then generated through the computational process. We inherit the illusion process with our context-independent behavior; both are products of our unique

4D experience. It is a confusing existence, for which we have created many expressions that expose the illusionary process. It is exposed, but irresistible; personal, and thus our reality.

Our daily life creates many situations that cause us to make statements that reflect the confusion surrounding our process of illusion. We speak of a stream of thought that we may become swept up in. We say things that indicate our absence of control over where our thoughts take us, such as "I don't know why I started thinking about it"; "I wish I could get that thought out of my head"; "I can't stop thinking about it"; or "Sometimes my mind has a will of its own." When we do something that, upon reflection, does not fit the social context, we say such things as, "I was on autopilot"; "I don't know why I did that"; "I didn't want to do that"; "I did it without thinking"; "I had no choice"; "I didn't mean to do that"; "What my mother did to me made me do it"; "You made me do it"; "They made me do it"; "Society made me do it"; " I'm out of control"; or "I was out of my mind." All people say things like this at times, but for individuals with extreme personalities who are consistently in opposition to the social context (e.g., so-called sociopaths or psychopaths), this class of response defines their daily lives. Some individuals may also invoke religious or spiritual concepts to describe their actions and say things like "The devil made me do it"; "The Lord guided my hand"; "I gave myself to a higher power"; "I surrendered my will to the gods"; or "The spirit moved me."

We have less of an illusion of control over our behavioral responses to sensory information generated within our internal visceral-autonomic world. We tend not to have a problem assessing the temporal order of information that involves some of our homeostatic mechanisms or extremes of external sensory stimuli. We don't perceive ourselves as having much of a choice about feeling pain when an arm is broken. If our bladder reaches a threshold state of distention, we typically don't say that we are willing ourselves to go to the restroom. If temperatures reach extremes or if oxygen becomes scarce, we do not perceive that it is our force of will that is making us move toward a milder temperature gradient or a higher oxygen concentration. We would acknowledge that the environment contained the sensory energy patterns (or information) that caused us to behave the way we did.

The illusion of will and control is exposed when we learn very new behaviors that involve situations that we have not previously encountered. In these contexts, we must be shown the learning steps and be led by the instructor. We have no illusions about who is controlling whom. We mimic, parrot, or ape the actions of the teacher. Because we do not already have a similar 4D sequence in our knowledge library, we cannot feel that we are choosing our actions or controlling the flow of behavior toward a known future. But the power of our learning by constructing a 4D sequence and the inseparable process of illusion soon reestablish their dominance. As we observe ourselves performing the new behaviors (i.e., as we transduce the moments of bodily movements that we may see, the sounds that we may make, our musculoskeletal motions, and our internal visceral-autonomic sensory state), these new sensory representations flow into our memory system before they reach the prefrontal regions and enter the prefrontal dominant modules to construct the full 4D sequence of multimodal experience. Once the 4D flow of experience comes back from the memory system, in only seconds (or minutes for extremely long learning sequences), the disparity computation now contains the internal experience. When this loop is completed and the *now* PIMs are comparing the current external learning situation with the remembered similar situation (even though it began only a few minutes ago or less), we begin to sense control.

At this point, we feel that we have regained our free will and that we may now exert it to guide our (remembered) behavior. This illusion process may flicker as new information that we have not incorporated into our memory is presented. We may surrender our will again, but only until the memory of the new behavior matches the ongoing external situation. From the frame of reference of the instructor, we may hear the comment, "Slow down, you don't have it yet" or, "You're acting as if you know what to do, but you must let me show you the next step." These comments may reflect the observation that we have begun to behave along the internal time dimension built from the new learning. From our internal experience in thought, we have regained our rightful, albeit illusionary, control!

For many decades, Benjamin Libet and his colleagues have painstakingly explored the human experience of sensation, time, and control.[11] Irrespective of the theoretical constructs and data interpretations, the basic finding is that individuals cannot exert their will (or, from our perspective, experience the illusion of control) until several hundred milliseconds following a particular sensory stimulus. These are fascinating results from very difficult research methodologies, and they are not inconsistent with the fundamental principles and biophysical parameters of our model.

Along the flow of daily events, we typically do not dwell on the subjects of illusions, animism, anthropomorphism, contiguity and causality, or free will and control. The demands of our lives keep us very busy just surviving. The prefrontal generated thought effect exerts its influence to inhibit or reinforce ongoing behavior. We tend not to sit around wondering who or what made us choose a doughnut and coffee for lunch! (Well, some might actually wonder about that.) Few of us spend time thinking about whether we really had a choice not to read that sentence in the last section.

Illusions in thought and mind are of critical concern to science and medicine, however. They determine our theories, our diagnoses, and our treatments. Furthermore, they determine the paths toward the discovery of new and better treatments. If we work from a basis of illusion, this may hinder great advances, the information for which may already exist and just be waiting for the veil of illusion to be lifted. When the illusion of the Earth's position in the universe was slightly refined, the awaiting cosmos was ours to understand. When Einstein penetrated the illusion of absolute measures of space and time, the era of modern physics and technology immediately became available to our minds. What may happen if the illusion of will and control, within the context of the thoughtful mind, is couched in a more accurate framework?

We create the illusion of the temporal order of information not only for ourselves, but for all life and for nonliving objects in motion. We may correct some of these errors in our daily experience and formal learning. The scientific method of illusion reduction allows us to peer more accurately into nature's processes, but we still feel illusions at nearly every moment of our private experience. We still construct our sentences to reflect these illusions and behave in reaction to them. We may always feel that computers are thinking, that trees and animals are feeling, and that we are in control of our self and of all things around us. It is our birthright and our constraint in thought and consciousness. We cannot go back across the evolutionary threshold that brought a 4D representational order to neural computation. We are at once both privileged and sentenced to move forward in time and create new information in consciousness. We have no choice but to interpret the world.

Final Constraints in Consciousness: Language, Information, and Boundaries

Consciousness is a frame of reference, an entire field of discrete local systems (brains) producing 4D information products (thoughts) that are propagated along an internal temporal dimension (thinking). Consciousness is a property, but it is not a force or power that can have an effect back on the local systems or on the background referent frames of life and the biosphere. Life is a frame of reference that gave rise to the consciousness field. All forms of life follow the paths of motions created by the 4D informational structure or the shape of the background biosphere. All cells, plants, and animals are fully immersed in the structure of the biosphere. Every moment of living behavior follows the changing informational shape of the background field, while maintaining a thermodynamically disconnected 4D existence.

If we could accurately account for the information in the local background field and in the internal environment of a cellular system, we could predict the next moment of behavior. Unfortunately, our ability to collect and analyze the necessary information is overwhelmed by the sheer complexity of the task. Nevertheless, the principle holds. Each of us, as a thinking participant in the life field, follows the paths of fluctuating matter-energy created by the background biosphere, and also the dynamic information shape of the life field created by the behavior of all living things, including one another. The interacting forces and information external and internal to each of us that create the shape of the pathway that determines our next moment of behavior are complicated indeed! Even so, we can do a fair job of predicting human behavior in the case of large-scale behaviors and high-magnitude sensory events.

Despite its constraints, the consciousness frame of reference has endowed humanity with three great advantages. Our *first great advantage in the consciousness frame of reference is the fusing of moments of background sensory information that provides us with the knowledge of all the 4D processes of the biosphere and life.* The emergent order of internal 4D sensory representation also endowed humanity with a memory structure of fused 4D moments of behavior and information. The growth and development of this 4D information space (our library of facts and processes) added a new level of flexibility to human behavior that is not seen in any other living animal. The internal sequences of behavior and thought move with each of us from place to place, and in time. A partial informational structure in the external or internal world may elicit complex sequences of behavior and thought that contain their own, internal temporal dimension. These fused moments of action or thought may be further combined with new sensory information derived in novel environmental situations, and then reentered into the memory structure.

The reiterative, recombinant refinement and growth of information define a second great advantage in the consciousness frame of reference. Our behavior may be fully determined by the complex information structure of the two background fields and our internal world, but our thoughts and actions become amazingly rich and diverse as we move through a lifetime. Finally, *our third great advantage in the consciousness frame of reference is the thought effect.* As our 4D knowledge space is expressed through efferent systems in motor actions, the resultant behavior causes changes in the background fields: the biosphere and life. The very outcomes or effects of human-caused changes are subsequently transduced as new sensory information, integrated into new thoughts, and then sent back again as actions that change the world. This is the engine of thought-action-transduction-thought that drives the reiterative, recombinant refinement and growth of the internal information space and all physical changes that we impose on the world. This principal set of fundamental processes are possible only in the consciousness field function not just across an individual's lifetime, but also across each successive generation, because the information and environmental changes left behind by the prior generation provide the foundation upon which the next generation's accomplishments (and failures) are created. The story of humanity, as the biophysical engines of every thought in the consciousness field, is manifest in the multigenerational creation and modification of all literature, art, music, science, technology, and society.

These three great advantages in the frame of reference of consciousness, all derived from the generation of the biophysical information product of thought, in turn predict the bounding limits and constraints of the referent frame. The brains that generate thought, thought-memory, and the 4D information space of knowledge are limited in the amount of sensory representation that they can integrate in each operational cycle of a prefrontal module. The sheer quantity of information that must be integrated to derive a complete sensory moment of the background stimulus energy patterns that surround an individual is far beyond the capabilities of our nervous systems. Even if we were able to grow more sensory receptors in every sensory organ and have them send more axons into the brain, the limits of information that can enter into disparity computation are set.

We may process only a limited number of *bits* (the word was derived from *binary*, 1-0, and *digit*, finger, as in counting with) per computation cycle of ≈ 200-ms duration. This limit is also influenced by the biophysical parameters of the cortical modules. In addition, there is a wealth of information that cannot be transduced by our sensory receptors because it is of the wrong energy type, at the wrong frequency of occurrence, or below a certain threshold of intensity. We cannot form a thought that has anywhere near the total amount of information that is available in the external world and the internal world at any single moment. A limit on the information in each thought also sets a limit for a sequence of thoughts, for any combination of sequences of thoughts, and for the growth rate of the 4D information space. In fact, it sets a limit on how much knowledge one could amass in a lifetime of thought. And, as we have discussed, the Piagetian progression gives great insight into the limits of knowledge growth in thought, as does our human history of discoveries and insights. There is so much about the information shape of the local context that we cannot assess that we are led to real-time misinterpretations about what forces are guiding the process or behavior of any living system, and illusion prevails. We cannot derive more information per moment about ourselves than we can about anything else!

However, the defining factor for each person in the consciousness frame of reference is that we do our own thinking, build our own mind, and follow our own context-defined paths through time. This is the operational definition of the individual, unique experience in consciousness. No two of us can be alike. Each of us has her or his own genetic structure, thought patterns, memory library, and internal world. We each participate in the dynamic creation of the internal and external information shape that determines our path, our behavior, in time. Our presence adds to the shape, and thus our moment-to-moment thoughts, actions, memories, and internal states are unique, even while the cumulative information guides our next moment of existence. We are each a unique moment in the universe, a moment of life and thought in the consciousness frame of reference. We cannot be compared along any single or multiple scaling continuums or standards. We are subjective. The universe expands, the world moves on, life behaves in generational time, and we, as living beings, are limited, but our presence and thoughts, in the form of actions, words, songs, ideas, constructions, and inventions, may live on in the memories of other thinking individuals and be shared across generations of humanity—our unique, individual, subjective, expression in thought, eternal.

Boundary Lines

Thoughts, and all permutations and aggregations of thoughts, are biophysical products. They exist in 3D structures of brain tissues and 3D structures of axon arrays. They are regions of biochemical and bioelectric structure that have energy, mass, and force. They are 3D structures whose unique order *is* a sensory representation of 4D information. They are propagated across time as the process of thinking, the generation of mind, in the consciousness frame of reference. A 4D process can be expressed only by collapsing the temporal dimension to zero and describing a component of the process. For the individual, we demonstrated how any sensation, perception, emotion, or the self, as a 4D process in consciousness, may be expressed as a place or point along an S-curve. But this act of depiction forfeits the 4D aspect of the process. We also showed that an individual has a nearly infinite number of unique states, operationally defined as dynamic products of expression for any sensory information, as the individual develops his or her unique 4D knowledge library. The attempt to name each state becomes not only difficult but also nearly irrelevant at some point in the infinite regression of subjective differentiation during a lifetime of experience.

We have come to the boundaries of our frame of reference: the limits and constraints of consciousness, as we can express them in thought. We cannot think quantitatively differently (with more speed, information, or functions) or qualitatively differently (as a nonhuman or superhuman something). Our brains cannot grow larger or more complex. At the boundaries of our frame of reference, at the biophysical walls that constrain and contain us, even our language fails. We introduce the phrase *bouncing off our biophysical walls* to give a visual analogy for this difficult, but fundamental, concept. It denotes the behavior we engage in when we are at the edge of our existence, when we are looking at ourselves reflected back from our thermodynamic barrier of energy, order, information, dimension, and time. We cannot write, speak, sing, dance, paint, draw, build, or think in any of its forms (e.g., conceptualize, hypothesize, image, dream, wish, hope, etc.) anything that shows the 4D experience of our thought processes as they are propagated in consciousness—just as we cannot express anything that shows the 4D process of any life function.

The critical insight and differentiating factor lies in the fact that only in the consciousness field can one transduce and derive the 4D sensory information of the life frame of reference. We can and do express a 4D process of a system in life by 4D representations that we construct within the flow of our own thoughts. We can express metabolism, migration, play, walking, talking, neurotransmission, or space flight by constructing sentences, drawings, or pictures and then either speaking or displaying depictions in rapid succession (flicker-fusion) to create the time dimension of the process *in our thoughts*! In other words, only along the flow of our internal temporal dimension may the temporal dimension of life be expressed. This is the process of human communication as the real-time exchange of 4D process information. These are the constraints on our ability to communicate any 4D process that exists in nature.

When we introduced the general categories of thought propagation in *consciousness, sensation, perception, emotion, self,* and *illusion,* we knew that such 4D constructs could not really be adequately, completely expressed. We used them for convenience and expediency, as condensed language for complex subjects. If we employ our model in a strict manner (as we would for a scientific or medical application), it is erroneous language. But, as we have tried to convey consistently, in our daily lives, our language and our illusions cannot be written away, nor should they be. We took time to show how the individual expression of any state of being, along any named or unnamed continuum, becomes profoundly complex as one matures in thought and life. We saw that although the words *sensation*, *perception*, *feelings*, and *emotion* were employed to describe the processes of thought, the complexity of the unique individual was being expressed exclusively as 3D descriptions of states for a collapsed 4D process, not as a process of thought that embodied the temporal dimension. We actually cannot express anything about a 4D process created in the consciousness frame of reference.

This brings us to a difficult concept to express, as we now firmly stand at the biophysical boundary of consciousness: We do not have any method in nature to transduce and integrate any sensory information about a 4D process that might be occurring as a result of the propagation of thought. For example, we cannot express a sensation, a perception, an emotion, the self, or an illusion by talking about it, writing about it, or even attempting to make a movie of it. Any movie we make in which an individual is shown behaving in 4D is depicting only a process of the life frame of reference (e.g., any motion or metabolic functions). We may experience the 4D reference systems of life within our ongoing perspective in the 4D reference system of consciousness. We may claim to have made a movie of someone experiencing the emotion of affection (somewhere on the S-curve), but we actually have shown only a fused sequence of 4D processes that are fully contained in the life field. Our movie may show smiles, hugs, heart rate changes, breathing rate increases, or other processes of life of which we can transduce the sensory information by our nervous system. However, nothing, nothing (!) in the movie transduced by our sensory systems is a biophysical process called affection that may, in turn, be experienced by the observer. Affection and all the other concepts of sensation, perception, emotion, self, and illusion are subjective. They are unique constructs in each of us, and they cannot be experienced as a sensory representation by anyone else's nervous system! Just to be clear, all behaviors in the life field are biophysical events that can be experienced, to some degree, by more than one individual. For example, if we show a film of a person falling (or watch it in real time), our sensory receptors can transduce the multimodal stimulus energy associated with each 3D sensory moment of the ongoing event in the flickering wavefronts of neural impulses and fuse them into 4D thoughts. We can then express what a fall may entail by our condensed language of speech, art, music, or math. We cannot, however, do the same with the pain or fear that the falling person may have experienced in thought.

Thus, in reality, any observation of a 4D biological process that we may assign a name to can be occurring only in the life frame of reference. If we say that someone looks very happy, we are collapsing the 4D behavior of the person into the word *happy*, not expressing anything about a 4D process of *emotion*. We cannot experience another person's 4D existence in consciousness. There are no receptors or devices by which to perform that function! And since we cannot transduce anything about a 4D process in consciousness, we cannot condense or collapse the temporal dimension to express it. *Note the error in the above sentence caused by the limits of our language and knowledge.* Our model proposes that we cannot know or even speculate if there is a temporal dimension in another's internal experience to be collapsed. These two sentences demonstrate a severe limitation on our ability to analyze our place in existence: We cannot gain a perspective on our perspective! When we enter into discussions such as this one, biological relativity draws a line and allows us to acknowledge that we are beginning to *bounce off our biophysical walls*.

The philosophical discussions of a concept called identity, filled with many definitions and contradictions, are related to this boundary.[12] Basically, our model states that we cannot differentiate between a collection of 4D metabolic processes or other processes in the life field and a hypothetical internally generated 4D thought process in the consciousness field. There is no way to project or map the 4D experience in consciousness onto the 4D processes of life. The position of biological relativity, however, is not one of semantics, metaphor, or lack of enough conferences to discuss it. It is a boundary in nature, a constraint of our frame of reference. Whatever else we experience in our subjective world of thought propagation is beyond our biophysical capacity and our thermodynamic barrier. *There is nothing more that can be said that will move or break the barrier*. We bounce off our biophysical walls as we persist in trying to think more deeply about what we are experiencing. We must note, however, that bouncing off thermodynamic barriers—that is, studying the boundary lines in nature—has often resulted in profound insights into limits, constraints, and illusions (as in special relativity). It certainly is a natural phenomenon.

It is important to know when we are engaging in circular behavior, when we are at the edge of consciousness and are beginning to reflect back on ourselves, so that this does not interfere with an effort to solve a problem, improve communication, construct scientific hypotheses, interpret data, diagnose patients, or design and conduct medical treatments. Getting stuck in a logical and language loop at the boundary of knowledge in consciousness may waste time or lives. First, let's look at a simple conversation between two individuals, while keeping in mind the S-curves for *emotions*. Two friends, Sam and Dave, are walking along a winding road. Sam turns to Dave and says, "You must be very angry!" Dave pauses, and then replies, "No, I'm frustrated." Sam continues, "You must be very frustrated!" "No, I'm just pretty frustrated," states Dave in further reply. Sam and Dave are in infinite regression along the S-curve path. They may reach agreement on a term before the walk is over, but Dave does not know anything about Sam's 4D process of emotion. And Sam cannot know either. He has learned a set of terms that are associated with a variety of sensory information states as frozen moments of collapsed information about life processes. He has no apparatus to learn more about anything beyond what resides in his biophysical products of thought. It is not that their discussion should not have taken place the way it did; they are friends, and they may communicate their concern, attraction, or affection for each other in many ways. We will always have dialogues like this. From a strict scientific or medical application of biological relativity, we may say that Dave learned about Sam's differential association predisposition and abilities with respect to internal states and external situations. We don't tend to talk like that with our friends, but that is perhaps a more accurate description of Sam's expressions. Thus, from our perspective at the edge of consciousness, we can now begin to identify our bouncing or reflective behavior. We can learn about the behavior.

In many times and in many ways, the struggle with concepts of consciousness, will, control, and other related terms has been described circularly. Consciousness, mind, and will have been described in such ways as choosing a choice, deciding to decide, willing a voluntary action, controlling the mind with the mind, awareness of consciousness, sensing our sensations, perceiving our perceptions, feeling our emotions, experiencing our experience, self-guiding the self, or I willing I. Another way in which these concepts are routinely phrased is to say that a force of free will determines all mental functions, which, in turn, produce a force of free will. Other examples invoke outside, superhuman forces at work. We may hear it said that a force or intelligence produced by a controlling spirit (a god or gods) chose to create human minds, so that we produce a free will that is actually under the control of the force that created it.

The infinite reflection in our thermodynamic mirror is perhaps what defines our so-called duality (the historical dual nature of mind and body).

Perhaps our reflection at the boundary of consciousness is a perfect symmetry that cannot be broken to initiate a new order, a new time, or a new existence. Would that hyperexistence be one that could observe and perhaps control the process of consciousness? Exercising thought at the boundaries of existence can be useful, but we will always learn only about our referent frame and nothing about one that is beyond our capacity. Every thought, every sentence ever written about other dimensions, other realities, or other consciousnesses is only a novel juxtaposition of the contents of thoughts, which are created by and wholly constrained to the referent frames we can transduce by our nervous system. We cannot think beyond the 4D existence from which we were created, and any device we invent to peer through the thermodynamic barrier to something would have to collapse the information into a form that we can integrate in our prefrontal neural modules.

Evolution as a function of entropy created a new 4D information existence by deriving the temporal dimension of the life referent clock, instead of being paced by it, within brain tissue that compares two moments of background time at a threshold level of order. Thus was created an emergent order of organic existence, a new 4D system, a new temporal dimension, a new biophysical referent system, with new (expensive) thermodynamic boundaries. We cannot experience what may come next in evolution's path, as we have no capacity to extrapolate another dimension of space or time. And we cannot know what came before the 4D universe in which we were created. We cannot know what came before space, time, dimension, or information.

Where does this leave us? At the beginning of this section, we restated the three great advantages in the frame of reference of consciousness. Collectively, these define the thought effect. Thoughts do have effects on the biosphere, on life, and thus on people. They are biophysical constructs of our brains that also exist in our memory. They are unique to each individual and, in that sense, subjective. And over time the unique internal 4D information space grows and matures through the reiterative, recombinant refinement process of thought and thought-memory. Biological relativity, therefore, considers the thought effect as the construct that may have utility in science and medicine. Our model indicates that we must begin to look for the biophysical parameters that brought thought to the human brain at around the age of 16 to 24 months. Human-based clinical research, with a frame of reference point of view, is the application. An explicit shift in our formal use of language in the laboratory and in the clinic is thus necessary in order to reduce the illusions of consciousness.

Thought will eventually be quantified. The biophysical parameters and informational content of thought will be measured. Therefore, thought will become more accessible for control and manipulation. When thought is changed, then anything else that thought might produce in consciousness will also be changed. We can observe this in metabolic shifts and structural damage. Advances in our understanding of thought and the thought effect will help in our efforts to treat any illness—genetic, metabolic, or structural—that alters the normal thought process and thereby affects memory and behavior. We can better understand the generation of thought, its memory, and its behavioral effects if we do not become distracted about what else consciousness may or may not produce. The quantification of thought, as operationally defined by biological relativity, presents an agenda for science and medicine.

The Frame of Reference Approach

We derived this model by applying a frame of reference approach to the organization of organic systems. With it we can see the thermodynamic boundaries that exist in nature, with respect to emergent 4D systems. Identifying these threshold boundaries in order and information also provided a framework for the language used to describe scalar quantities and 4D processes within each referent frame. We may now understand that the various state and phase transitions that may occur within a particular referent frame (e.g., water to steam, wind to tornado, nerve impulse wave, or group behavior in an ant colony) do not denote *emergent properties* as defined by biological relativity. Within a frame of reference, a set of terms may describe a behavior in a manner that is unnecessary or inappropriate in another referent system. For example, to say that a frog thought about whether he was going to choose a mate or eat a bug not only may be inaccurate, but may also confuse the understanding of the consciousness referent frame. Likewise, from the perspective of biological relativity, to say that ants display thought, mind, or consciousness in their coordinated behavior is equivalent to proposing that a group of billiard balls expresses a collective consciousness about a game of 8-ball by their patterns of movement.

Defining the context for behavioral observation, and accounting for the information available and its temporal flow, allows us to better determine the distinction between the pre-thought and thought conditions. As we have stressed, *context is everything*. Proposing that life and consciousness are frames of reference in nature gave us thermodynamic boundaries for each system that cannot be overcome. Life cannot think, and in consciousness we may not know what is beyond. We were also able to define the point at which our language fails when we try to describe any 4D process that may occur within the referent frame of consciousness. We can now identify the use of reflective, circular phrases and concepts as we begin to bounce off our biophysical walls.

Einstein held the referent system model in his thoughts as he derived special relativity. With this model, he saw deeply into the limits and constraints of the 4D universe by understanding the relative nature of each dimension within thermodynamically distinct referent systems. As he continued to contemplate the universe with special relativity and referent systems churning in his mind, he realized that another adjustment in perspective had to be made. He was also interested in behavior, the behavior of matter and energy in the space-time continuum of the electromagnetic field. Einstein thus described the behavior of every referent system relative to the background field. In his thoughts, he brought together information and his imagination to form a novel internal 4D construct in moments of disparity computation. He saw what no one had seen before, because he viewed the universe as a multitude of referent systems relative to one another. When he did this, he saw the frame of reference of the electromagnetic field, the structure-function of space-time, and the behavior or motion of all participants within it. His radical new vision changed everything, again! We will now examine the relationship between his view of space-time's shape and the model of biological relativity.

12

Einstein's Vision of the Universe II: The Structure of Space-Time

The frame of reference approach was first applied to the universe of inorganic matter and energy in the special theory of relativity. The discussion of reference systems in Chapter 1 allowed us to better identify the evolutionary emergent thresholds to organic life and consciousness and to understand how the illusions of force and will have been applied to both referent systems. We proposed that the 4D structure of the biosphere determines the next metabolic moment in each cell, and that as a direct extension the 4D structure of the information, space determines the next moment in nervous system sensory representation, and thus each thought product and behavior. Now we look back across the threshold to life to the larger universe of the electromagnetic field, atoms, planets, and galaxies for an understanding of how the 4D structure of space-time determines the next moment of behavior for every particle in nature. Einstein defined this model of the universe in his general theory of relativity.[1]

The towering vision that Einstein expressed in general relativity remains the best description of the known universe. Before Einstein, Sir Isaac Newton had written the guidebook for understanding nature.[2] Newton's insight and mathematical invention (he was a major figure in the formulation of calculus) gave us the laws of inertia and force. In his time, within the limits of knowledge available, he proposed the existence of an absolute (invariant) space and an absolute time. However, as we presented in Chapter 1, Einstein's vision revealed the relativity of all the parameters of nature by applying a frame of reference approach.

An important aspect of Newton's principles involved the force of gravity. The idea that there is such a force that guides all matter in all its motions and keeps all planets in their orbits presented great problems for

Newton. His observations and mathematical derivations appeared to reflect the true nature of this force, but it was indeed mysterious, and he was well aware of its oddity. Gravity was believed to be a force generated by each particle of matter, and this force could reach across the universe to exert an effect on other masses. That a force could have an instantaneous action at a great distance and that it pulled with just the right strength to match the mass of a distant object did not seem right. The Earth, for example, appeared to *know* how much gravity force to send out in order attract objects that came close enough, and not to pull more on smaller objects than on larger ones. It seemed that the Earth would have to have the information about the mass before it sent out its attractive force! It was mysterious. Perhaps the information was in some way already present in the context, and the observation that the Earth knew *a priori* what to do was in error. Einstein also had difficulty with this oddity, as it seemed a discordant way for the universe to work, and his belief in the harmony of nature is well documented.

We return to Einstein's vehicle, as it were, for his thought experiments: an elevator with no windows that contains two people (observers) and measuring devices (a scale and a clock). The elevator is gently moved out into a region of space that is very far away from any matter that may be sending out the force of gravity to tug on it. It is in *empty* space (a theoretical construct) and at rest. Inside the elevator, the observers and their instruments are floating, as are their pens, their papers, and anything else around them. From the limited perspective of the observers, either they are falling down a very long elevator shaft or they are out in empty space. They have no way to tell the difference. *Free fall* effects are the same in both situations. If they were to try to weigh each other on a scale, they would find that *they have no weight (a measure of the pull of gravity) in this region of* space.

Special relativity showed that local four-dimensional (4D) systems experience a change in the metric of their dimensions as they accelerate to a speed near that of light, the limit of the universe. And the changes in scale can be measured or experienced only relative to another referent system or the background system of the larger space-time environment. The spatial dimension of length contracts with respect to the direction vector of the acceleration (as observed from another referent frame). No such change may be determined within the moving system, however, as its measuring devices all undergo the same transformation. The time dimension expands, and thus the interval between the ticks of any type of clock, mechanical or biological, becomes longer in the accelerating system. And, finally, the mass of the system (its relative weight and its gravity) is increased. Einstein showed that the speed of light waves was the boundary limit for this effect and that if you could accelerate a 4D system (a particle, a rocket, or an elevator with people in it) to the speed of light (c), you would hit a thermodynamic barrier—time would stop, the motion vector length would go to zero, and inertial mass, and thus gravity, would be infinite! The so-called black holes are natural phenomena in which it appears that particles and larger-matter systems are accelerated to close to this barrier (perhaps smashing right into it), and they probably populate the center of each galactic system.

Einstein understood that the acceleration (inertial change) of any mass near c causes an increase in both mass and gravity. The Newtonian hypothesis was that mass generates a force of gravity, but Einstein saw the deeper relationship: that mass is the equivalent of gravity. Furthermore, in his thought experiment, the elevator that is either at rest in empty space or falling down an elevator shaft on the Earth is amazingly utterly immune to any apparent force of gravity. That is, within the elevator, it is impossible to measure any mass or weight; hence, it and all objects within are suspended. Thus, the equivalency of mass and gravity appeared to hold in the zero condition: Without gravity, there would be, in effect, no weight or mass.

With respect to the imaginary elevator, the logical question arises: What in this universe must happen to get some mass, to be able to detect a weight, and thus to create a unit of measure from nothing? Well, we know from relativity theory that if the elevator were instantaneously accelerated to near c, the increase in mass would be measurable. So, some unit of mass within the elevator system is detectable when the elevator is accelerated at this incredible rate; thus, acceleration appears to induce a change in mass equivalent to its magnitude. But this presents a peculiar situation, a conundrum in nature: At one moment there was no way to tell if any mass existed, but then at the very next instant there is a great amount of mass near c. What happens between the zero point and the near-c acceleration?

If we compare the set of equivalency statements that we developed above, we see that acceleration is equivalent to mass, and that mass is equivalent to gravity. When the common term *mass* is cancelled out, acceleration is seen to be equivalent to gravity (if $a = m$ and $m = g$, then $a = g$). The zero condition for this equivalency may be also imagined as no acceleration equals no gravity. These relationships imply that there is no difference between the effect of acceleration and that of gravitation upon any object and that this effect is unique to each and every system undergoing any amount of acceleration or gravitational influence that is greater than zero and less than c. This is Einstein's principle of equivalence of gravitation and inertia.

Motion, the last physical property of the world that had been considered invariant since Newton, now became a relative concept. There was no standard, absolute force of nature guiding the motion of all objects. In the mind of Einstein, the elevator sat in empty space with no acceleration, no gravity, and no units of mass. Applying his new thought structure to the imagined scene, he saw that if the elevator were accelerated (by any means, in linear or rotational motion) by any amount greater than the zero point, there would be gravity. And if there is gravity, then there must be mass. Therefore, gravity is only the acceleration of matter. As we accelerate the elevator in space and the observers inside are pressed to the floor opposite the direction of the motion, they will begin to experience mass and thus gravity.

The final and crucial question thus emerged: From what did the force of gravity emanate? Who or what was generating the mysterious magnetic-like attraction on the elevator or any system in motion? Who or what was watching the behavior of matter and at the exact moment of acceleration began to pull with a force equal to the changing movement? Who or what was controlling the force of gravity? From the perspective of the observers inside the elevator, if the acceleration was very gradual, they might not even know that they were moving. All they could measure or know was that they were getting heavier, more massive.

Einstein understood that no one and nothing was watching from a distance and perfectly matching a force of gravity with acceleration. The relationship between acceleration and mass was all that one needed to know in order to fully describe the behavior of matter systems in motion. The mysterious force of gravity, despite having been accepted as a fact for centuries, was not a force; it was just a descriptive word that related the acceleration of matter in one system relative to another, or to the entire background space-time continuum. Einstein's vision of the universe was of the entire background field of electromagnetic energy as a structure with force, within which all matter is immersed. As any particle or particles of matter accelerate—electrons, atoms, elevators, people, planets, stars, galaxies—relative to the background field or to any other system of particles, mass increases. This happens not just near the speed of light, but with any relative motion. Gravity was not a force reaching out across space-time with invisible power to bind together all matter in the universe. Gravity was the property of 4D systems in relative motion.

Based on his knowledge of quantum phenomena, field theory, the reality of a space-time continuum and its limits in acceleration, the relativity of all dimensions in local systems, and the geometric principles of curved objects and geodesic paths that span their surfaces, Einstein imagined a model of an active and dynamic universe that brought all observations and theories into harmony. The background field of electromagnetic waves (which defines the boundaries of the known universe at this level of organization) may be conceptualized as a homogeneous structure of undulating energy, in which local systems distort or warp the field in all four dimensions! From special relativity we know that each system has its own matter-energy ($m = E/c^2$) and creates a unique 4D referent frame. The interaction between any two systems will be observed as the one with less matter-energy falling (accelerating) toward the one with more matter-energy. In the universe of Einstein's unveiling, the larger the matter-energy system, the more the distortion, or the deeper the 4D warp (Figure 12-1). And in perfect congruity, the greater the acceleration (linear or rotational), the deeper the warp.

In the 3D interpretation that is used to describe this image, each electron, planet, and galaxy creates a well in the space-time continuum. The 4D continuum is itself in motion, expanding outward from the initial moment of existence at a rate (c) that determines the processes and limits of all metrics that we may detect. Within this grand expansion, local matter-energy systems emerged out of the electromagnetic background. The larger matter-energy systems warp the field to a degree such that smaller systems appear to accelerate toward them. The acceleration effect is due to the fact that all four dimensions are relative to the local system, and mass systems warp the temporal dimension as well. Smaller mass systems are influenced by larger-magnitude dimensional contractions, and their dimensions begin to change to reflect the metrics of the local region of space-time.

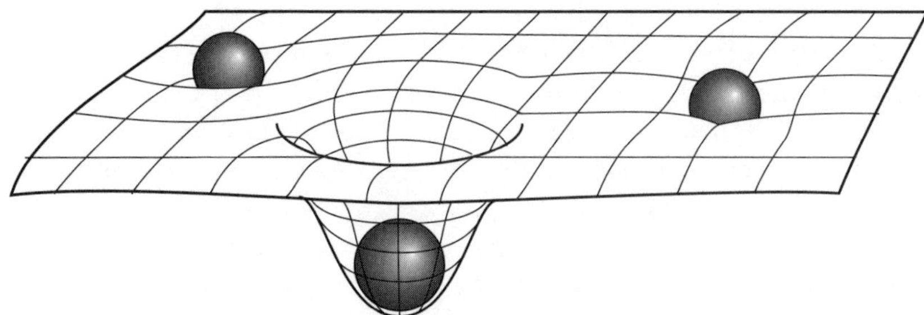

Figure 12-1 The four-dimensional electromagnetic field warped by particles and bodies of matter. The very shape of the universe, including its temporal coordinate system, is defined by the distribution of its particles. All matter follows paths in the structure of space-time.

In Einstein's dynamic universe, there is no longer any such thing as empty space; there is only the full 4D fabric of the electromagnetic field. If one local system (body) is in motion relative to a larger one, the smaller system will appear to alter its path through space-time. It is not that the larger body is emitting a mysterious force with some sort of magneticlike property; rather, the shape of space-time that the larger body creates may be large enough to physically involve the path of the smaller body so that it must follow a geodesic curved path through that region of space-time. From the perspective of the smaller body, it is moving along a straight line across space. No new force has caused a change in the path of the system, and thus the principle of inertia is preserved. The smaller body is just falling along a curve in space-time created by the mass of the larger body.

On the Earth, we are not being drawn to the ground by a force; we are constantly falling into our moving local warp. The rate of fall, the acceleration or gravity constant, is set by the mass of the Earth and its linear and rotational velocity, thus creating the warp. We immediately notice this effect whenever we try to move against the focal point of the gravity well (the center of the Earth) by jumping, climbing stairs, or flying in an airplane. A moving body, however, is not falling, in a relative sense, when its motion matches the rate of acceleration that is set by the local warping mass and is in a direction toward the center of the warp field. For each moment in time that a body accelerates toward the center of the warp at the exact rate set by the larger body, there is no relative difference in the acceleration of the two bodies, and thus there is no relative change in speed that would result in a detection of mass. This explains why we may experience weightlessness (free fall) in an airplane that dives toward the Earth (center of warp) at a certain rate. If the acceleration becomes greater than the warp constant, we experience an increase in mass that exactly matches the amount of acceleration above that of the warp.

So what became of gravity? Where did it go? Einstein effectively reduced one of the great pillars of human belief to an illusion of cause-effect. He was able to see the electromagnetic space-time structure fold around each system, however small or large that system might be. He was able to see that the mysterious force of gravity was actually a manifestation of one local system interacting with another or with the background field across moments in time. *Gravity became the behavior of 4D systems immersed in and indivisible from the shape of the electromagnetic energy field.* There is no quantity of a gravity effect. There is no independent unit of measure. There is no more gravity in Earth than there is in the moon. Gravity describes the behavior of Earth, the moon, and all bodies in the universe as relative rates of acceleration. The gravity term in mathematical expressions was always just the rate constant, derived by the ratio of the warps in space-time.

Einstein's vision of the universe changed everything, again. With the general theory of relativity, he proposed a view of the structure-function of the electromagnetic field and all the forms of matter-energy within it. He eliminated an illusionary force by understanding that gravity was just describing the behavior of matter within the warped space-time continuum. The three fundamental forces of electromagnetism (electromagnetic, weak nuclear, strong nuclear) that we can measure and observe do act upon all matter that emerges from the background field. All these forces are indivisible from all forms of matter and energy, and each local system has its own irreducible four dimensions relative to other systems and to the background field. (Indeed, all forces of nature are interactions, and we will eventually have a formulation that encompasses them as well.) From our perspective in consciousness, we view the inorganic world of particles and waves and classify them by many names. The behavior of all the local matter-energy systems, no matter how small or large, is described in terms of gravity. Gravity has no units of its own, has no action back on the system, and is thus not a force. Gravity is the 4D frame of reference of the entire electromagnetic field.

Since the time of Faraday and Maxwell, we have conceived of the electromagnetic field as one that is in some way creating effects on surrounding regions. It is well known that the arclike shape of the invisible magnetic field created by the poles of a bar magnet is revealed when particles of iron filing are scattered around the magnet. Thus, the iron particles conform to the background shape of the force field. The shape of a background field determines the behavior of systems emerging from that field.

As another example, picture Earth as a 3D sphere whose surface is curved, and upon which a straight line is actually an arcing geodesic (Figure 12-2). The lines drawn on the sphere in the figure show the separate paths that two imaginary travelers take as they head due north from starting positions thousands of miles apart along the equator. From the point of view of each traveler, he or she is walking a straight line and never wavering. At a point near the north pole, the travelers encounter each other. If they indeed kept to their straight course, what force of nature or fate brought them together? What pulled them nearer to each other as they proceeded north? Again, from our perspective far above Earth, the answer is obvious, because we can see the entire shape of the space within which the behavior took place. The two travelers were following their own straight lines, but on the curved surface of a sphere these lines are geodesics. The travelers' encounter

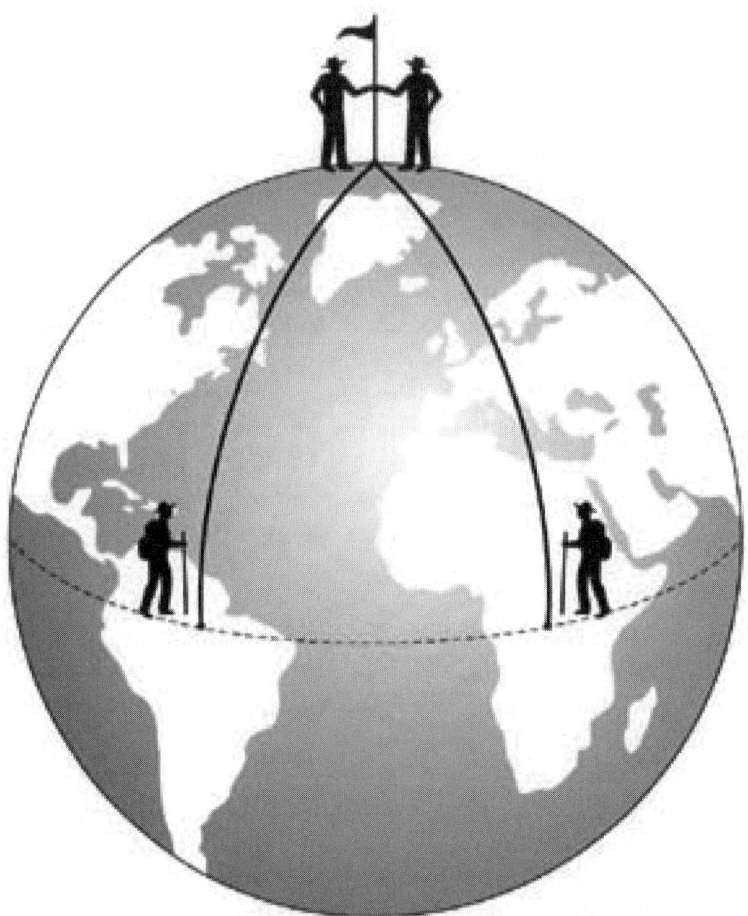

Figure 12-2 Earth is a 3D sphere upon which a straight line is actually an arcing geodesic. Two travelers may begin a "straight-line" trek heading north from widely spaced points along the equator, but they will meet at an intersecting point near the north pole.

was not due to an outside force of attraction or desire, but was a predetermined fact created by the shape of the background physical context.

The Structure of Space-Time and the Biological Earth

The entire 4D matter-energy fabric of the universe may be considered the gravity field. This referent system defines and predicts the behavior of all matter systems that emerge from the electromagnetic background. If we now change our focus and look toward the organic world again, we see that relative to the gravity field, the life field is the frame of reference of all cellular systems that emerged out of the background biosphere, which itself is a participant and forms the local gravity warp. The consciousness field, in turn, is the frame of reference of all thought-producing brain systems that emerged out of the background life field. In thought, we can look across all scales of organization in nature and see these relationships between emergent 4D systems in organic and inorganic fields. Gravity is the emergent property for all local systems interacting or behaving in the 4D landscape of the electromagnetic field. A gravitating planet is like a living cell is like a human in consciousness.

Our proposed arrangement of referent systems now extends from the grand gravity field (which is the electromagnetic field) to the local space-time warp of the Earth and its two relatively infinitesimal biological referent systems, life and consciousness. The three emergent fields of our existence can be visualized as three concentric spheres: the light-years expanse of the gravity field, the Earth-bound life field, and the brain-bound consciousness field. Outside the boundary of the electromagnetic energy field is the so-called quantum world or other unnamed existence, and inside the boundary of the consciousness field is the unnamed, unknown, and unimaginable. When matter-energy emerges across the thermodynamic threshold of the electromagnetic field, it creates a 3D order and 1D time. Only when we can observe and measure a spatial organization of energy for even a brief (how brief?) time will we be able to conceptualize a physical framework for its behavior, as Einstein did for gravity. Thus, we have not been able to understand the potential field of quantum phenomena as a system with structure or time. What produces energy, how energy becomes matter, and how matter returns to energy are not known to a sufficient degree to allow us to conceptualize or see the system. It is a mystery, defined by mysterious phenomena and even more mysterious hypotheses about what it all means.

The Earth creates a local space-time warp. Within this region of space-time, all the components that collectively add up to the mass of the Earth have one rate of acceleration in a vacuum condition (variations do exist with large local masses and with elevation). Galileo was the first to systematically derive this insight. If we built a large cylinder and created an absolute vacuum inside, a car and a feather would drop toward the ground (toward the center of the warp) at exactly the same rate. This rate, the Earth's gravitational constant, which is far less than the universal limit (*c*), sets an Earth limit (we could call this *e*; in the terminology of gravity constants it is 1 *g*, and it is measured at 9.8 m/s^2). This limit is the upper boundary for all processes of the inorganic and organic biosphere, the life field, and the consciousness field. All behavior, from reaction rates to metabolic pathways, to cell division, to jumping, to nerve cell activities, to thought generation, is constrained by the local system warp constant.

The evolution perspective is important here in that the rate *e* is a constraint on the process of evolution in our world, as is *c* on the unfolding of the larger universe. The time lines of each emergent order are thus also limited by the local background clock. Life is thus constrained in the propagation of its generations to a certain maximum rate. Life cannot live more rapidly. Again, this is not a semantic concept, but a thermodynamic limit determined by the structure of nature. Evolutionary processes thus are constrained in terms of how fast any genetic mutation can be expressed in a population of living cells, plants, or animals. The pace of evolution has a local limit of *e*.

The nervous system and its activities are likewise bounded by our local space-time warp. All sensory representations, and thus all the information that the prefrontal modules can process, can flow only within the limits of the system. We cannot be encouraged or motivated to see faster, hear more quickly, think faster, remember faster, or create new ideas, insights, and technological marvels faster than a certain upper limit. Of course, within the maximum rate allowed by *e*, the complex nervous system may at times work more slowly or less efficiently than it might, and so the rate of new insight and new technologies is also dependent upon the internal juxtaposition of information into novel patterns. Even with these important considerations, there remains a boundary on the basic processes of thought and the reiterative, recombinant refinement that cannot be surpassed. Again, perhaps Piaget was peering deeply into these constraints of nature as he observed the ongoing, but temporally constrained, development of human concepts and abilities of thought. Our very existence, the pace of our daily functions, and long-term evolutionary modifications are tied inseparably to the Earth and its local shape in the background of electromagnetic energy.

In general relativity, Einstein showed us the structure of the space-time continuum of electromagnetic energy and the shapes produced by its interaction with the emergent matter of the universe. The magical force of gravity was thus seen to be an illusion. This illusion is exactly the same one that our normal process of disparity computation will always perform, and it occurred only because the information entering our prefrontal modules contained the wrong temporal order. If we had known that the information was preexisting in the local region of space-time that the warp created, then any behavior of a system participating in the warp and the behavior of any system coming near the warp could have been predicted. When the concept of general relativity was introduced, it affected our thought processes, and the illusion vanished! However, many continued to accept the illusion, even responding with emotion to the idea that they were operating under an illusion. Others rejected the idea, but weren't sure what the actual reality was.

Information as entropy, order, and patterns in matter and energy at all levels of organization may be derived from the context. The information contained in the structure of space-time is the dynamic, churning interplay of matter and energy forming a shape in the local field. The shape of the information determines the next moment of behavior for all matter-energy systems in motion. The living world exists within this information space, and the local shape created by the interplay of life and the background field determines and predicts the next moment of any living organism.

If we do not see this clearly, then we create an illusion that cellular life, in any form, is generating a force that moves it along its path into the future, and that this force must know where to go before it gets there. This illusion disappeared when we learned that biological life was not generating a new force, but was following the shape of the information structure in the local context (including the intracellular environment, as it too is derived from the background materials).

When the illusion of a life force faded into the background, we lost the animism and much of the anthropomorphism that had served as the reality of humankind for centuries. It could now be understood that a flower bloomed when the internal and external conditions determined that behavior, or that a lion pursued prey as a result of internal and external stimuli. More importantly, we began to understand that we could control the pathways of living things by manipulating the information in the internal and external worlds. We are in the infancy of our ability to stack the deck, to shape the information context in ways that will give us a degree of exquisite control over all life.

In the field of consciousness—the final emergent order of organic systems—our thoughts are created by information derived from internal and external sources of matter-energy. They are the most complex patterns in the known universe and may forever remain so, but they are biophysical constructs nonetheless. At the edge of our existence, we remain convinced that we have a novel force of nature—our will and control—that by its very actions must be able to view the viewer, look ahead in time, and then decide what to do. In this illusion, we see a self-generated force guiding us through

Table 12-1 Principle of Equivalence in Biological Relativity

Proposed: Three 4D Frames of Reference Have Emerged in Nature's Evolution			
Field Property	Field Process	Field Products	Elemental Systems
Gravity	Gravitating	Waves–particles	Matter
Life	Living	Organic molecules	Cells
Consciousness	Thinking	Thoughts	Modules

our pathways of behavior. We must ask whether the shape of the information space created by all the incomprehensible complexities of the external and internal sensory environments and the patterns of information entering the *now* prefrontal modules from the memory system determine the next moment of behavior for us as a system in nature. Can we see that perhaps there is no force that knows the future and thus determines our thoughts, hopes, and dreams? The illusion is a product of the limitations and constraints of our biophysical existence. At the boundary, we begin to bounce off the biophysical walls, and language becomes circular and mystical, involving timelessness, spacelessness, hyperdimensionality, and superhuman forces that have knowledge about future time over great distances. The exposure of the illusion process allows us to correct for the temporal order of information in circumstances when it is important to do so, as in the fields of science and medicine.

Biological relativity proposes a unified principle of equivalence that relates gravity, life, and consciousness as 4D referent systems (Table 12-1). All properties, processes, and products of each frame of reference may be understood within the thermodynamic boundaries imposed by evolution and entropy. The illusions of force for gravity, life, and consciousness are eliminated when we view the behavior of local systems from a frame of reference perspective.

The Structure of Space-Time, Matter, and Energy

At the electromagnetic-quantum boundary, we have questions that cover a wide variety of unknowns. What is energy, and how is it produced? How does it become matter, and when it does, why does it return to an energy state? From an evolutionary perspective, we ask, What was the original force, the original particles or waves from which the universe expanded? Twelve years after the introduction of general relativity, Heisenberg (1927) proposed the principle of uncertainty, which appeared to focus on the limits and constraints of gathering information about another system.[3] He proposed that any attempt to observe the location of an electron (an elementary particle that also propagates as a waveform) would necessitate directing some energy into the system, and thus any information about its velocity would be contaminated by the act of observation. Conversely, if you allow the electron wave to behave freely so that you may gather information about its velocity, you cannot know, with certainty, its exact location. It is a wave, and therefore it does not exist as a stable, measurable 3D particle until you hit it with another energy source or stop it. The limits of information lie at this level of the organization of the universe, according to this theory and others that have followed.

This theory immediately generated a great debate that continues to rage today, with no end in sight. Alternative explanations of the proposed limitation have been devised that allude to hidden variables, for which we are not accurately accounting (as expressed in the work of David Bohm[4]). Uncertainty and other explorations at the boundary between pre-energy, energy, and matter have led to various hypotheses centered on the temporal order of information. The basic position expressed is that if we are uncertain about nature at this level of organization, perhaps we should be uncertain about nature in the mechanical world as well. Further articulation of this position includes basic questions of cause-effect relationships. In a simplification of experimental designs and theories under the heading of quantum linear superposition, we find interesting behaviors described for certain strictly conducted demonstrations. In one such type of demonstration, a single photon is generated and then is split into two parallel waves that will reach recording devices on both paths of travel. If the design is preset so that the path of one photon is always allowed to reach the target, the other split product will not. Then, if the path that is always open to the split photon is blocked, the other split photon will reach its target!

From the human observer's point of view, it appears that the split photons have reached out into the future to see which path was open, then decided which wave could go on to the open target in order to register the energy hit. Where did this mysterious force that looks ahead and then makes a decision come from? In addition to our uncertain, unpredictable future, we now have a basic uncertainty as to what order a cause-effect relationship really takes. The temporal order of information at this fundamental level of nature's organization may not be what we think it is at all! Thus, the arguments that follow this line of reasoning propose that what we experience as our 4D existence in nature may be wrong, that there is no real way to predict anything with a reasonable degree of certainty, that what we think causes something to happen may also be in error, and that we may have no way of knowing.

The application of the uncertainty principle (and other concepts such as instantaneous action at a distance, found in superposition theories) to all levels of behavior poses the same problem as did gravity. What force, what intelligence is looking into the future and making a decision about what to do or not do next? If all actions are really an expression of some type of quasi-randomness, then why do so many patterns exist at all levels of nature, and why do they follow a course of evolutionary change? The answer from those who propose such theories is that we, as humans, are misperceiving the true reality of nature. Such theories typically state that if we could only understand the uncertainty and quasi-randomness of nature, then we would know the mysterious force that transcends all 4D conceptualizations of space, time, and dimension. When we reach that level of human knowledge, we may know why we have free will! The current discourse that surrounds these various hypotheses is certainly not new.

The 1920s were abuzz with the deterministic, albeit relativistic, universe created by Dr. Einstein. Since that time, it has been fashionable to attempt a deconstruction of this worldview. Our current round of speculation on the randomness of nature, coupled with the idea that the answer to human consciousness and free will involves so-called quantum solutions, thus actually began well over 60 years ago.

> *For by dealing in terms of statistics and probabilities it abandons all idea that nature exhibits an inexorable sequence of cause and effect between individual happenings. And by its admission of margins of uncertainty it yields up the ancient hope that science, given the present state and velocity of every material body in the universe, can forecast the history of the universe for all time. One by-product of this surrender is a new argument for the existence of free will. For if physical events are indeterminate and the future is unpredictable, then perhaps the unknown quantity called 'mind' may yet guide man's destiny among the infinite uncertainties of a capricious universe.*

Barnett penned this observation in his book *The Universe and Dr. Einstein*, first published in 1948![5]

At the boundaries of the consciousness frame of reference, our language reflects our reflection off the thermodynamic mirror and expresses our inability to know anything beyond our 4D nervous system function of sensory transduction, representation, computation, thought production, and dynamic memory organization. We may be observing the same phenomenon at the boundaries of the electromagnetic frame of reference. The quantum world, whatever it is, may actually lie beyond a barrier, so that we can know nothing about it. If the quantum world has no expression of a 3D structure over a moment of 1D time, then we have no apparatus, no capacity, to convert that *something* into a structure that we can enter into our brain function.

The nervous system doesn't care what type of information it receives; that information just has to be of an energy form that we can transduce, transmit, and perform biomathematical transformations upon to enter it into our 4D information space. This is our limit and our constraint. As we stated in Chapter 11, reaching into the next hypothetical frame of reference is a vital exercise of our thoughts. We can learn much about our existence, our 4D existence, by doing so. The quantum experimentation and the application of devices that take advantage of quantum effects are superb examples. It must be noted, however, that our experimentation takes place and our devices are designed, built, and function in the 4D space-time continuum. Whatever happens in them that makes us think and say, "That was a quantum event" may not necessarily be an event of the *something* of the quantum world. Instead, we simply may have more to learn about the shape of the information space in the local context of the electromagnetic frame of reference.

In the field of high-energy particle physics, we see the amazing convergence of theory and technology. Our current theories of the evolution of the universe have brought the three forces of electromagnetism into an alignment. Reasoning back toward the origins of our cosmic expansion, we think that in the early moments, there was an incredible high-energy, and thus high-temperature, environment in which no particles as we know them now could exist. As expansion proceeded through time and distance, the cooling of the energies of origin began the condensation process that we may view as the evolution of the entropy path of our universe. As wavelengths expanded and particles began to emerge out of the subatomic void, this set off the organization of stars, black holes, galaxies, planets, and all the other forms of matter-energy. To research questions about the validity of theories of origin, a technique was devised wherein two atomic particles, such as protons and antiprotons, are collided into each other at near-*c* speed. This atom smashing creates brief moments of incredibly high energy and annihilates the participating atoms. In this process, the new particles that are created in the high-energy environment may include those that could have existed only near the first moments of our universe's time line. These experiments have been overwhelmingly successful, and many new particles, albeit with a fleeting 4D material existence, have been discovered.

The point of this description is that even at this fundamental level of investigation into the origins of our universe, the only way we, as observing, thinking, computing, and remembering humans, can gather and understand the information from these marvelous events is by the physical trace left by the particles as they flicker into a fused 4D existence before returning to the energy world. Moreover, because the sensory receptors of our nervous systems cannot even come close to transducing such a brief, pinpoint moment of existence (in nanoseconds or picoseconds), we must view these events only as memories, created first in the collection sensors of the particle accelerator, then in the computer memory, and then finally in our memory. It is ultimately only 3D sensory information that enters into our brains to become fused into a 4D series of thoughts.

The inherent complexity of the universe is so great that we have glimpsed only fleeting shadows of its intricate structure and function. Even within the bounds of special and general relativity, Einstein and others thereafter conceived of black holes, gravitational lenses, and gravitational waves. We can imagine the ride to the limit of the universe, to *c*. In the moment we go from near-*c* to *c*, our mass becomes infinite, our length in the direction of acceleration becomes zero, and the time interval between each tick of our biological processes becomes infinite. In consciousness we can think these things. We may not have a choice in the matter; we may not be able to control our actions or feelings or be able to reach out ahead to guide our destiny. But we can think about it.

13

Beyond Behaviorism and Mentalism: Toward a Framework for Biological Relativity

Biological relativity proposes an emergent threshold model of nature that creates an organizing framework by which to view *within*-reference-system functions and *between*-reference-system functions for the three frames of reference in nature: gravity, life, and consciousness. The gravity frame of reference contains all the actions and reactions of matter and energy, including those of carbon-based molecules, up to the threshold of life. Life contains all the actions and behaviors of cells and cellular systems, including nervous systems, up to the threshold of consciousness. Consciousness contains all the actions and behaviors of humans in thought. Within each four-dimensional (4D) field, any and all combinations of reactions, interactive behaviors, and complex events or processes may be understood, measured, and classified as occurring in the same background system of spatial and temporal limits and constraints. Thus, no phase change, state transition, or collective event marks the emergence of a new level of order, information, or threshold system. Only the changes from nonmatter to matter, from nonlife to life, and from nonconsciousness to consciousness define emergent phenomena that contain novel, internally generated dimensions of space and time.

Any model of inorganic, organic, or nervous system behavior that lacks operational definitions for 4D thresholds of order and information may therefore define virtually any observed behavior that appears unexpectedly or is complicated, collective, nonlinear, chaotic, mystical, magical, or just plain odd as an emergent property. In fact, most of the current discourse on complex brain function and consciousness lacks a coherent approach to an integrated biophysical nature and is nearly devoid of sound operational definitions that can be examined by scientific methods.

Models of thought, mind, and consciousness permeate our daily existence and have a significant effect on our scientific endeavors and our medical treatment of patients. To presuppose insect thought or animal consciousness directly affects how scientists design investigations, interpret behavior, and report findings. To presuppose a force of consciousness or disembodied free will has profound implications for the biomedical theory of brain function and the diagnosis and treatment of illnesses that affect the central nervous system. Moreover, models of thought, mind, and memory significantly influence the basic design and testing of new medications for treatment of virtually all brain disorders. The future course of neuroscience and central nervous system medicine will be guided by the dominant theories of brain function and the relationship of complex neural processes to the larger biophysical world.

Two well-known models bound the spectrum of theories on brain function and consciousness: behaviorism and mentalism. Matson (1973) expressed the differences between these two models as a "without-within" problem, indicating the primary focus of behavioral control that each position postulates.[1] Behaviorism, very simply, formulates the actions of all animals based on the observable stimuli of the context and the reaction patterns of the subjects. It does not entertain theories of mind and consciousness that infer that there are disembodied forces with special qualities. Mentalism, as the other extreme, describes animal behavior in terms of forces that cannot necessarily be quantified, and motivations that cannot necessarily be linked to the biophysical world. We propose that biological relativity encompasses both of these models and provides a set of principles that bind together the critical tenets of each.

Modern behaviorism perhaps began with Konrad Lorenz and Oskar Pfungst. Lorenz, in his much-celebrated role as a surrogate parent to young geese, taught us about the power of early learning (imprinting) of basic associations.[2] He also showed us that the nervous system does not care about the information it receives. It transduces without prejudice the sensory patterns in space and time. The goslings didn't think about whether or not Lorenz was their mother—such contemplations are beyond their referent frame. Pfungst (discussed in Chapter 8) demonstrated the great ability to expose illusion by careful observation of the temporal order of information in the context of behavior.[3] Hans the horse could not count or remember the names of people. The information was already present, and Pfungst demonstrated that Hans was just responding to the context in the only way he could.

The formal examination of the basic rules by which we learn and the things that drive us to behave the way we do became a behavioral science.

The knowledge that we have gained, and continue to gain, by the study of all behavior under the controlled conditions required by the scientific method of illusion reduction has given us amazing insights into the basic mechanisms of learning and memory. The entire lexicon of behavioral science came from the early decades of research by scientists such as Pavlov, Watson, Clark, Hull, Thorndike, and perhaps most notably Skinner.[4] Today, there is no single experimental design produced in any research setting that measures an aspect of animal or human behavior that does not utilize the knowledge of basic behavioral science. Implicitly or explicitly, the principles of classic and instrumental conditioning are embedded in every investigation of the behavior of nervous systems. Skinner, standing on the shoulders of Mendel, Lorenz, Pfungst, and others, gave us the language of operant conditioning and the ability to properly assess the information in the context, manipulate it, and, to a certain degree of reliability, predict the behavioral outcome.[5] Skinner was able to understand the contingencies of reinforcement and to gain insight into the power of a variable rate of reward, and these were monumental achievements. Importantly, these mechanisms apply with a certain degree of reliability to all nervous systems in action, from that of the flatworm to that of the human.

The fundamental theoretical basis of the mentalist approach to learning, memory, education, and the advancement of our knowledge of the human condition is predicated on the existence of an independent force of free will and control.[6] No matter how it is articulated or what level of scientific explanation is applied, in the final analysis, a mental process—a so-called cognitive ability—must include a self-controlled intent, volition, will, or choice. Under the mentalist agenda, the who, what, when, where, and how of the multitudes of hypotheses become the important research issues. And, as we have noted throughout this book, if one starts with a hypothesis of a mysterious force, whether it is gravity, life, or consciousness, it will to some degree determine the design, methods of conduct, data analysis, and conclusions drawn in any scientific or pseudo-scientific effort.

The primary, if not the sole, argument that the mentalist point of view has with the extreme of behaviorism is that the internal processes of the nervous system are ignored when we examine only the external contingencies of reinforcement. And from the behaviorist perspective, it may be argued that the entire wide range of current cognitive theories may be understood as a set of hypotheses that examine the particulars of the internal processing of the contingencies of reinforcement and the neural and special mental transformations that are performed before a behavior is expressed.[7] This represents an important distinction from classic behavioral experimental designs, which are concerned only with the real-time observable chain of events in the external context.

This is the basis of the within-without dichotomy of behaviorism and mentalism. Does the internal world of sensory stimuli and memory function play an incredibly important role in behavior? Of course it does. Does the internal world of sensory stimuli and memory function add such a great amount of complexity, nonlinearity, and quantum chaos that we must invoke a force of free will and control as a guide to our behavior into the future? Not necessarily, and absolutely not as a default hypothesis in the world of careful, systematic, scientific and medical exploration of our existence. Furthermore, the distinctions among who, when, where, what, and how with respect to hypotheses of cognition and free will become glaringly murky in the absence of operational definitions when this default approach is adopted. In life and love, it may not matter. In science and medicine, it may make the difference between knowledge and illusion.

If we strip away the social and political (and, frankly, financial) aspects of the history of this duel of dualism in this country, we may encompass these extremes within the framework of biological relativity. Simply stated, our internal, 4D information space, while it is the source of illusions, is also the source of our freedom, dignity, and humanity. The emergence of thought and its propagation in consciousness as a frame of reference has endowed humankind with the ability to transform the environment and manipulate the forces of nature. We domesticate (genetically engineer) plants and animals. We train dogs to help the blind and chimps to push buttons. We also teach, train, educate, indoctrinate, and manipulate one another. And we do most of this entirely without any notice of, or regard for, concepts of free will or self-control.

Fundamentally, at the level of the neuron and the nervous system across evolutionary time, information is information, disparity computation is disparity computation, and memory is memory. From the hydra to the human, the biophysical mechanisms remain virtually identical. The revolution in understanding this, in applying a scientific methodology to the study of these basic principles, came in the form of behaviorism. Historically, in prescientific times, the process began as soon as human thought emerged on this planet. Manipulating the environment as a result of the three great advantages of the thought effect is a form of behaviorism. Fashioning clothes and weapons and making a fire are all abilities that the internal generation of a temporal dimension brought to us. Crops and pets are genetically engineered mutations of the natural flow of genetic material across generations and are expressions of human control of living behavior. These examples are fundamentally identical to any genetic design and cloning studies conducted in laboratories today and in the future.

Biological relativity draws lines at the thermodynamic boundaries of emergent systems. It acknowledges the limits and constraints of observation and knowledge at the edges of our existence, as do the nonbiological formulations of relativity theory. The inherent difficulties at the limits of our 4D existence, our bouncing off the biophysical walls, the circularity of argument, the breakdown of concept and language will always be with us. The efforts to prove the existence of a force of gravity or of life may have been replaced by the efforts to prove that quantum uncertainty and free will are the same force of nature. In between these mirror images reflected from the two extremes of our thermodynamic barriers, a biological relativity may have utility in organizing our observations as they relate to thinking and nonthinking organic systems. In other words, we may be able to see new patterns of behavior and develop more accurate assessments of brain functions and thus new treatments of brain disorders if we can distinguish between the frames of reference of life and consciousness by detecting the thought process and its effects. If there is a utility in this approach to life and mind, it involves maintaining an awareness of the boundaries of thought and knowledge. In this approach, it is the vision that moves us beyond behaviorism and mentalism—for it is, at the most fundamental level of analysis, all about freedom, dignity, and humanity.

At the foundation of biological relativity is the proposition that an emergent order of existence results from brain activity in humans as they approach the second year of life—the emergent twos. In the hypothetical prefrontal integration module (PIM), we listed the potential sensory representations that may undergo a disparity computation in pre-thought and in emergent thought processes. The simple formulaic expression of the biomathematical transformation of the cumulative information from the external sensory environment, the internal sensory environment, and the memory system was $f(R_a t_n, R'_a t_{n-1}, R''_a t_{n-x})$. Contained within the afferent projections of the 3D sensory representations of $R_a t_n$ are all the patterns of transduced stimulus energies of the external and internal worlds. Their partial representations in the afferent arrays of axons and wavefronts of neural impulses for the immediate past and the more distant past are expressed in $R'_a t_{n-1}$ and $R''_a t_{n-x}$, respectively.

We proposed that, in fact, it is the internal sensory information that sets the tone for and thus creates the basic waves of our emotional experience in consciousness. This effectively drives our thought processes to certain spheres of information in the ongoing interaction with the memory system and in many situations determines complex behavior that is virtually in direct opposition to the immediate external environmental influences. However, as we discussed, there is no choice in the matter. This certainly indicates the relative importance of our internal world of visceral-autonomic sensory experience and the memory system in our behavior. But at the same time, it does not require us defer to the cognitive formulations of free will, intent, and self-control.

The crucial differences in our model, with respect to the extreme behavioralist or mentalist position, come at the threshold between pre-thought and thought—at the emergence of the context-independent, internal 4D information space and its maturation through the Piagetian progression of reiterative, recombinant refinement. At this biophysical threshold, we may find a path between the feared loss of freedom, dignity, and humanity that comes with extreme behavioral theory and the mysterious force of free will and control that is so determinedly demanded, but so doggedly unexplained, by the cognitive theories—a path that avoids bouncing off of our biophysical walls.

In evolution and in human development prior to the emergence of the consciousness frame of reference, each moment of sensory representation processing by the nervous system is a discrete event in background time. In highly developed primates such as chimps and human infants, great amounts of high-resolution sensory information converge in the prefrontal modular regions at each flux of afferent synaptic zone activity, sending waves of unimaginably complex patterns of biochemical and bioelectrical energies through the most complicated and interconnected arrangements of organic tissues in the known universe. Indeed, it is a dance that makes the single intracellular waltz look like a drunken stagger.

But for all its intricate informational integrity, each computational transformation in pre-thought contains only the temporal dimension set by the background neural activity. Each moment in pre-thought time is an extension of the life field of biological existence. Each association made, each behavior learned, each refinement of action between the genetically determined homeostasis-maintaining biases of positive and negative, approach and avoidance, is linked in time to the pulse of neural activity. These pre-thought constraining parameters set the limits to what can be learned, how long and complicated a sequence of behavior can be entered into the memory system, and in what contexts these learned association patterns can be expressed in future behavior.

From our position in consciousness, we have manipulated the world in one basic fundamental manner. We have imposed our internal temporal dimension of existence—our thoughts in propagation across time—onto every system of nature with which we come into contact. We arrange the order of information in the external world that leads, determines, and predicts the outcomes of behavior in nonliving systems such as rivers, molecules and atoms, and in all living systems. We supply the temporal order of information for our pets and infants whenever we train, teach, or guide their learning and subsequent behavior. We stack the deck of information; we manipulate the contingencies of reinforcement in the exact manner in which Skinner understood nature to work. We do not necessarily induce hunger in our pets or babies to promote learning, but when they are hungry, we certainly take advantage of it, knowingly or not, to reinforce certain behaviors and to create the associations that will lead to new ones. We most definitely manipulate the affection that our babies and young infants have for us in order to guide their learning and thus produce new behaviors that we want. We mostly do this out of love and to great mutual benefit, but unfortunately the world is full of examples of those who do this with ill intent, with tragic outcomes.

When the human infant crosses the threshold to consciousness, she forever leaves behind the nearly equal chimp. The thermodynamic disconnect between the temporal dimensions of background neural activity and the fusion of sensory representation in the prefrontal modules endow the child with the power of thought and its effects. The simple example of toilet training underscores this emergent order of existence for any parent who has watched the transition between chained sequences of near misses and infrequent hits to the revelation moment (the celebration day) when the child appears to have known this all along! It is also with the emergence of an internal, context-independent 4D representation of the world that the child may begin to express opposition to the real-time contingencies of reinforcement, dashing all attempts to train him or her to obey or to do something new.

In thought, the development of the internal 4D information space brings flexibility to behavior that is unseen in nature. At any moment in time, in any setting in space, the integration of the three informational components of each thought may produce a behavior that does not appear to follow the current conditions in the local environment. As a child experiences and learns, the internal 4D information space matures in terms of the breadth and depth of its behavioral options and its biases. A new point along an S-curve of reaction or behavior is created for each of a nearly infinite number of patterns of sensory representation of the internal world (the visceral-autonomic state) in combination with the ever-growing number of patterns of external sensory representation placed in memory through thought. A nearly infinite number of S-curves come into existence that define individual continuums of positive-negative, like-dislike, good-bad, and so on for almost any combination of external and internal sensory representations that have been created in the reiterative, recombinant refinement process leading to the maturation of 4D information space. At virtually any moment in time, in any situation, a sensory representation from memory, and thus a behavioral sequence of prior learning, may be expressed that appears to be completely at odds with the demands of the environment.

This is the illusion of free will, choice, opposition, and control. However—and this is the crucial point—in the maturation of the 4D information space, the near-infinite refinement of points along the S-curves of bias and behavior brings the complexity of the behavioral expression of the individual to a level that cannot be easily manipulated, controlled, or predicted by an observer in another referent system (e.g., a parent). When our ability to control a child's behavior by manipulating the contingencies of reinforcement fades (e.g., when we can no longer get the child to do exactly what we want by offering the typical rewards), this marks the point in that child's internal 4D experience at which a level of complexity has virtually removed the child from the strict control of the real-time external environment. And, for better or worse, that includes the influences of parents, teachers, and other interested parties. The child is said to be developing a mind of her own.

In thought, each of the trio of afferent sensory representations that we may express as external, internal, and memory—or more commonly as sensation, emotion, and memory—creates a stream of 4D internal reality. The developing subtleties of this reality produce the illusion of free will, volition, and choice. They also create an internal world of intricate proportions that may not be understood by any means available in a real-time analysis or attempted manipulation. This is the unique, individual, subjective experience of each and every person as he or she matures in thought and consciousness. At a level of biophysical reality, the history and real-time shape of the information space determine each moment as it is integrated from this trio of sources. At the level of human interaction, in our experience of serial time, divided into ≈ 200-ms intervals, we observe only a freely behaving individual for whom we cannot always predict what will happen next. The behavior that we begin to observe in 2-year-old children, the opposition to outside attempts to control them, is only the precursor of things to come.

Each person opposes attempts by outside forces to guide his behavior to a degree set by such individual factors as genetically inherited bias patterns for homeostatic parameters, developmental patterns of growth and maturation, effects of illness and trauma, abilities of learning and memory, and subjective experience in time. When the memory component of a series of thoughts creates a mismatch between sensory representation and the current external environment, when some individual, subjective homeostatic subtlety associated with external information is challenged by real-time contingencies of reinforcement, a behavior of opposition, shutdown, revolt, or revolution may occur. In other words, when we feel that something isn't quite right with what's happening around us, we stop, pause, disagree, oppose, flee, or sometimes fight. At the original level of basic neural operations, this is a homeostatic reaction, albeit the most complex one in the known universe.

This is the path between behaviorism and mentalism. Simply stated, there is always one more point that can be added along any one of our individual, subjective S-curves. When sensation, emotion, and memory meet in human thought, the disparity computation of the 4D coordinates of the information sequences may produce a mismatch. This is new learning, new experience, and it may result in behavior that is new, unexpected (to an outside observer), and in direct opposition to any planned learning or indoctrination that may have been working to impose a temporal order on the information in the background external context. This is an operational definition of freedom, dignity, and humanity that may reflect a closer approximation of the true nature of behavior, without resorting to a reliance on unseen forces or overly simplified stimulus-response formulations.

In the model of biological relativity, we do not have to impose a mystical force of free will or control to appreciate the unique individual reaction to any situation. The thought function in the consciousness frame of reference provides humans with the unique ability to refine context-independent behavior to a degree that separates each individual in so many ways that it is impossible to find any two people who will always react identically in all situations. This is the relativistic effect in the consciousness field of human behavior. The 4D experience, the information patterns that flow through propagated thought, is unique to the individual and must be different from that for any other individual. In pre-thought, behavior may be more easily manipulated and controlled, although this can become quite difficult as fully and consistently determining an adequate shape of the information space in time can consume great amounts of time and energy. Therefore, in the application of our model, we can at once acknowledge the absolute biophysical limits, constraints, and illusions of our 4D existence and the absolutely unique, subjective, individual experience at each moment of time. No free will and control does not equate with loss of freedom, dignity, and humanity.

It is our unique, internal 4D experience, as it matures in time, that defines our freedom, dignity, and humanity. For some, the realization that each individual's experience and knowledge defines the freedom of our behavior and our sense of choice provides a greater feeling of liberation and humanity than does the proposition that we and all other animals (and perhaps inorganic matter) generate a force of will that leads us into the future—irrespective of what we know or what we learn. If the model of biological relativity has merit, then the processes of reiterative, recombinant refinement of our internal 4D information space ensure that we will continue to be in opposition, to revolt, to create revolution—and thus to be creative. We will always find a way to be free of disharmonious control and maintain a dignity of individuality. We will always be human.

We have come full circle, back to the ideas expressed in the introduction. The utility of providing a set of organizing principles that relates behavior to neural function and draws lines at thresholds for emergent systems comes from the fact that theories about thought, mind, and consciousness pervade our everyday existence in science and medicine. Mostly, they are implicit in the manner in which experiments are designed and conducted. The science and medicine of human brain function have been in a state of atheoretical free fall that has led to a myriad of approaches to the diagnosis and treatment of a wide range of illnesses that affect thought, mood, and memory. When there are no boundaries for the definitions of thought, mind, and consciousness, then virtually any approach to the diagnosis and treatment of disorders of these entities can be adopted. Perhaps this helps to explain the several hundred forms of psychotherapy being practiced today. We need a basic framework for our daily thinking about illnesses of the human central nervous system that will have real utility in the development of better assessment instruments and treatment medications. Neuroscience and central nervous system medicine are among the youngest of scientific and medical fields, and we should keep our eyes open as we enter into what is certain to be a future involving a quantitative approach to thought and mind.

We must also remain aware of important factors that create a resistance to the scientific approach to behavior. In part, the fear of control and of the loss of free will drives some of the mentalistic or cognitive thinking. It reflects a search for the security of private absolutes that defy the limits and constraints of our universe. The progression of science is indeed only a reflection of the current social context. It can be no other way. As we continue to walk into a future that brings together digital speed and biological determinism, the resistance will mount, the fear will increase, and more eyes will close. Humanity, collectively, cycles through periods of great expectation and wonderment at its own scientific revelations and the subsequent technological applications, into moments of mysticism and resentment of the control and perceived loss of freedom and dignity that these things also appear to bring. This is the pendulum of opinion, the waves of emotion across generational time. In our fleeting moment of existence, as we enter into more exacting control of biological processes and a deeper understanding of their deterministic realities, the questions of control, judgment, and ethics come to the fore, and the specter of eugenics is revived as quickly as any deep tendon reflex.

The typical question is posed as follows: "If we are able to control thought and understand brain function to an exacting degree, along with our rapidly advancing knowledge of genetics, would not we begin to decide who is eligible to live and who is not good enough?" The model presented here stands in strong, direct opposition to this argument. Most simply, we must maintain the highest degree of variation possible in order to generate novel thoughts. Variation of information, whether we call it good or bad, healthy or unhealthy, is the fuel of thought. And we must always remain aware of the relative nature of information, in that what we call desirable today may become the very opposite tomorrow. Variation of experience determines the range and scope of each of our thoughts, and thus determines all we can think and all our actions. If we did not have a certain number of experiences in life that are unpleasant, difficult, unhappy, or even harrowing, we would lose the ability to adequately respond to crisis situations. Any aspect of biology—human or nonhuman, plant or animal—may be a vital source of information that will create a novel answer to a problem in health, art, music, or technology that needs a solution. We cannot know which of life's offerings are the ones that we will need to help us though the generations. Diversity in biology is paramount for our survival and growth.

Biological relativity indicates how our study of an illness may lead to a cure, through the reiterative, recombinant cycle of thought and thought-memory. This biological engine of knowledge takes information and time. We cannot know *a priori* what information it requires, or how long it will take. To think that we know what the future needs of an entire species would be an extreme illusion that some may create in thought; it is an error of temporal flow and knowledge development. We must learn from Einstein and Piaget about the time that is required for insight. We must learn from Pavlov, Lorenz, and Skinner about not being sheep. Anyone who says that he or she can tell us which individuals, plants, or animals are not needed in our joint venture into the future is speaking in gross illusion.

We will always be forced to make hard decisions about life and health in certain instances. Decisions about the quality of life and the right to death will continue to change in time and across different local cultures. That is the way it has always been. We will always draw some lines concerning terminal illness and chronically debilitating states, and these should always be hard decisions. We must always take the true scientific stance that we do not know the answers *a priori*. We must always take the true scientific path to understanding the rich depth of nature at its most infinitesimal organization and at its most complex systems of thought function.

Anyone who defines the word *reductionism* with a negative connotation does not understand the real danger. It has always been in those times when we feel comfortable with our current knowledge that we get into trouble. When we think we know enough, we tend to make decisions based on inadequate information, and this includes the horror of past cultural decisions about who is adequate and who is disposable. It is when we hear that the study of nature at its most difficult levels of organization is just a reductionistic exercise that we must become alarmed and concerned about such things as eugenics. It is when we hear that we have enough information about life and nature and thought and behavior, and that no further investigation or information gathering is necessary, that we must be truly on the alert. The rejection of knowledge and information marks the end of new experiences that may improve our chances of continued survival and growth.

The continued saga of the depth and beauty of nature that comes from our inquisitive minds has no equal. The story is not lacking in any human quality or emotion. Natural reductionism is the process of thought refinement; it is the engine by which we learn, understand, and explore. The process of discovery in our human search is an unfolding, an opening, an unveiling of nature's full majesty. The only negative reductionism is the call to reduce our information to what we have right now, and add no more. The true scientific adventure is one of constant questioning of our own knowledge: whether we are doing the right thing, in the right manner, and drawing the right conclusions. If we continue to employ the formal methods of scientific conduct that have been with us for the last several hundred years, we will never conclude that we have enough information to decide what the perfect world will look and feel like, and who and what should populate it. We must be wary only of those who claim to have *a priori* information that they did not work to obtain, did not take the time to understand or test, and have simply accepted as ultimate truth.

Jacob Bronowski, the renowned physicist and mathematician, made a profound comment on these issues in what was perhaps the single most compelling, thoughtful, and heartrending moment that modern television has produced with respect to science and humanity. Dr. Bronowski stood in a pool of mud, placed his fingers in it, and said with great personal eloquence,

> *It is said that science will dehumanize people and turn them into numbers. That is false, tragically false. Look for yourself. This is the concentration camp and crematorium at Auschwitz. This is where people were turned into numbers. Into this pond were flushed the ashes of some four million people. And that was not done by gas. It was done by arrogance. It was done by dogma. It was done by ignorance. When people believe that they have absolute knowledge, with no test in reality, this is how they behave. This is what men do when they aspire to the knowledge of gods. Science is a very human form of knowledge. We are always at the brink of the known, we always feel forward for what is to be hoped. Every judgement in science stands on the edge of error, and is personal. Science is a tribute to what we can know although we are fallible. . . . I owe it as a scientist to my friend Leo Szilard, I owe it as a human being to the many members of my family who died at Auschwitz, to stand here by the pond as a survivor and a witness.*[8]

We feel that the model presented in this book, the lines drawn, and the conclusions posed are in complete agreement with the spirit of Bronowski's remarks. What biological relativity says is that we—the only animals that can think about life—cannot know anything beyond our limited moments in time. We may have great insightful vision of Einsteinian proportion, but such constructs in our own personal information space must be tested, examined, and shared with others to ensure that they are not illusions, no matter how simple and benign, or potentially world-shattering.

We do this testing from the moment we step across the threshold to thought. We reinvent the entire universe and our place in it. Each individual does this. No individual or group has an ultimate source of knowledge or truth. There is not one person who did not discover in his or her unique development the differences between up and down, light and sound, three dimensions and four dimensions, and right and wrong. There is not one person who has not had to go through the thought and thought-memory cycles that each of us must experience in order to build an information store upon which our words and actions are wholly based. It takes time and information to mature this information space, and there are strict limits to the operating parameters. No one can get around them. If someone studies a narrow area of life or nature for 50 years, she or he has a certain amount of information about that subject. No one who has studied it for ten minutes or one hour can have the same information, knowledge, or insight, unless the 50 years are reduced to symbolic language and expressed in the form of a lecture or a book. Even then, certain important aspects of the long learning process are lost.

We must strive to keep and revere the diverse life around us so that we and all life may benefit from our experiences in a rich world of plants, animals, and people. It is our solemn responsibility as the only ones who can place our fingers in a mud pond and understand the meaning of that act—as a young girl discovering math, writing, and the letter *I* as something that represents her self, or as a great scientist and man feeling and knowing the tragedy and the unspeakable horror that the claim of ultimate truth and knowledge may bring to humanity. Perhaps it is the same pond, at different times in our history of illusions and truths.

The history of the world contains many stories of good and evil men and women who shaped their times. In the century just past, we have had the singular fortune of being graced by the presence of a man whom many consider to be the personification of dignity and humanity. He is nearly as renowned and respected for his radical positions on the freedom of thought and the fight against all forms of absolute truth as he is for his science. Albert Einstein showed us in his writings and in his deeds that to understand our limitations, constraints, and illusions in no way leads to a loss of our humanity. It may be just the opposite. He once wrote,

> *A human being is a part of the whole, called by us "Universe," a part limited in space and time. He experiences himself, his thoughts and feelings, as something separated from the rest—a kind of optical delusion of his consciousness. This delusion is a kind of prison for us, restricting us to our personal desires and to affection for a few persons nearest to us. Our task must be to free ourselves from this prison by widening our circle of compassion to embrace all living creatures and the whole nature in its beauty. Nobody is able to achieve this completely, but the striving for such achievement is in itself a part of the liberation and a foundation for inner security.*[9]

A humanistic reverence for life is embodied within the biological relativity point of view. Perhaps the best we can do in our personal, unique thoughts is to associate our richest emotions of love with perceptions of the beauty that nature provides, remembered as moments in which we sense the truth of existence.

Notes

Introduction Toward a Framework for Consciousness

1. A. Einstein, E. P. Adams, and E. G. Straus, *The Meaning of Relativity*, Princeton University Press, Princeton, N.J.,1945.
2. E. Muybridge, *Muybridge's Complete Human and Animal Locomotion: All 781 Plates from the 1887 Animal Locomotion*, Dover Publications, New York, 1979.
3. L. K. Barnett, *The Universe and Dr. Einstein*, W. Sloane Associates, New York, 1957.

Chapter 1 Einstein's Vision of the Universe I

1. A. Einstein and R. W. Lawson, *Relativity: The Special and General Theory*, H. Holt and Company, New York, 1920.
2. I. Newton, I. B. Cohen, and A. M. Whitman, *The Principia: Mathematical Principles of Natural Philosophy*, University of California Press, Berkeley, 1999; H. Poincaré, *Science and Hypothesis*, Dover Publications, New York, 1952; G. F. Wheeler and L. D. Kirkpatrick, *Physics: Building a World View*, Prentice-Hall, Englewood Cliffs, N.J., 1983; G. L. Naber, *The Geometry of Minkowski Spacetime: An Introduction to the Mathematics of the Special Theory of Relativity*, Springer-Verlag, New York, 1992.
3. M. Born, *Einstein's Theory of Relativity*, Dover Publications, New York, 1962, pp. 1, 2.
4. A. Einstein and L. Infeld, *The Evolution of Physics, from Early Concepts to Relativity and Quanta*, Simon and Schuster, New York, 1938, p. 198.
5. Born, *Einstein's Theory of Relativity*, p. 5.
6. Einstein and Infeld, *The Evolution of Physics*, p. 207.
7. Ibid.
8. L. K. Barnett, *The Universe and Dr. Einstein*, W. Sloane Associates, New York, 1957, p. 117.

Chapter 2 Evolution and the Emergence of Life

1. A. G. Cairns-Smith, *Seven Clues to the Origin of Life: A Scientific Detective Story*, Cambridge University Press, Cambridge and New York, 1990; J. A. V. Butler, *The Life of the Cell: Its Nature, Origin, and Development*, Basic Books, New York, 1964; S. W. Fox, *The Emergence of Life: Darwinian Evolution from the Inside*, Basic Books, New York, 1988; M. Eigen and R. Winkler, *Steps towards Life: A Perspective on Evolution*, Oxford University Press, Oxford and New York, 1992; J. H. Postlethwait and J. L. Hopson, *The Nature of Life*, McGraw-Hill, New York, 1995; S. Bengtson, *Early Life on Earth*, Columbia University Press, New York, 1994.
2. E. Schrödinger, *What Is Life? and Other Scientific Essays*, Doubleday, Garden City, N.Y., 1956; A. I. Oparin, *Life, Its Nature, Origin and Development*, Academic Press, New York, 1961; J. Brooks and G. Shaw, *Origin and Development of Living Systems*, Academic Press, London and New York, 1973; B.-O. Küppers, *Information and the Origin of Life*, MIT Press, Cambridge, Mass., 1990; R. Rosen, *Life Itself: A Comprehensive Inquiry into the Nature, Origin, and Fabrication of Life*, Columbia University Press, New York, 1991; M. P. Murphy and L. A. J. O'Neill, *What Is Life? The Next Fifty Years: Speculations on the Future of Biology*, Cambridge University Press, Cambridge and New York, 1995; N. Lahav, *Biogenesis: Theories of Life's Origin*, Oxford University Press, New York, 1999; F. Crick, *Life Itself: Its Origin and Nature*, Simon and Schuster, New York, 1981.
3. International Society for the Study of the Origin of Life, *Origins of Life and Evolution of the Biosphere: The Journal of the International Society for the Study of the Origin of Life*, Reidel, Dordrecht and Boston, 1984; A. G. Cairns-Smith and H. Hartman, *Clay Minerals and the Origin of Life*, Cambridge University Press, Cambridge and New York, 1986; D. L. Rohlfing, A. I. Oparin, and S. W. Fox, *Molecular Evolution: Prebiological and Biological*, Plenum Press, New York, 1972; A. I. Oparin, *The Chemical Origin of Life*, Charles C Thomas, Springfield, Ill., 1964.
4. J. W. Gibbs, *Scientific Papers*, Dover Publications, New York, 1961; L. P. Wheeler, *Josiah Willard Gibbs: The History of a Great Mind*, Ox Bow Press, Woodbridge, Conn., 1998.
5. M. Goldman, *The Demon in the Aether: The Story of James Clerk Maxwell*, P. Harris, A. Hilger, Edinburgh and Bristol, 1983; J. C. Maxwell, E. Garber, S. G. Brush, and C. W. F. Everitt, *Maxwell on Molecules and Gases*, MIT Press, Cambridge, Mass., 1986.
6. R. M. Gray, *Entropy and Information Theory*, Springer-Verlag, New York, 1990; B. H. Weber, D. J. Depew, J. D. Smith, and California State University Fullerton, School of Natural Science and Mathematics, *Entropy, Information, and Evolution: New Perspectives on Physical and Biological Evolution*, MIT Press, Cambridge, Mass., 1988; S. A. Kauffman, *The Origins of Order: Self-organization and Selection in Evolution*, Oxford University Press, New York, 1993; R. F. Fox, *Energy and the Evolution of Life*, W. H. Freeman, New York, 1988.
7. B. Kursunoglu, A. Perlmutter, L. F. Scott, and University of Miami Center for Theoretical Studies, *The Significance of Nonlinearity in the Natural Sciences: Proceedings*, Plenum Press, New York, 1977; D. Jou and J. E. Llebot, *Introduction*

to the *Thermodynamics of Biological Processes*, Prentice-Hall, Englewood Cliffs, N.J., 1990; Kauffman, *The Origins of Order*; H. M. Pinsker, W. D. Willis, and University of Texas Medical Branch at Galveston, Department of Physiology and Biophysics, *Information Processing in the Nervous System*, Raven Press, New York, 1980; T. F. Weiss, *Cellular Biophysics*, MIT Press, Cambridge, Mass., 1996.

8. Oparin, *The Chemical Origin of Life*; S. L. Miller, H. C. Urey, and J. Oro, *J Mol Evol* 9:59–72, 1976.
9. S. L. Miller and L. E. Orgel, *The Origins of Life on the Earth*, Prentice-Hall, Englewood Cliffs, N.J., 1974.
10. *Early Life on Earth*, Columbia University Press, New York, 1994; Cairns-Smith, *Seven Clues to the Origin of Life.*
11. Cairns-Smith and Hartman, *Clay Minerals and the Origin of Life.*
12. Fox, *The Emergence of Life.*
13. L. E. Orgel, *J Theor Biol* 123:127–149, 1986; L. E. Orgel, *Trends Biochem Sci* 23:491–495, 1998.
14. *Early Life on Earth*; J. Maddox, *Nature*, 371:101, 1994.

Chapter 3 The Reference System of Life

1. L. K. Barnett, *The Universe and Dr. Einstein*, W. Sloane Associates, New York, 1957.

Chapter 4 Development and Systems of Neurons

1. M. Jacobson, *Foundations of Neuroscience*, Plenum Press, New York, 1993; R. S. Creed, D. Denny-Brown, J. C. Eccles, E. G. T. Liddell, and C. S. Sherrington, *Reflex Activity of the Spinal Cord*, Clarendon Press, Oxford, 1932; B. Katz, *Nerve, Muscle, and Synapse*, McGraw-Hill, New York, 1966; C. S. Sherrington, *The Brain and Its Mechanism*, Cambridge University Press, Cambridge, 1933; S. Ramón y Cajal, J. DeFelipe, and E. G. Jones, *Cajal on the Cerebral Cortex: An Annotated Translation of the Complete Writings*, Oxford University Press, New York, 1988.
2. E. Neher, B. Sakmann, and J. H. Steinbach, *Pflugers Arch* 375:219–228, 1978; D. J. Nelson and F. Sachs, *Nature* 282:861–863, 1979; F. J. Sigworth and E. Neher, *Nature* 287:447–449, 1980.
3. J. R. Cooper and F. E. Bloom, *The Biochemical Basis of Neuropharmacology*, Oxford University Press, New York, 1996; I. Törk, D. J. Tracey, G. Paxinos, and J. Stone, *Neurotransmitters in the Human Brain*, Plenum Press, New York, 1995; C. A. Sandman and New York Academy of Sciences, *Neuropeptides: Structure and Function in Biology and Behavior*, New York Academy of Sciences, New York, 1999; L. L. Iversen, S. D. Iversen, and S. H. Snyder, *Neuropeptides*, Plenum Press, New York, 1983.
4. E. R. Kandel, J. H. Schwartz, and T. M. Jessell, *Principles of Neural Science*, McGraw-Hill, New York, 2000; L. Deecke, J. C. Eccles, V. B. Mountcastle, and H. H. Kornhuber, *From Neuron to Action: An Appraisal of Fundamental and Clinical Research*, Springer-Verlag, Berlin and New York, 1990; P. S. Churchland and T. J. Sejnowski, *The Computational Brain*, MIT Press, Cambridge, Mass., 1992; W. J. Freeman, *Mass Action in the Nervous System: Examination of the*

Neurophysiological Basis of Adaptive Behavior through the EEG, Academic Press, New York, 1975; F. Rieke, *Spikes: Exploring the Neural Code*, MIT Press, Cambridge, Mass., 1997; C. Koch and J. L. Davis, *Large-Scale Neuronal Theories of the Brain*, MIT Press, Cambridge, Mass., 1994.

5. D. R. Brooks and E. O. Wiley, *Evolution as Entropy: Toward a Unified Theory of Biology*, University of Chicago Press, Chicago, 1988; R. Baddeley, P. J. B. Hancock, and P. Földiák, *Information Theory and the Brain*, Cambridge University Press, Cambridge and New York, 2000; R. U. Ayres, *Information, Entropy, and Progress*, AIP Press, New York, 1994.
6. C. E. Shannon and W. Weaver, *The Mathematical Theory of Communication*, University of Illinois Press, Urbana, 1949; N. Wiener, *Cybernetics: Control and Communications in the Animal and the Machine*, John Wiley & Sons, New York, 1948.
7. W. S. McCulloch and W. H. Pitts, *Bull Math Biophys* 5:115–113, 1943; J. Mira, W. S. McCulloch, and R. Moreno-Díaz, *Brain Processes, Theories, and Models: An International Conference in Honor of W. S. McCulloch 25 Years after His Death*, MIT Press, Cambridge, Mass., 1996; A. M. Turing, "Computing Machinery and Intelligence," *Mind* 49:433–460, 1950; A. M. Turing, P. J. R. Millican, and A. Clark, *The Legacy of Alan Turing*, Clarendon Press, Oxford University Press, Oxford and New York, 1996; J. Von Neumann, *The Computer and the Brain*, Yale University Press, New Haven, 1958.
8. M. Newborn, *Kasparov versus Deep Blue: Computer Chess Comes of Age*, Springer, New York, 1997.
9. L. N. Cooper, *How We Learn, How We Remember: Toward an Understanding of Brain and Neural Systems: Selected Papers of Leon N. Cooper*, World Scientific, Singapore and River Edge, N.J., 1995; Koch and Davis, *Large-Scale Neuronal Theories of the Brain*; Churchland and Sejnowski, *The Computational Brain*; G. M. Edelman, V. B. Mountcastle, and Neurosciences Research Program, *The Mindful Brain: Cortical Organization and the Group-Selective Theory of Higher Brain Function*, MIT Press, Cambridge, Mass., 1978; T. Kohonen, *Associative Memory: A System-Theoretical Approach*, Springer-Verlag, Berlin and New York, 1977.

Chapter 5 The Brain and Sensory Information

1. P. Rakic, *Brain Res* 33:471–476, 1971; R. L. Sidman and P. Rakic, *Brain Res* 62:1–35, 1973.
2. Lorente de No, "The Structure of the Cerebral Cortex," in J. F. Fulton (ed.), *Physiology of the Nervous System*, Oxford University Press, Oxford and New York, 1949.
3. V. B. Mountcastle, *J Neurophysiol* 20:408–434, 1957; V. B. Mountcastle, *Medical Physiology*, C. V. Mosby Co., St. Louis, 1974.
4. D. H. Hubel, *Eye, Brain, and Vision*, Scientific American Library, distributed by W. H. Freeman, New York, 1988.
5. M. A. Arbib, P. Érdi, and J. Szentágothai, *Neural Organization: Structure, Function, and Dynamics*, MIT Press, Cambridge, Mass., 1998; J. Szentágothai, *Brain Res* 95:475–496, 1975.

6. S. W. Kuffler, J. G. Nicholls, and A. R. Martin, *From Neuron to Brain: A Cellular Approach to the Function of the Nervous System*, Sinauer Associates, Sunderland, Mass., 1984; D. H. Hubel and T. N. Wiesel, *Nature* 221:747–750, 1969; D. H. Hubel and T. N. Wiesel, *Sci Am* 241:150–162, 1979; D. H. Hubel and T. N. Wiesel, *Neuron* 20:401–412, 1998.
7. W. Penfield and T. Rasmussen, *The Cerebral Cortex of Man: A Clinical Study of Localization of Function*, Macmillan, New York, 1950; W. Penfield and H. H. Jasper, *Epilepsy and the Functional Anatomy of the Human Brain*, Little, Brown, Boston, 1954.
8. E. G. Jones and T. P. Powell, *Brain* 93:793–820, 1970.
9. D. H. Hubel and T. N. Wiesel, *Nature* 225:41–42, 1970; Hubel, *Eye, Brain, and Vision*; I. P. Howard and B. J. Rogers, *Binocular Vision and Stereopsis*, Oxford University Press, New York, 1995.
10. Hubel, *Eye, Brain, and Vision*.
11. B. Julesz, *Foundations of Cyclopean Perception*, University of Chicago Press, Chicago, 1971; D. Marr and T. Poggio, *Science* 194:283–287, 1976; D. Marr, *Vision: A Computational Investigation into the Human Representation and Processing of Visual Information*, W. H. Freeman, San Francisco, 1982; J. A. Anderson, E. Rosenfeld, and A. Pellionisz, *Neurocomputing*, MIT Press, Cambridge, Mass., 1988; T. Poggio, V. Torre, and C. Koch, *Nature* 317:314–319, 1985; S. Zeki, *A Vision of the Brain*, Blackwell Scientific Publications, Oxford and Boston, 1993.
12. D. Brewster, C. Wheatstone, N. Wade, and Experimental Psychology Society, *Brewster and Wheatstone on Vision*, Academic Press, London and New York, 1983.
13. C. Blakemore and B. Julesz, *Science* 171:286–288, 1971.
14. Penfield and Rasmussen, *The Cerebral Cortex of Man*.
15. G. A. Ojemann, *Neuropsychologia* 12:1–10, 1974; G. Ojemann and C. Mateer, *Science* 205:1401–1403, 1979; W. H. Calvin and G. Ojemann, *Inside the Brain: Mapping the Cortex, Exploring the Neuron*, New American Library, New York, 1980; I. Fried, C. Mateer, G. Ojemann, R. Wohns, and P. Fedio, *Brain* 105:349–371, 1982; G. Ojemann, *Adv Neurol* 57:361–368, 1992.
16. A. W. Toga and J. C. Mazziotta, *Brain Mapping: The Methods*, Academic Press, San Diego, 1996; M. I. Posner and M. E. Raichle, *Images of Mind*, Scientific American Library, New York, 1994; J. R. Binder, S. M. Rao, T. A. Hammeke, F. Z. Yetkin, A. Jesmanowicz, P. A. Bandettini, E. C. Wong, L. D. Estkowski, M. D. Goldstein, V. M. Haughton, et al., *Ann Neurol* 35:662–672., 1994; P. T. Fox, R. J. Ingham, J. C. Ingham, F. Zamarripa, J. H. Xiong, and J. L. Lancaster, *Brain* 123:1985–2004, 2000.
17. G. W. Van Hoesen, D. N. Pandya, and N. Butters, *Science* 175:1471–1473, 1972; D. L. Rosene and G. W. Van Hoesen, *Science* 198:315–317, 1977; G. W. Van Hoesen, *Ann N Y Acad Sci* 444:97–112, 1985; A. Solodkin and G. W. Van Hoesen, *J Comp Neurol* 365:610–617, 1996.
18. J. W. Papez, *J Neuropsychiatry Clin Neurosci* 7:103–112, 1995.
19. P. Gloor, *The Temporal Lobe and Limbic System*, Oxford University Press, New York, 1997.

20. P. Glees and H. B. Griffith, *Monastschr Psychiat Neurol* 123:193–204, 1952.
21. W. B. Scoville and B. Milner, *J Neurol Neurosurg Psychiatry* 20:11–21, 1957.
22. B. Milner, *Clin Neurosurg* 19:421–446, 1972; B. Milner, S. Corkin, and H.-L. Teuber, *Neuropsychologia* 6:215–234, 1968.
23. N. J. Cohen and L. R. Squire, *Science* 210:207–210, 1980; S. Zola-Morgan, N. J. Cohen, and L. R. Squire, *Neuropsychologia* 21:487–500, 1983; L. R. Squire, *Memory and Brain*, Oxford University Press, New York, 1987; L. R. Squire and N. Butters, *Neuropsychology of Memory*, Guilford Press, New York, 1992.
24. J. O'Keefe and J. Dostrovsky, *Brain Res* 34:171–175, 1971.
25. J. O'Keefe and L. Nadel, *The Hippocampus as a Cognitive Map*, Clarendon Press, Oxford University Press, Oxford and New York, 1978.
26. E. C. Tolman, *Purposive Behaviour in Animals and Men*, Century, New York, 1932; E. C. Tolman, *Psychol Rev* 55:189–208, 1948.
27. D. S. Olton, *Sci Am* 236:82–84, 89–94, 96, 98, 1977; D. S. Olton, J. A. Walker, and F. H. Gage, *Brain Res* 139:295–308, 1978.
28. R. M. Pico and J. L. Davis, *Behav Neural Biol* 40:5–26, 1984; R. M. Pico, L. K. Gerbrandt, M. Pondel, and G. Ivy, *Brain Res* 330:369–372, 1985.

Chapter 6 The Emergence of Consciousness

1. P. S. Goldman, H. E. Rosvold, and M. Mishkin, *Exp Neurol* 29:221–226, 1970; W. J. Nauta and M. Feirtag, *Sci Am* 241:88–111, 1979; M. Mishkin, *Philos Trans R Soc Lond B Biol Sci* 298: 83–95, 1982; D. T. Stuss and D. F. Benson, *The Frontal Lobes*, Raven Press, New York, 1986; H. S. Levin, H. M. Eisenberg, and A. L. Benton, *Frontal Lobe Function and Dysfunction*, Oxford University Press, New York, 1991; R. E. Passingham, *The Frontal Lobes and Voluntary Action*, Oxford University Press, Oxford and New York, 1993; J. C. Eccles, *Evolution of the Brain: Creation of the Self*, Routledge, London and New York, 1995; J. M. Fuster, *The Prefrontal Cortex: Anatomy, Physiology, and Neuropsychology of the Frontal Lobe*, Lippincott-Raven, Philadelphia, 1997; N. A. Krasnegor, G. R. Lyon, and P. S. Goldman-Rakic, *Development of the Prefrontal Cortex: Evolution, Neurobiology, and Behavior*, P. H. Brookes Pub. Co., Baltimore, 1997.
2. Fuster, *The Prefrontal Cortex.*
3. P. S. Goldman-Rakic and M. L. Schwartz, *Science* 216:755–757, 1982.
4. K. H. Pribram and A. R. Luria, *Psychophysiology of the Frontal Lobes*, Academic Press, New York, 1973; P. S. Goldman-Rakic, *Neuron* 14:477–485, 1995; Fuster, *The Prefrontal Cortex.*
5. J. M. Fuster and G. E. Alexander, *Science* 173:652–654, 1971.
6. Fuster, *The Prefrontal Cortex.*
7. R. B. Goldberg, J. M. Fuster, and R. Alvarez-Pelaez, *Physiol Behav* 25:425–432, 1980.

Chapter 7 The Thought Effect

1. D. O. Hebb, *The Organization of Behavior: A Neuropsychological Theory*, John Wiley & Sons, New York, 1949.

2. D. O. Hebb, *Essay on Mind*, L. Erlbaum Associates, Hillsdale, N.J., 1980; L. R. Squire and E. R. Kandel, *Memory: From Mind to Molecules*, Scientific American Library, distributed by W. H. Freeman and Co., New York, 1999; A. D. Baddeley, *Essentials of Human Memory*, Psychology Press, Hove, England, 1999; E. R. Kandel, J. H. Schwartz, and T. M. Jessell, *Principles of Neural Science*, McGraw-Hill, New York, 2000; H. Eichenbaum and N. J. Cohen, *From Conditioning to Conscious Recollection: Memory Systems of the Brain*, Oxford University Press, Upper Saddle River, N.J., 2000; E. Tulving and F. I. M. Craik, *The Oxford Handbook of Memory*, Oxford University Press, Oxford and New York, 2000.
3. D. P. Todes, *Ivan Pavlov: Exploring the Animal Machine*, Oxford University Press, New York, 2000.

Chapter 8 Insect Thoughts and Animal Minds

1. O. Pfungst and R. Rosenthal, *Clever Hans, the Horse of Mr. Von Osten*, Holt, Rinehart and Winston, New York, 1965.
2. I. M. Pepperberg, *The Alex Studies: Cognitive and Communicative Abilities of Grey Parrots*, Harvard University Press, Cambridge, Mass., 1999.
3. D. Premack and A. J. Premack, *The Mind of an Ape*, Norton, New York, 1983; J. Goodall, *My Life with the Chimpanzees*, Pocket Books, New York, 1996.
4. F. Patterson and R. H. Cohn, *Koko's Story*, Scholastic Inc., New York, 1987.
5. R. A. Gardner and B. T. Gardner, *Science* 165:664–672, 1969.
6. H. S. Terrace, *Nim*, Columbia University Press, New York, 1986.
7. D. M. Rumbaugh, *Language Learning by a Chimpanzee: The Lana Project*, Academic Press, New York, 1977.
8. Premack and Premack, *The Mind of an Ape.*
9. E. S. Savage-Rumbaugh and R. Lewin, *Kanzi: The Ape at the Brink of the Human Mind*, John Wiley & Sons, New York, 1994.
10. G. G. Gallup, *Science* 167:86–87, 1970.
11. Ibid.
12. B. F. Skinner, *Science* 173:752–753, 1971.

Chapter 9 Human Thought and the Emergent Twos

1. R. W. Wrangham and Chicago Academy of Sciences, *Chimpanzee Cultures*, Harvard University Press in cooperation with the Chicago Academy of Sciences, Cambridge, Mass., 1994; D. Peterson and J. Goodall, *Visions of Caliban: On Chimpanzees and People*, Houghton Mifflin, Boston, 1993.
2. E. S. Savage-Rumbaugh, S. Shanker, and T. J. Taylor, *Apes, Language, and the Human Mind*, Oxford University Press, New York, 1998.
3. J. Dobbing and J. Sands, *Arch Dis Child* 48:757–767, 1973.
4. J. P. Schade and W. B. Van Groenigen, *Acta Anat* 47:74–111, 1961.
5. L. Mrzljak, H. B. M. Uylings, C. G. Van Eden, and M. Judas, "Neuronal Development in Human Prefrontal Cortex in Prenatal and Postnatal Stages," in H. B. M. Uylings, C. G. Van Eden, J. P. C. De Bruin, M. A. Corner, and M. G. P.

Freenstra (eds.), *The Prefrontal Cortex: Its Structure, Function and Pathology*, Elsevier, Amsterdam, 1990.

6. A. N. Schore, *Affect Regulation and the Origin of the Self: The Neurobiology of Emotional Development*, L. Erlbaum Associates, Hillsdale, N.J., 1994.
7. P. M. Thompson, J. N. Giedd, R. P. Woods, D. MacDonald, A. C. Evans, and A. W. Toga, *Nature* 404:190–193, 2000.
8. R. W. Thatcher, *Brain Cogn* 20:24–50, 1992.
9. H. T. Chugani and M. E. Phelps, *Science* 231:840–843, 1986.
10. Schore, *Affect Regulation and the Origin of the Self.*
11. J. Kagan, *The Nature of the Child*, Basic Books, New York, 1994; J. M. Fuster, *The Prefrontal Cortex: Anatomy, Physiology, and Neuropsychology of the Frontal Lobe*, Lippincott-Raven, Philadelphia, 1997; S. I. Greenspan and B. L. Benderly, *The Growth of the Mind: And the Endangered Origins of Intelligence*, Perseus Books, Reading, Mass., 1998; A. N. Meltzoff, *J Commun Disord* 32:251–269, 1999.
12. L. Rescorla and J. Mirak, *Semin Pediatr Neurol* 4:70–76, 1997.
13. Greenspan and Benderly, *The Growth of the Mind.*
14. P. H. Mussen, J. J. Conger, and J. Kagan, *Child Development and Personality*, Harper & Row, New York, 1969.
15. I. Bretherton, S. McNew, and M. Beeghly, "Early Person Knowledge in Gestural and Verbal Communication: When Do Infants Acquire a 'Theory of Mind?'" in M. Lamb and L. Sherrod (eds.), *Infant Social Cognition*, L. Erlbaum Associates, Hillsdale, N.J., 1981; A. M. Leslie, *Psych Rev* 94:411–426, 1987; Schore, *Affect Regulation and the Origin of the Self.*
16. Greenspan and Benderly, *The Growth of the Mind*, pp. 69–73.
17. Kagan, *The Nature of the Child.*
18. J. Chasseguet-Smirgel, *The Ego Ideal*, Free Association Books, London, 1985.
19. M. Radke-Yarrow and C. Zahn-Waxler, "Roots, Motives, and Patterns in Children's Prosocial Behavior," in E. Staub, J. Bar-Tai, J. Karylowski, and J. Reykowski (eds.), *Development and Maintenance of Prosocial Behavior*, Plenum Press, New York, 1984, pp. 81–99.
20. M. Lewis, J. Jaskir, and M. Enright, *Intelligence* 10:331–354, 1986.
21. A. N. Meltzoff, *Ann N Y Acad Sci* 608:1–31, 1990; A. N. Meltzoff, *J Commun Disord* 32:251–269, 1999.
22. J. Piaget and B. Inhelder, *The Child's Conception of Space*, Routledge & Kegan Paul, London, 1956; J. Piaget, *The Child's Construction of Reality*, Routledge & Kegan Paul, London, 1954.
23. J. A. Usher and U. Neisser, *J Exp Psychol Gen* 122:155–165, 1993.

Chapter 10 Reference Systems of Consciousness I

1. W. Penfield and T. Rasmussen, *The Cerebral Cortex of Man: A Clinical Study of Localization of Function*, Macmillan, New York, 1950; D. O. Hebb, *A Textbook of Psychology*, Saunders, Philadelphia, 1958; A. R. Luria, *Higher Cortical Functions in Man*, Basic Books, New York, 1966; R. W. Sperry, *Science and Moral Priority: Merging Mind, Brain, and Human Values*, Praeger, New York, 1985; H. S. Levin, H. M. Eisenberg, and A. L. Benton, *Frontal Lobe Function and Dysfunction*, Oxford University Press, New York, 1991; B. Milner, *Adv Neurol* 66:67–81,

1995; M. S. Gazzaniga, *The Mind's Past,* University of California Press, Berkeley, 1998; A. C. Roberts, T. W. Robbins, L. Weiskrantz, and Royal Society (Great Britain), Discussion Meeting, "The Prefrontal Cortex: Executive and Cognitive Functions," Oxford University Press, Oxford and New York, 1998.
2. M. S. Gazzaniga and E. Bizzi, *The Cognitive Neurosciences,* MIT Press, Cambridge, Mass., 1995.
3. H. Keller, *The Story of My Life,* Dover Publications, Mineola, N.Y., 1996.
4. W. B. Scoville and B. Milner, *J Neurol Neurosurg Psychiatry* 20:11–21, 1957.

Chapter 11 Reference Systems of Consciousness II

1. L. K. Barnett, *The Universe and Dr. Einstein,* W. Sloane Associates, New York, 1957.
2. E. R. Kandel, J. H. Schwartz, and T. M. Jessell, *Principles of Neural Science,* McGraw-Hill, New York, 2000.
3. B. S. McEwen and H. M. Schmeck, *The Hostage Brain,* Rockefeller University Press, New York, 1994; J. E. LeDoux, *The Emotional Brain: The Mysterious Underpinnings of Emotional Life,* Simon & Schuster, New York, 1996; A. R. Damasio, *The Feeling of What Happens: Body and Emotion in the Making of Consciousness,* Harcourt Brace, New York, 1999; E. T. Rolls, *The Brain and Emotion,* Oxford University Press, Oxford and New York, 1999.
4. G. W. Hohmann, *Psychophysiology* 3:143–156, 1966.
5. A. Schweitzer, *Reverence for Life,* Harper & Row, New York, 1969.
6. C. G. Jung and R. F. C. Hull, *The Archetypes and the Collective Unconscious,* Princeton University Press, Princeton, N.J., 1980.
7. K. W. Fischer and S. P. Rose, *Dynamic Development of Coordination of Components in Brain and Behavior,* in G. Dawson and K. W. Fischer (eds.), *Human Behavior and the Developing Brain,* The Guilford Press, New York, 1994.
8. N. A. Fox, *Am Psychol* 46:863–872, 1991.
9. R. T. Knight, M. F. Grabowecky, and D. Scabini, *Adv Neurol* 66:21–34, 1995.
10. C. A. Nelson, "Neural Correlates of Recognition Memory in the First Postnatal Year," in G. Dawson and K. W. Fischer (eds.), *Human Behavior and the Developing Brain,* The Guilford Press, New York, 1994.
11. B. Libet, E. W. Wright, Jr., B. Feinstein, and D. K. Pearl, *Brain* 102:193–224, 1979; B. Libet, C. A. Gleason, E. W. Wright, and D. K. Pearl, *Brain* 106: 623–642, 1983; B. Libet, *Neurophysiology of Consciousness: Selected Papers and New Essays,* Birkhäuser, Boston, 1993.
12. U. T. Place, "The Identity Theory," in W. G. Lycan (ed.), *Mind and Cognition,* Basil Blackwell, Cambridge, Mass., 1990; S. A. Kripke, "The Identity Thesis," in N. Block, O. Flanagan, and G. Guzeldere (eds.), *The Nature of Consciousness: Philosophical Debates,* MIT Press, Cambridge, Mass., 1998.

Chapter 12 Einstein's Vision of the Universe II

1. A. Einstein, E. P. Adams, and E. G. Straus, *The Meaning of Relativity,* Princeton University Press, Princeton, N.J., 1945.
2. I. Newton, I. B. Cohen, and A. M. Whitman, *The Principia: Mathematical Principles of Natural Philosophy,* University of California Press, Berkeley, 1999.

3. D. C. Cassidy, *Uncertainty: The Life and Science of Werner Heisenberg,* W. H. Freeman, New York, 1992.
4. D. Bohm, *Causality and Chance in Modern Physics,* Routledge & Kegan Paul, London, 1984; D. Bohm, *Quantum Theory,* Dover Publications, New York, 1989.
5. L. K. Barnett, *The Universe and Dr. Einstein,* W. Sloane Associates, New York, 1957.

Chapter 13 Beyond Behaviorism and Mentalism

1. F. W. Matson, *Without Within: Behaviorism and Humanism,* Brooks/Cole Publishing Co., Monterey, Calif., 1973.
2. K. Lorenz, *The Foundations of Ethology: The Principal Ideas and Discoveries in Animal Behavior,* Simon and Schuster, New York, 1982.
3. O. Pfungst and R. Rosenthal, *Clever Hans, the Horse of Mr. Von Osten,* Holt, Rinehart and Winston, New York, 1965.
4. B. F. Skinner, *Science and Human Behavior,* Macmillan, New York, 1953.
5. B. F. Skinner, *Beyond Freedom and Dignity,* Knopf, New York, 1971.
6. H. Gardner, *The Mind's New Science: A History of the Cognitive Revolution,* Basic Books, New York, 1987.
7. M. S. Gazzaniga and E. Bizzi, *The Cognitive Neurosciences,* MIT Press, Cambridge, Mass., 1995.
8. J. Bronowski, *The Ascent of Man,* Little, Brown, Boston, 1974.
9. L. K. Barnett, *The Universe and Dr. Einstein,* W. Sloane Associates, New York, 1957.

Index

About the Author

Richard M. Pico, Ph.D., M.D. is past director of inpatient psychiatric services at The Mount Sinai School of Medicine, New York, and is currently Vice President of Research and Development and Chief Medical Officer of NexxtHealth, Inc. He is the founder and President of 4THOUGHT, Inc., a medical and biotechnology consulting company, and has served on the antipsychotic medication advisory panel for Eli Lilly and Co. His many areas of expertise include electron microscopy, electrophysiology, memory systems, statistics, electronics, psychopharmacology, quantitative brain imaging, and human thought disorders.